Orofacial and Head Pain

Ghabi A. Kaspo • Gary D. Klasser
Editors

Orofacial and Head Pain

Imaging Selection and Strategies

Springer

Editors
Ghabi A. Kaspo
Henry Ford Health Systrem
Henry Ford Hospital
Department of Otolaryngology
Royal Oak, Michigan, USA

Wayne State University
Department of Psychiatry
Detroit, Michigan, USA

Gary D. Klasser
School of Dentistry
Louisiana State University Health
Science
New Orleans, LA, USA

ISBN 978-3-032-08274-9 ISBN 978-3-032-08275-6 (eBook)
https://doi.org/10.1007/978-3-032-08275-6

This Springer imprint is published by the registered company Springer Nature Switzerland AG
The registered company address is: Gewerbestrasse 11, 6330 Cham, Switzerland

Contents

Contributors

Utkarsh Agarwal Henry Ford Health – Henry Ford Hospital, Detroit, MI, USA

Christos Angelopoulos Oral Diagnosis and Radiology, National & Kapodistrian University, Athens, Greece

Jerold E. Armstrong Henry Ford Health – Henry Ford Hospital, Detroit, MI, USA

Michigan State University, East Lansing, MI, USA

Benjamin T. Barbetta Henry Ford Health – Henry Ford Hospital, Detroit, MI, USA

Michigan State University, East Lansing, MI, USA

Steven D. Bender Texas A&M College of Dentistry, Dallas, TX, USA

Mirela Cerghet Henry Ford Health, Department of Neurology, Wayne State University, Detroit, MI, USA

School of Medicine, Department of Neurology and Ophthalmology, Michigan State University, East Lansing, MI, USA

Carla Y. Falcon, DMD, MDS Diplomate, American Board of Endodontics, Department of Endodontics, Rutgers School of Dental Medicine, Newark, NJ, USA

John J. Frazier Department of Diagnostic Sciences, Oral and Maxillofacial Radiology, Louisiana State University Health Sciences Center, School of Dentistry, New Orleans, LA, USA

Mohamed Ali Garada Henry Ford Hospital, Detroit, MI, USA

Ali Ghanem Department of Neurology, Henry Ford Health System, Detroit, MI, USA

Zahid Iqbal Henry Ford Health, Department of Neurology, Wayne State University, Detroit, MI, USA

Brad M. Hong Division of Oral and Maxillofacial Radiology, University of Pennsylvania School of Dental Medicine, Philadelphia, USA

Ghabi A. Kaspo Henry Ford Health Systrem, Henry Ford Hospital, Department of Otolaryngology, Royal Oak, Michigan, USA

Wayne State University, Department of Psychiatry, Detroit, Michigan, USA

Bassam M. Kinaia, DDS, MS Diplomate, American Board of Periodontology, Diplomate, International Congress of Oral Implantology, Graduate Periodontics Program, University of Detroit Mercy, Detroit, MI, USA

Gary D. Klasser Louisiana State University Health Sciences Center, School of Dentistry, Department of Diagnostic Sciences, New Orleans, LA, USA

Irene H. Kim Division of Oral and Maxillofacial Radiology, University of Pennsylvania School of Dental Medicine, Philadelphia, USA

Mel Mupparapu Division of Oral and Maxillofacial Radiology, University of Pennsylvania School of Dental Medicine, Philadelphia, USA

Chew Lip Ng Department of Otolaryngology-Head and Neck Surgery, Ng Teng Fong General Hospital, National University Health System, Singapore, Singapore

Kaan Orhan Department of Oral and Maxillofacial Radiology, Faculty of Dentistry, Ankara University, Ankara, Türkiye

Medical Design Application and Research Center (MEDITAM), Ankara University, Ankara, Türkiye

Cameron J. Szelesi Henry Ford Health – Henry Ford Hospital, Detroit, MI, USA

Gurkan Unsal Department of Oral and Maxillofacial Radiology, Schulich School of Medicine & Dentistry, Western University, London, ON, Canada

Sandeep Uppal The ENT Clinic, Singapore, Singapore

Robert Utsman Department of Biomedical and Community Health Sciences, Division of Diagnostic Sciences & Services, James B. Edwards College of Dental Medicine, Medical University of South Carolina, Charleston, SC, USA

Iram F. Zaman, DO Department of Neurology, Wayne State University School of Medicine, Detroit, MI, USA

Department of Neurology & Ophthalmology, Michigan State University College of Human Medicine, East Lansing, MI, USA

Department of Neurology, Henry Ford Health System, Detroit, MI, USA

Dace Zvirbulis Wayne State University, Department of Psychiatry, Detroit, Michigan, USA

Fundamentals of Orofacial Pain

1

Gary D. Klasser and Steven D. Bender

1.1 Introduction

According to the American Academy of Orofacial Pain (AAOP) "Orofacial Pain is the specialty of dentistry that encompasses the diagnosis, management, and treatment of pain disorders of the jaw, mouth, face, head, and neck" and "is dedicated to the evidenced-based understanding of the underlying pathophysiology, etiology, prevention, and treatment of these disorders and improving access to interdisciplinary patient care" [1]. Orofacial pain (OFP) is a broad category encompassing a number of associated disorders which include, but are not limited to, temporomandibular muscle and joint disorders, jaw movement disorders, neuropathic and neurovascular pain disorders, and vascular and sleep disorders [1]. One of the most frequently encountered OFP conditions, although it is difficult to assess true prevalence given the broad diagnostic criteria, is temporomandibular disorders (TMDs). TMD is a subgroup of conditions within the broad classification of various OFP disorders. In essence, it is also an umbrella term for a group of disorders that result specifically from pain and functional limitation of the masticatory structures, including the temporomandibular joint (TMJ), associated musculature, or a combination of the two. There are more than 30 conditions that can be identified as a TMD and may include, but are not limited to, arthralgia, myalgia, local myalgia, myofascial pain with or without referral, articular disc disorders, degenerative joint disease, subluxation, and headache attributed to TMD [2, 3]. Furthermore, TMDs have been identified as a major cause of non-dental pain in the stomatognathic system often associated with difficulties involving mastication and speaking due to pain and/or dysfunction [4, 5]. TMD may also manifest or be comorbid with several other health conditions such as fibromyalgia, back pain, irritable bowel syndrome, and headache [6]. TMD is most commonly observed in individuals between the ages of 20 and 40 years. Approximately 33% of the population has at least one TMD symptom and 3.6% to 7% of the population has TMD with sufficient severity to cause them to seek treatment [7–9].

1.2 Classification of Orofacial Pain (Including TMD)

Classification systems for OFP conditions are an important undertaking since they assist clinicians to pinpoint the specific entity regarding the condition's etiology, pathophysiology, symptomatology, diagnosis, and therapeutic

G. D. Klasser (✉)
Louisiana State University Health Sciences Center, School of Dentistry, Department of Diagnostic Sciences, New Orleans, LA, USA
e-mail: gklass@lsuhsc.edu

S. D. Bender
Texas A&M College of Dentistry, Dallas, TX, USA

G. A. Kaspo, G. D. Klasser (eds.), *Orofacial and Head Pain*,
https://doi.org/10.1007/978-3-032-08275-6_1

approaches. The definition and terminology employed also serve to facilitate communication with the patient, who then may feel more comfortable belonging to a specific group that is recognized and for which a diagnostic and therapeutic process is available. Terminology and classification are also extremely helpful instruments in providing correct communication for researchers when discussing or comparing their data. The ultimate goals for an ideal classification system are to organize objects and group them together, establish a link between the objects, provide an overview and maximize understanding, highlight similarities and differences, draw attention to the grouping and contrasting of objects, and encourage reflection on what direction collections should take. In other words, an ideal classification system ensures that the information is coherent and homogenous.

Over the years, OFP classification systems have been presented by several organizations such as the International Headache Society, International Association for the Study of Pain, American Academy of Craniofacial Pain, and American Academy of Orofacial Pain in the form of guidelines or criteria. Furthermore, individual articles from various individuals or groups of authors have also been published on this very same topic. Despite not yet developing a universal and uniform consensually agreed upon and evidence-based classification system for OFP, each contributes its own unique definitions and diagnostic criteria albeit with various inherent advantages, strengths and limitations. A discussion of such is beyond the scope of this chapter.

The first classification system to implement a dual-axis diagnostic framework for the provision of operationalized diagnostic algorithms for the most common TMD was the Research Diagnostic Criteria for Temporomandibular Disorders (RDC/TMD) published in 1992 [10]. The aim was to utilize this empirically derived approach for clinical and epidemiological research purposes while incorporating and accounting for psychosocial and behavioral considerations. In an evolutionary progression, the Diagnostic Criteria for Temporomandibular Disorders (DC/TMD) was published in 2014 [3]. The DC/TMD provides reliable and validated evidence-based diagnostic criteria for the most common pain and non-pain-related TMDs. Similar to the RDC/TMD, the DC/TMD follows a dual-axis assessment, by employing both a physical and psychosocial diagnosis. The expanded DC/TMD was also published in 2014 [11]. The purpose for the development of this international expert consensus-based classification system was to standardize the diagnostic algorithms for the less common TMDs not addressed in the DC/TMD for clinical and research applications. Despite the global acceptance and adoption of the DC/TMD, this classification system is only focused on adults. Therefore, in 2023, the DC/TMD for adolescents and children was developed [12, 13]. The purpose of this initiative was to adapt the pre-existing DC/TMD for adults and revise it to be more applicable to the adolescent and child populations for implementation in clinical and research settings. In 2024, due to the complexity and excessively time-consuming physical exam, as well as the difficulty of implementing psychosocial diagnosis associated with the DC/TMD [14, 15], the brief DC/TMD (bDC/TMD) was developed [16]. Although the validity, reliability, and utility of the bDC-TMD has not yet been tested, the aim is to have this classification system expedite clinical diagnosis and initial management in non-specialist clinical settings to the benefit of patients by earlier recognition of TMD, thereby improving prognosis [16].

1.3 Evolution of Orofacial Pain

In 1975, the AAOP was formed as the professional membership organization representing the field of OFP. AAOP is an organization of dentists and other health professionals dedicated to alleviating pain and suffering through the promotion of excellence in education, research, and patient care in the field of OFP and associated disorders. One of the goals of this organization was to have the discipline of OFP recognized as a specialty. Unfortunately, despite several attempts in achieving this goal, all efforts for being recognized as a specialty were rejected. However, in March 2020, this situation changed when the AAOP's request to recognize OFP as a dental specialty was granted by the National Commission on Recognition of Dental Specialties and Certifying Boards (NCRDSCB) based on compliance with the Requirements for Recognition of Dental Specialties as determined by the american dental association (ADA).

The ADA states that, "Dental specialties are recognized by the National Commission on Recognition of Dental Specialties and Certifying Boards to protect the public, nurture the art and science of dentistry, and improve the quality of care. Specialties are recognized in those areas where advanced knowledge and skills are essential to maintain or restore oral health (Association policies are contained in the ADA Principles of Ethics and Code of Professional Conduct)" [17]. Due to this landmark decision by organized dentistry, as of September 2020, OFP is currently considered a specialty of dentistry.

In another significant event, in March 2022, the NCRDSCB recognized the American Board of Orofacial Pain (ABOP—founded in 1994 in response to the need for a valid certification process for OFP practitioners), as the national certifying board for OFP. This decision entrusts the ABOP as the sole recognized national certifying board. It bestows upon the ABOP the responsibility of administering the board certification examination certifying qualified practitioners as Diplomates in the specialty of OFP.

Overall, these momentous acts of recognizing this specialty strengthen the connection between dentistry and medicine, acknowledging that the orofacial region, oral cavity, and masticatory system are an integral part of total patient care [18]. The benefits of these relatively recent but rather significant events are numerous and include the following: improved access to care by providing a resource for referral of patients not responding to basic therapy; the maintaining of educational standards for postgraduate OFP training programs thereby educating and providing a supply of properly trained clinicians and faculty; the ability to emphasize the importance of OFP in predoctoral dental education resulting in enhanced patient care through OFP training for newly graduating dentists; providing protection and service to the public by identifying qualified dentists who recognize and are knowledgeable in managing OFP including TMD; and ensuring a standard of care through a certified credentialing process administered by a recognized board [19].

1.4 Importance of History and Clinical Examination

One the most important aspects of OFP practice is the establishment of an accurate diagnosis for the presenting patient. Many individuals experiencing OFP have previously consulted with numerous providers and have received ineffective and, in some cases, inappropriate treatment, based on an incomplete or incorrect diagnosis. The complexity of the numerous, extensively innervated structures located in the oral, facial, and head region adds to the complexity of the diagnostic process. Because of this, the OFP clinician can benefit by adopting a systematic approach to the diagnostic process. In addition to a comprehensive history, an appropriate thorough clinical evaluation is necessary to avoid missing important data. Additional laboratory tests and imaging studies should be initiated only when deemed necessary to confirm a differential diagnosis formulated from the findings of the history and clinical examination.

A comprehensive history will help guide the clinician to conduct the most relevant physical examination. The components of a comprehensive history for the patient with OFP include the chief complaint, medical history, dental history, and psychosocial history. Obtaining the report of the chief complaint or chief presenting concern gives the patient the opportunity to provide the clinician, in their own words, a description as to why they are seeking care. Other data to be gathered as components of the chief complaint include the date of onset, previous consultations/treatments, associated symptoms, location of the pain, quality, intensity, aggravating and alleviating factors, and whether and how the pain has changed over time.

The medical and dental history should reveal data concerning any previous or current illnesses and be weighed in relation to the patient's presenting pain. Any history of trauma, especially to the head and face, should be noted. Other components of the medical/dental history should include the patient's current medications, including supplements, tobacco, alcohol, caffeine, and any recreational drug use. While considered a sensitive topic of discussion, any history of emotional, sexual, or physical abuse is an essential component of the history [20]. A discussion of sleep quality as well as awareness of disturbances such as snoring and other sleep-related breathing disorders such as obstructive sleep apnea should be a routine inclusion in the history-gathering process [21]. Ascertaining the patient's history of dental treatment may reveal information impacting their current presenting pain.

A review of systems may reveal systemic entities that are, at least in part, contributing to the patient's pain experience. These may include connective tissue disorders, endocrine disorders, cardiovascular disease, autoimmune disease, and neurologic disorders.

Psychosocial factors may play a significant role in the initiation, maintenance, or intensification/ chronification of OFP complaints [22]. The psychosocial history will help the clinician understand the patient's mental status and coping skills that may be relevant in eventual therapy recommendations. It is important to include questions concerning depression, anxiety, and stressors, either past or present. The clinician may choose to use validated screeners, such as the 4-item Patient Health Questionnaire (PHQ-4) [23].

The physical examination should begin with a general inspection of the head and neck, evaluating the general appearance and looking for any evidence of current or previous trauma, asymmetries, swellings, abnormal posture, or involuntary movements. It may be preferable to begin the examination positioned in front of the patient. This allows for the opportunity to observe the patient's facial expressions and affect as the process proceeds. Because of the complexity of many OFP complaints, the physical examination also should include an inspection of the ears, both superficially and otoscopically, a nasal examination, and an examination of the oropharynx. It is useful, especially in patients experiencing a new onset of headache, to include a fundoscopic examination. A neurologic screening, to include a cranial nerve review, may reveal issues of the nervous system that are either primary or secondary factors to the patient's concern. Other structures to evaluate would include the lymph nodes and blood vessels involving the carotid, facial, and superficial temporal arteries. Pain to palpation of these blood vessels may indicate a vascular entity contributing to the pain complaint. Examinations of the masticatory system and the cervical region, as well as an intraoral examination, are also necessary components of the comprehensive examination. The masticatory muscles should be palpated and assessed for "familiar pain" [3]. This would be pain that is like or similar to the pain that the patient has been experiencing, leading to the consultation. Any referral of pain distant from the site of palpation should be noted. Along with palpation of the TMJs to assess for pain, noises emanating from these structures should be recorded as well. The noise also can be characterized based on the nature: whether it is a popping noise or more of a crepitus or grinding noise. Joint noises, as well as irregular movements of the mandible, could indicate internal derangements or pathology of the structures. However, it is important to note that these noises do not necessarily correlate with the pain presentation, nor do they provide an indication for therapeutic intervention [24]. Measuring the range of mandibular movement is also important in assessing the health of the masticatory structures. An opening of less than 40 mm is considered to be limited [3].

The intraoral examination should be guided by the presenting complaint and history. The soft tissues should be routinely inspected for lesions, suspicious swellings, masses, or ulcerations. Although the role of occlusal factors in orofacial pain disorders lacks scientific creditability [25], relationships may be documented as a part of the comprehensive examination to monitor for any changes due to potential disease progression during the therapeutic process or with observation. If the patient's pain complaint mimics pain of odontogenic origin, appropriate studies such as pulp vitality testing, periodontal probing, radiographic surveys, percussion, and thermal response testing should be used. Milking of the parotid, submandibular, and sublingual glands can assess for overall functional status of these glands.

1.5 Adjunctive Diagnostic Tests

The purpose of a diagnostic test is to establish the presence (or absence) of disease as a basis for management decisions in symptomatic individuals. All diagnostic tests are not indicated for every patient presenting with OFP complaints. The application of the diagnostic test must be based on the individual's unique presentation after a comprehensive history and physical examination have been performed and the results contemplated. The value of the test should be weighed against evidence-based protocols, with consideration given to whether it will have a meaningful impact on the diagnosis and subsequent course of management. If the test does not fulfill these criteria, it should not be ordered. Testing methods for OFP complaints may include imaging, laboratory studies, and diagnostic analgesia. Laboratory tests should not be considered a routine part of the evaluation of patients with OFP. The test should be ordered only to evaluate for certain conditions.

When indicated, imaging can serve as an essential adjunct to diagnostic testing in OFP patients, providing the clinician a deeper understanding of the anatomical and pathological factors contributing to pain that are often not easily discerned through clinical evaluation alone. Imaging techniques such as panoramic radiography, cone-beam computed tomography (CBCT), magnetic resonance imaging (MRI), computed tomography (CT), and ultrasonography can provide essential visual information that supplements the clinical evaluation. Each of these modalities offers unique advantages depending on the suspected pathology, and the choice of imaging technique is determined by the specific clinical presentation.

Panoramic radiography is often used as an initial diagnostic tool because it provides a broad view of the jaw, teeth, and surrounding structures. This modality may reveal gross anatomical abnormalities such as fractures, impacted teeth, or extensive bone pathologies that may be contributing to pain. However, while panoramic radiography offers a general overview, its limited resolution and two-dimensional nature may obscure finer details, necessitating more advanced imaging techniques for complex cases.

CBCT can offer a three-dimensional, high-resolution image of bone structures, making it ideal for evaluating bony pathologies such as TMJ osteoarthritis, jawbone fractures, and cysts.

MRI is used primarily for soft tissue evaluation. Unlike CBCT, which is optimal for hard tissue visualization, MRI provides detailed images of tissues including muscles, ligaments, and the articular disc of the TMJ, as well as structures in the central nervous system. MRI is the gold standard for diagnosing conditions like disc displacement or TMJ capsular effusion.

Computed tomography (CT) uses computer processing to produce detailed cross-sectional images. In OFP practice, CT imaging can be used to visualize the facial bones, teeth, and surrounding soft tissues, enabling clinicians to identify abnormalities that may not be visible on traditional radiographs. In cases of OFP, CT imaging can help identify issues such as TMJ disorders or fractures. In cases where MRI is contraindicated, CT imaging can also be used to visualize some soft tissue structures.

In some cases, ultrasonography can also play a role in the diagnostic process, especially for assessing superficial soft tissues like muscles and glands. This noninvasive technique may be useful in identifying sialolithiasis (salivary stones) or muscle inflammation, both of which can manifest as OFP.

1.6 Diagnosis

As mentioned previously, arriving at an accurate diagnosis is critical to successfully managing the OFP patient. In many cases, failure to properly diagnose the source of the pain can lead to inappropriate treatment choices potentially exacerbating the presenting problem, leading to a more chronic pain condition. Therefore, a comprehensive and stepwise diagnostic approach is essential for guiding effective management approaches, ensuring more optimal outcomes and improving the overall quality of life for the patients.

From the history and physical examination, one can gather key information about the onset, location, intensity, and duration of the pain, as well as any associated symptoms such as clicking, jaw locking, or aberrant nerve sensations, in order to focus upon potential etiologies. For instance, pain associated with chewing or jaw movement may point toward TMD, while sharp, electrical, burning, or tingling pain triggered by light touch could suggest a neuropathic pain condition.

One of the key challenges in diagnosing OFP is that many different disorders can produce similar symptom presentations. For example, TMD, trigeminal neuralgia (TN), odontogenic pain, and headaches can all cause facial pain. However, the underlying mechanisms of these conditions are very different. Each requires a distinct management approach. TMD, for instance, often involves problems with the jaw joint or surrounding muscles, which may require management strategies such as behavior modification, physical therapy, or in some cases oral appliance therapy. TN, on the other hand, is a neuropathic pain condition that involves dysfunction/dysregulation of the trigeminal nerve. Most trigeminal neuropathic pains are typically initially managed with pharmacotherapy. A misdiagnosis not only delays appropriate management but may also lead to unnecessary interventions, such as dental extractions or invasive surgeries, that could further complicate the patient's condition.

Imaging and other diagnostic instruments will also play a crucial role in confirming or ruling out potential diagnoses. When odontogenic pain is suspected, appropriate diagnostic radiographs can be utilized to augment clinical testing of the suspected teeth. While the diagnosis of TN is primarily clinically based, MRI of the brain and brainstem can help differentiate primary from secondary causes. Panoramic imaging, and even more so CBCT, can be utilized to help differentiate degenerative joint disease from conditions such as osteonecrosis dissecans and synovial chondromatosis of the TMJ. The implementation of this approach will result in enhanced and appropriate patient care and outcomes.

1.7 Management Principles

OFP conditions including TMD are multifactorial and multi-etiological in nature, meaning there are many complex factors that promote disease presentation and progression. Therefore, it is important to recognize and have a thorough understanding of the various contributing factors to these conditions. This approach will be helpful in subsequently addressing the disease process and promoting pain reduction. Acknowledgement of predisposing (elements that are present prior to disease manifestation), precipitating (specific events that lead to the onset of disease), and perpetuating (maladaptive behaviors that individuals develop in relationship to their disease symptoms) factors—those biological, psychological, and socio-environmental factors that contribute to a disease state—is critical in the development and implementation of management strategies [26].

Effective management is aimed at addressing acute pain in order to prevent the transformation to a chronic condition. The chronification of pain results in a myriad of nociplastic changes ultimately resulting in central sensitization. Central sensitization is essentially an amplification of central nervous system processing that contributes to pain hypersensitivity [27]. Once this amplification occurs, the management strategies require a thorough reevaluation and reconceptualization. Both the peripheral components of the disease process and alterations in the central nervous system need to be addressed in chronic painful conditions [27]. Patients that are refractory to initial management strategies should be considered for referral to a clinician with appropriate knowledge and training in complex OFP conditions such as an OFP specialist. The reasons for the possible lack of patient response to management may be an incorrect diagnosis, ineffective etiological assessment, or inappropriate management strategies. An OFP specialist will provide expert consultation, potentially utilize adjunctive measures such as advanced imaging, and may provide alternative management modalities while working with both an interdisciplinary (integration of multiple disciplines through collaboration toward coordinated patient-centered care) and multidisciplinary (the utilization of the skills and experience of individuals from different disciplines, with each discipline approaching the patient from their own perspective) team. This team management approach, with its abilities to provide multimodal and multicomponent interventions encompassing both supportive and definitive care, often is the ideal strategy. Supportive care is considered any form of management provided to a patient to prevent, control, or relieve complications and side effects and to improve the patient's comfort and quality of life. Definitive care implies the development and implementation of a management plan for a disease or disorder that has been chosen as the best one for a patient after all other choices have been considered. Therapies are directly targeted at either the elimination or the alteration of the etiologic factors responsible for the disorder. Ultimately, these strategies assist in the prevention of overtreatment and/or inappropriate/inadequate or harmful treatment, individualize management needs, and focus on physical, behavioral, social, and psychological functioning for overall holistic patient-centered care [27].

1.8 Conclusion

The specialty and practice of OFP encompass a very diverse range of conditions. As such, a clear understanding of its classifications, historically and especially current, is essential for accurate diagnosis and effective management. As the specialty has evolved, advancements in diagnostic and management strategies have emphasized the importance of multidisciplinary and interdisciplinary collaboration. However, at the very heart of successful management is the taking of a patient history and performing a clinical examination, which serve as the foundation for diagnosis and guide the selection of appropriate adjunctive diagnostic tests to potentially confirm our findings. A comprehensive approach that integrates these components ensures the application of sound diagnostic and management principles, enabling personalized recommendations that addresses biological, social, and psychosocial factors. With continued research and innovation, the field of OFP will further enhance patient care and outcomes.

References

1. American Academy of Orofacial Pain. What is orofacial pain? 2024. https://aaop.clubexpress.com/content.aspx?page_id=22&club_id=508439&module_id=107327. Accessed 20 Dec 2024.
2. National Institute of Dental and Craniofacial Research. Prevalence of TMJD and its signs and symptoms. National Institutes of Health, United States Government. Updated. July 2018. https://www.nidcr.nih.gov/research/data-statistics/facialpain/prevalence. Accessed 8 Feb 2024.
3. Schiffman E, Ohrbach R, Truelove E, Look J, Anderson G, Goulet JP, et al. Diagnostic Criteria for Temporomandibular Disorders (DC/TMD) for clinical and research applications: recommendations of the International RDC/TMD Consortium Network and Orofacial Pain Special Interest. J Oral Facial Pain Headache. 2014;28:6–27.
4. Greene CS. Managing the care of patients with temporomandibular disorders: a new guideline for care. J Am Dent Assoc. 2010;141:1086–8.
5. Okeson J. Bell's oral and facial pain. 7th ed. Chicago: Quintessence; 2014.
6. Klasser GD, Bassiur J, de Leeuw R. Differences in reported medical conditions between myogenous and arthrogenous TMD patients and its relevance to the general practitioner. Quintessence Int. 2014;45:157–67.
7. Klasser GD, Romero Reyes M. Orofacial pain: guidelines for assessment, diagnosis, and management. 7th ed. Batavia: Quintessence Publishing Co. Inc; 2023.
8. Wright EF, Klasser GD. Manual of temporomandibular disorders. 4th ed. Hoboken: Wiley Blackwell; 2020.
9. Okeson JP. Management of temporomandibular disorders and occlusion. 8th ed. St. Louis: Mosby; 2019.
10. Dworkin SF, LeResche L. Research diagnostic criteria for temporomandibular disorders: review, criteria, examinations and specifications, critique. J Craniomandib Disord. 1992;6:301–55.

11. Peck CC, Goulet JP, Lobbezoo F, Schiffman EL, Alstergren P, Anderson GC, et al. Expanding the taxonomy of the diagnostic criteria for temporomandibular disorders. J Oral Rehabil. 2014;41:2–23.
12. Ekberg E, Nilsson IM, Michelotti A, Al-Khotani A, Alstergren P, Rodrigues Conti PC, et al. Diagnostic criteria for temporomandibular disorders-INfORM recommendations: comprehensive and short-form adaptations for adolescents. J Oral Rehabil. 2023;50:1167–80.
13. Nilsson IM, Ekberg E, Michelotti A, Al-Khotani A, Alstergren P, Conti PCR, et al. Diagnostic criteria for temporomandibular disorders-INfORM recommendations: comprehensive and short-form adaptations for children. J Oral Rehabil. 2023;50:99–112.
14. Haggman-Henrikson B, Ekberg E, Ettlin DA, Michelotti A, Durham J, Goulet JP, et al. Mind the gap: a systematic review of implementation of screening for psychological comorbidity in dental and dental hygiene education. J Dent Educ. 2018;82:1065–76.
15. Sharma S, Breckons M, Bronnimann Lambelet B, Chung JW, List T, Lobbezoo F, et al. Challenges in the clinical implementation of a biopsychosocial model for assessment and management of orofacial pain. J Oral Rehabil. 2020;47:87–100.
16. Durham J, Ohrbach R, Baad-Hansen L, Davies S, De Laat A, Goncalves DG, et al. Constructing the brief diagnostic criteria for temporomandibular disorders (bDC/TMD) for field testing. J Oral Rehabil. 2024;51:785–94.
17. Council on Ethics, Bylaws and Judicial Affairs. Principles of Ethics and Code of Professional Conduct. American Dental Association, 2021. https://www.ada.org/about/principles/code-of-ethics. Accessed 18 Sept 2022.
18. Heir GM. Orofacial pain, the 12th specialty: the necessity. J Am Dent Assoc. 2020;151:469–71.
19. Klasser GD, Abt E, Weyant RJ, Greene CS. Temporomandibular disorders: current status of research, education, policies, and its impact on clinicians in The United States of America. Quintessence Int. 2023;54:328–34.
20. Curran SL, Sherman JJ, Cunningham LL, Okeson JP, Reid KI, Carlson CR. Physical and sexual abuse among orofacial pain patients: linkages with pain and psychologic distress. J Orofac Pain. 1995;9:340–6.
21. Klasser GD, Almoznino G, Fortuna G. Sleep and orofacial pain. Dent Clin N Am. 2018;62:629–56.
22. Nicholas MK. The biopsychosocial model of pain 40 years on: time for a reappraisal? Pain. 2022;163(Suppl 1):S3–S14.
23. Kroenke K, Spitzer RL, Williams JB, Lowe B. An ultra-brief screening scale for anxiety and depression: the PHQ-4. Psychosomatics. 2009;50:613–21.
24. Tallents RH, Hatala M, Katzberg RW, Westesson PL. Temporomandibular joint sounds in asymptomatic volunteers. J Prosthet Dent. 1993;69:298–304.
25. Manfredini D, Lombardo L, Siciliani G. Temporomandibular disorders and dental occlusion. A systematic review of association studies: end of an era? J Oral Rehabil. 2017;44:908–23.
26. Wright CD, Tiani AG, Billingsley AL, Steinman SA, Larkin KT, McNeil DW. A framework for understanding the role of psychological processes in disease development, maintenance, and treatment: the 3P-Disease Model. Front Psychol. 2019;10:2498.
27. Nijs J, George SZ, Clauw DJ, Fernandez-de-Las-Penas C, Kosek E, Ickmans K, et al. Central sensitisation in chronic pain conditions: latest discoveries and their potential for precision medicine. Lancet Rheumatol. 2021;3:e383–e92.

2 Multidisciplinary Approach to Orofacial Pain Management

Steven D. Bender and Ghabi A. Kaspo

2.1 Introduction

Orofacial pain (OFP) encompasses a variety of painful conditions affecting the mouth, jaws, face, and related structures. The complexity of orofacial pain often necessitates a comprehensive, multidisciplinary approach for effective management. This chapter explores the collaborative strategies often necessary to appropriately address OFPs, emphasizing the contributions of various healthcare professionals and the significance of a well-coordinated treatment approach [1].

2.2 Understanding OFP

OFP may originate from multiple sources, including odontogenic, neurogenous, myogenous, and arthrogenous, while being influenced by psychosocial factors [2]. The potential overlap of many OFPs necessitates an intentional and thorough diagnostic process to be as precise as possible, identifying all potential contributing etiologic factors and ultimately developing a personal tailored therapy. Misdiagnosis or inadequate treatment can potentially lead to the chronification of pain which has the potential to significantly impact a patient's quality of life [3, 4].

2.3 Common Symptoms of OFPs

OFPs commonly manifest through a variety of symptoms that can affect the mouth, face, and jaws and may often overlap with other medical conditions. Patients may report persistent or intermittent aching, sharp, or throbbing pain in the jaw, cheeks, or around the eyes, sometimes radiating to the neck or ears. Some may express difficulty with chewing, speaking, or jaw movements accompanied by clicking or popping sounds in the temporomandibular joints (TMJs). Sensory disturbances such as numbness, tingling, or burning sensations in the mouth, tongue, or face are also OFP presentations that may be encountered in clinical practice. Headaches such as migraine, sometimes presenting in the facial or forehead region, can occur alongside other facial pains. Other symptoms may include tooth or periodontal sensitivity or pain without apparent pathology, clinically or radiographically. Some patients may also report ear pain, fullness, or ringing. Swelling, redness, or visible inflammation in the face or jaw may further complicate the clinical presentation. As one can easily infer, these diverse symptoms further emphasize the

S. D. Bender (✉)
Texas A&M College of Dentistry, Dallas, TX, USA

G. A. Kaspo
Henry Ford Health Systrem, Henry Ford Hospital, Department of Otolaryngology, Royal Oak, Michigan, USA

Wayne State University, Department of Psychiatry, Detroit, Michigan, USA

G. A. Kaspo, G. D. Klasser (eds.), *Orofacial and Head Pain*,
https://doi.org/10.1007/978-3-032-08275-6_2

importance of a comprehensive evaluation to identify the underlying etiologies and best guide effective management strategies.

2.4 The Multidisciplinary Team

As mentioned previously, the clinician who manages OFP patients often needs to integrate with a multidisciplinary team to deliver comprehensive care tailored to the complexities of managing pain in the head, neck, face, and jaw regions. This multidisciplinary team, besides an OFP specialist, will often include directly or indirectly the following specialists [3]:

1. Oral and maxillofacial surgeons: While most patients with temporomandibular disorders (TMDs) do not require surgical interventions, there are occasions when structural abnormalities or trauma do contribute to the presenting pain complaint. These situations may require the surgeon to perform invasive procedures like corrective jaw surgery, joint arthrocentesis, arthroplasty, or other joint-related procedures [5].
2. Chronic pain specialists: Pain specialists, including anesthesiologists and pain medicine physicians, focus mainly on managing chronic pain through various methods, including long-term medication management, nerve blocks, and other procedures such as nerve stimulator placement and biomodulation procedures.
3. Physical therapists: Physical therapists play a critical role in managing orofacial pain by addressing the musculoskeletal components of the condition. Physical therapists assist patients in managing pain through therapeutic exercises, manual therapy, and other modalities such as ultrasound and electrical stimulation. They will also help the patient by providing education and self-management techniques to address their musculoskeletal issues contributing to OFP.
4. Psychologists and psychiatrists: Psychologists and psychiatrists address the psychosocial aspects of pain, providing cognitive-behavioral therapy (CBT), counseling, and medication management for conditions like depression, anxiety, and other mood disorders which can negatively impact OFPs.
5. Neurologists: Neurologists can assist in cases that may involve primary or secondary headache presentations or other neurologic disorders that may be outside the scope of the orofacial pain practitioner [6, 7].
6. Otolaryngologist: Many OFP patients present with pain in the ears, sinuses, and throat areas. Otolaryngologists or Ear, Nose, and Throat Physicians (ENTs) can aid in the evaluation and treatment of conditions related to the sinuses, nasal passages, and throat that may contribute to orofacial pains [7, 8].
7. Radiologists: Radiologists play a vital role in the diagnostic process, providing and interpreting imaging studies such as radiographs, magnetic resonance imaging (MRIs), and computed tomography (CT) scans to identify structural abnormalities which help guide treatment planning.
8. Clinical pharmacists: A clinical pharmacist can help manage an OFP patient by optimizing medication therapy, ensuring proper dosing, minimizing drug interactions, and providing education on the safe and effective use of pain management medications.
9. Sleep medicine specialist: A sleep medicine specialist can optimize the diagnosis and management of an OFP patient by identifying sleep-related disorders, such as sleep-related breathing disorders or other sleep-related disorders that may underlie or aggravate the pain, and working with the practitioner to implement targeted treatments to improve both sleep quality and pain outcomes [9–12].
10. Rheumatologist: A rheumatologist plays a critical role in managing an OFP patient by diagnosing and treating autoimmune or inflammatory conditions, such as rheumatoid arthritis or other systemic entities that may contribute to or exacerbate OFP.
11. Functional medicine specialists: While often overlooked, a functional medicine specialist can help an OFP patient by addressing under-

lying systemic imbalances and dysbiosis, such as chronic inflammation, nutritional deficiencies, or hormonal dysregulation, to provide a holistic approach to pain management and overall well-being [13].

2.5 Diagnostic Approach

An accurate diagnosis is one of the most important and compassionate services provided for a patient with OFP. The diagnostic process will involve a thorough medical and dental history, a systematic clinical examination, and imaging and laboratory studies when appropriate. A detailed patient history can reveal patterns and triggers of pain and will guide the clinician through the physical examination process, while a clinical examination can identify signs of infection, inflammation, or structural abnormalities [3, 14, 15].

Imaging techniques play a crucial role in diagnosing OFP conditions. Radiographs help identify dental issues, bone fractures, and sinusitis, while magnetic resonance imaging (MRI) provides detailed views of soft tissues, including the brain and spinal cord, muscles and TMJ structures. Computed tomography (CT) offers comprehensive assessments of bone structures, making it valuable for complex cases, and ultrasound serves as a noninvasive tool for evaluating soft tissues and guiding interventions. In addition to imaging, specialized tests such as nerve conduction studies help assess peripheral nerve function in neuropathic pain conditions, and laboratory tests assist in ruling out systemic diseases like infections or autoimmune disorders [16–18].

A multidisciplinary approach to OFP management integrates various treatment modalities tailored to individual patient needs. Pharmacological treatments range from over-the-counter analgesics like acetaminophen and ibuprofen for mild to moderate pain to opioids for severe pain presentations, administered under strict supervision. Antidepressants and anticonvulsants are typically used for neuropathic pains, while muscle relaxants target musculoskeletal pain. Interventional procedures, including nerve blocks with local anesthetics with or without the addition of corticosteroids, botulinum toxin injections for muscle-related pain, and surgical interventions such as TMJ surgery or dental extractions, provide additional treatment options. Physical therapy aims to improve function and reduce pain through manual therapy techniques like massage and mobilization, exercise therapy for strengthening and stretching, and modalities such as ultrasound, electrical stimulation, and heat/cold therapy. Psychological interventions are equally important in comprehensive pain management, with cognitive-behavioral therapy (CBT) helping patients develop coping strategies, biofeedback assisting in controlling physiological functions like muscle tension, and relaxation techniques such as meditation and deep breathing aiding in pain reduction [14, 19]. A multidisciplinary care approach is exemplified in a patient with chronic orofacial pain due to TMD, neuropathic pain, and significant psychosocial stressors. Treatment may involve a dentist providing an oral appliance, a pain specialist prescribing medication and performing nerve blocks, a physical therapist designing an exercise program, a psychologist conducting CBT sessions, a neurologist monitoring pharmacological treatments, and a radiologist utilizing MRI to assess TMJ structures. However, challenges remain, including coordination of care, access to multidisciplinary teams, and insurance coverage limitations [15, 19]. Future directions in OFP management include expanding telemedicine to enhance access to care, advancing research into genetic and molecular pain mechanisms, uncovering of specific biomarkers, and improving education for healthcare professionals through interprofessional training programs to optimize patient outcomes.

2.6 Conclusion

Managing OFP requires a comprehensive, multidisciplinary approach to address the complex interplay of factors. By integrating the expertise of various healthcare professionals, patients can receive tailored, effective treatment that addresses both the physical and psychosocial aspects of their pain. This holistic approach not only alleviates pain but also improves the overall quality of life for individuals suffering from OFP. Embracing future advancements in telemedicine, research, and education will further enhance the effectiveness of multidisciplinary OFP management.

References

1. De Rossi SS. Orofacial pain: a primer. Dent Clin N Am. 2013;57(3):383–92.
2. Barad M, Romero-Reyes M. Orofacial pain. Continuum (Minneap Minn). 2024;30(5):1397–426.
3. Romero-Reyes M, Uyanik JM. Orofacial pain management: current perspectives. J Pain Res. 2014;7:99–115.
4. Sarlani E, Balciunas BA, Grace EG. Orofacial pain—part I: assessment and management of musculoskeletal and neuropathic causes. AACN Clin Issues. 2005;16(3):333–46.
5. Dimitroulis G. Management of temporomandibular joint disorders: a surgeon's perspective. Aust Dent J. 2018;63(Suppl 1):S79–s90.
6. Israel HA, Scrivani SJ. The interdisciplinary approach to oral, facial and head pain. J Am Dent Assoc. 2000;131(7):919–26.
7. Köling A. Neurologist, otolaryngologist...? Which specialist should treat facial pain? Lakartidningen. 1998;95(20):2320–5.
8. Benoliel R. Classifying head, face and oral pain. Cephalalgia. 2017;37(14):1315–6.
9. Thimma Ravindranath P, Smith JG, Niloofar RN, Ebelthite C, Renton T. Sleep disturbances are associated with pain intensity and pain-related functional interference in patients experiencing orofacial pain. J Oral Rehabil. 2023;50(10):980–90.
10. McCloy K, Herrero Babiloni A, Sessle BJ. Sleep disorders and orofacial pain: insights for dental practice. Aust Dent J. 2024;69:S5.
11. Klasser GD, Almoznino G, Fortuna G. Sleep and orofacial pain. Dent Clin N Am. 2018;62(4):629–56.
12. Almoznino G, Benoliel R, Sharav Y, Haviv Y. Sleep disorders and chronic craniofacial pain: characteristics and management possibilities. Sleep Med Rev. 2017;33:39–50.
13. Crandall JA. An introduction to orofacial pain. Dent Clin N Am. 2018;62(4):511–23.
14. Gremillion HA. Multidisciplinary diagnosis and management of orofacial pain. Gen Dent. 2002;50(2):178–86; quiz 87-8.
15. Patel K, Eley KA, Cascarini L, Watt-Smith S, Larkin M, Lloyd T, et al. Temporomandibular disorders-review of evidence-based management and a proposed multidisciplinary care pathway. Oral Surg Oral Med Oral Pathol Oral Radiol. 2023;136(1):54–69.
16. Whyte A, Matias M. Imaging of orofacial pain. J Oral Pathol Med. 2020;49(6):490–8.
17. Shintaku W, Enciso R, Broussard J, Clark GT. Diagnostic imaging for chronic orofacial pain, maxillofacial osseous and soft tissue pathology and temporomandibular disorders. J Calif Dent Assoc. 2006;34(8):633–44.
18. Hunter A, Kalathingal S. Diagnostic imaging for temporomandibular disorders and orofacial pain. Dent Clin N Am. 2013;57(3):405–18.
19. Li DTS, Leung YY. Temporomandibular disorders: current concepts and controversies in diagnosis and management. Diagnostics (Basel). 2021;11(3):459.

3 Overview of Radiographic Anatomy of Head, Face, and Neck Structures

John J. Frazier

3.1 Introduction

Imaging studies can play a crucial role in the evaluation of orofacial pain. A complete clinical history and examination will guide the clinician as to whether imaging is beneficial and to which imaging studies should be undertaken. Many imaging modalities are available for the evaluation of orofacial pain. The imaging modality that yields the most information for the evaluation of the anatomical regions and tissue types of interest should be selected [1]. Once an imaging study is acquired, a thorough read of all images is required. For a successful diagnostic interpretation, the clinician must have a thorough knowledge of normal imaging anatomy. This chapter presents the important normal intraoral and extraoral imaging anatomy present on plane radiographs, cone beam computed tomography (CBCT), and magnetic resonance imaging (MRI) used for the imaging analysis of orofacial pain [2].

J. J. Frazier (✉)
Department of Diagnostic Sciences, Oral and Maxillofacial Radiology, Louisiana State University Health Sciences Center, School of Dentistry, New Orleans, LA, USA
e-mail: jfraz2@lsuhsc.edu

3.2 Plane Radiographs

Plane radiographs use ionizing radiation in the form of X-rays. The X-rays are emitted at an anatomical region of the patient where the X-rays interact with the tissues. The density of the tissue determines the amount of X-rays that penetrate the different tissue types. The denser a tissue is, the more it will absorb the X-rays and decrease the quantity of X-rays exiting the patient that go on to interact with the X-ray sensor. The more X-rays that interact with the sensor, the brighter the image will be (radiopaque). Conversely, as fewer X-rays interact with the sensor, the darker the image will be (radiolucent). In the oral and maxillofacial region, plane radiographs are used for evaluation of hard tissues (teeth, dentin, and bone) and air spaces (maxillary sinus, pharyngeal). Soft tissue structures are poorly visualized, but evaluation of the hard tissues that contain the soft tissues is useful as a proxy for soft tissue evaluation. The two most common plane radiographs used in dentistry are the intraoral periapical radiograph and the extraoral panoramic radiograph.

3.3 Periapical Radiographs

The purpose of periapical (PA) radiographs is to capture all the tooth anatomy and the surrounding hard tissue structures and soft tissue spaces

G. A. Kaspo, G. D. Klasser (eds.), *Orofacial and Head Pain*,
https://doi.org/10.1007/978-3-032-08275-6_3

[3]. Tooth morphology captured on PA radiographs includes the crown, root(s), pulp chamber, root canal(s), and the landmark cemento-enamel junction (CEJ) (Fig. 3.1a). Surrounding the teeth is the periodontium. The radiographic structures of the periodontium consist of the following:

(a) *Periodontal ligament (PDL) space*: A thin, uniform radiolucent curvilinear line that surrounds the root(s). The PDL space contains the PDL ligament. The PDL space starts at the level of the CEJ and continues inferiorly toward the apex of the root. At the apex, the PDL space bends around the root apex and ascends superiorly along the root to the contralateral level of the CEJ. The PDL space is slightly wider coronally and then tapers toward the apex.
(b) *Lamina dura*: A thin, uniform radiopaque curvilinear line that surrounds the PDL space. Like the PDL space, the lamina dura starts at the level of the CEJ. The lamina dura is continuous with the cortical bone of the alveolar crest.

The teeth and periodontium are embedded in the bone of the maxilla and mandible, collectively called the alveolar bone. The alveolar bone is made up of an outer dense bone, the *cortical bone*, and a less dense inner bone, the *cancellous bone*. Anatomical structures of the alveolar bone are:

(a) *Alveolar crest*. The alveolar crest is the cortical bone that runs through the interradicular bone and connects the lamina dura of adjacent teeth. The alveolar crest is approximately 1.5–2 mm below the level of the CEJ. The architecture of the interradicular alveolar crest changes from the anterior teeth to the posterior teeth. Between the anterior teeth, the alveolar crest tends to a point in between the teeth. Going toward the posterior teeth, the alveolar crest becomes wider and horizontal. In the posterior teeth, the alveolar crest is at 90 degrees to the lamina dura.
(b) *Floor of the maxillary sinus*. The floor of the maxillary sinus is a thin radiopaque mean-

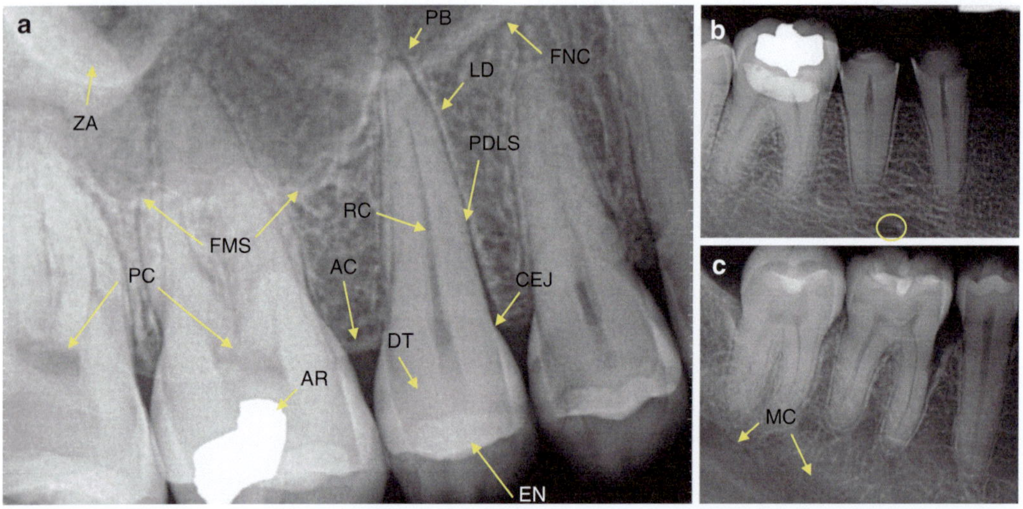

Fig. 3.1 (**a**) AC alveolar crest, AR amalgam restoration, CEJ cemento-enamel junction, DT dentin, EN enamel FMS floor of the maxillary sinus, FNS floor of the nasal cavity, LD lamina dura, PB periapicl bone, PC pulp chamber, PDLS periodontal ligament space, RC root canal, ZA zygomatic arch. (**b**) Yellow circle: mental foramen. (**c**) MC mandibular canal

dering line that is present on PAs of the maxillary molars. The floor of the maxillary sinus is present over the roots of the molars and can drape down between the roots of the molars. As it progresses anteriorly toward the second premolar, it sharply bends superiorly and radiographically crosses over the floor of the nasal cavity.

(c) *Floor of the nasal cavity.* The floor of the nasal cavity is a thin radiopaque horizontal line that is present in posterior PAs at the level of the apices of the premolars. At the distal end of the second premolar, the radiographic floor of the nasal cavity crosses the radiographic floor of the maxillary sinus.

(d) *Mental foramen.* The mental foramen is an oval radiolucent structure located around the apices of the mandibular premolars. The location of the mental foramen is variable as it depends on the angle the PA is taken. The mental foramen can be superimposed on the premolar root apices or inferior to the root apices. The location of the mental foramen in the anteroposterior direction can be from the mesial of the first premolar to the distal of the second premolar or anywhere in between (Fig. 3.1b).

(e) *Mandibular canal.* Posterior mandibular PAs can, on occasions, image the mandibular canal. When visible, the canal presents as a curvilinear radiolucent strip bordered by thin radiopaque lines both superior and inferior to the radiolucent strip. The canal when present on the radiograph will be between the root apices of the mandibular molars and the inferior border of the mandible, depending on the acquisition angle (Fig. 3.1c).

3.4 Panoramic Radiograph

A panoramic radiograph is an imaging modality that captures in a single image the gross osseous structures of the maxilla and mandible and the dentition of both arches (Fig. 3.2). Extra-oral structures are also imaged, but the visibility is generally of poorer radiographic quality than the images of the jaws. The anatomy of the anatomical structures viewed on a panoramic radiograph may differ significantly from radiograph to radiograph due to the inherent imaging physics (i.e., magnification), the patient's normal variation of anatomical structures, and patient positioning. However, the image quality is generally suffi-

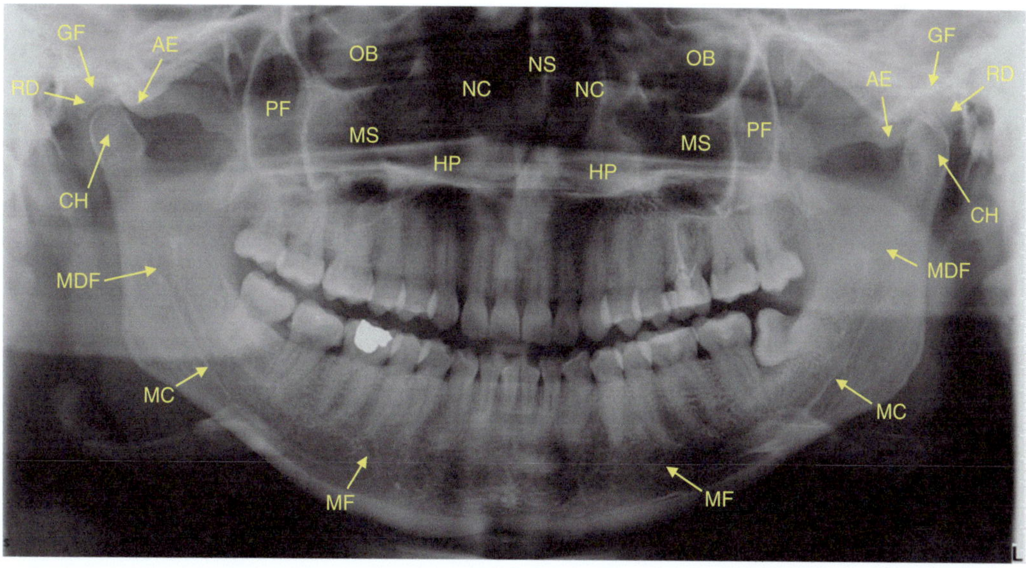

Fig. 3.2 AE articular eminence, CH condylar head, GF glenoid fossa, HP hard palate, MC mandibular canal, MDF mandibular foramen, MF mental foramen, MS maxillary sinus, NF nasal cavity, NS nasal septum, OB orbit, PF pterygopalantine fossa, RD radiographic disk space

cient to distinguish gross normal structures from abnormality. It is critical for the clinician doing the image analysis to have a strong understanding of normal anatomy imaged on panoramic radiographs. Moreover, it is crucial for the clinician to know what anatomical structures are not present in the radiograph. This is important when deciding if a panoramic radiograph is the best imaging modality for diagnosing or treatment planning. When doing an image analysis of a panoramic radiograph (or any other image), it is important that the clinician follows a structured pattern for viewing the image and that this pattern is done with each new image. This structured approach makes sure the entire image is analyzed and analysis is consistent from image to image [4]. The order in which this pattern is done is not critical, but it should be consistent and, most importantly, ensure that the entire image is viewed. For image analysis of orofacial pain, one structured pattern could be to (1) analyze the midface structures, (2) analyze the jaws, and (3) analyze the osseous structures of the temporomandibular joints (TMJ).

The anatomical structures of the midface include the orbits, maxillary sinuses, and the nasal cavity.

(a) *Orbits*. The orbits are circular to elliptically shaped paired structures that house the eyeballs. On panoramic radiograph, the orbits are radiolucent with blurred radiopacities from superimposed osseous structure. The floor of the orbit shares a bony wall with the roof of the maxillary sinus.
(b) *Maxillary sinuses*. The maxillary sinuses are paired, triangularly shaped air-filled structures that flank the nasal cavity. The internal structure of the sinuses is radiolucent. The maxillary sinus shares a medial wall with the nasal cavity; the roof of the sinus wall is shared with the floor of the orbit. The floor of the sinus projection undulates about the roots of the maxillary molars. Of note, the apices of the maxillary molars superimpose over the inferior region of the sinus. However, the roots do not project into the sinuses.
(c) *Nasal cavity*. The nasal cavity or nasal fossa is a midline, pyramid-shaped air-filled structure that contains the nasal septum and the inferior turbinates. The nasal septum divides the nasal cavity into two spaces. The inferior turbinates are paired osseous bones that are attached to the lateral wall of the nasal cavity and project into the lower portion of the nasal cavity. The lateral wall of the nasal cavity is shared as the medial wall of the maxillary sinus.

The anatomical structures of the jaws on a panoramic radiograph include the maxilla, mandible, and teeth. Although the condyles are part of the mandible, for image analysis of a panoramic radiograph for orofacial pain, it is better to include evaluation of the condyle in the analysis of the osseous structures of the TMJs as evaluation of the TMJs is a common procedure in orofacial pain [5].

(a) *Maxilla*. The normal anatomy of the maxilla on panoramic radiograph consists of a uniform trabecular pattern of the maxillary bone and a straight radiopaque horizontal line of bone, the hard palate, which denotes the roof of the oral cavity. The hard palate is also the floor of the nasal cavity.
(b) *Mandible*. The anatomy seen on the panoramic radiograph of the mandible includes the mandibular body, rami, condyles, mandibular foramen, mandibular canal, and mental foramen.
    1. The *mandibular foramen* is the entry point of the mandibular branch of the trigeminal nerve (V2). The foramen is located in the middle of the ramus and leads into the mandibular canal.
    2. The *mandibular canal* contains the inferior alveolar nerves. Radiographically, the canal is a uniform, curvilinear radiolucent structure bordered superiorly and inferiorly by thin radiopaque bone.
    3. The *mental foramen* is the exiting point for the mental nerve, which is a branch of the inferior alveolar nerve. The foramen's

location is variable in the region of the premolars. Radiographically, the foramen is a circular to elliptically shaped radiolucency that may or not be corticated.

(c) *Teeth.* Panoramic radiograph can be used to assess the number, overall shape, and morphology of the teeth. Detailed radiographic analysis of the teeth should not be done with panoramic radiographs.

A panoramic radiograph is a good screening tool for evaluation of the osseous structures of the temporomandibular joints [6]. Visualized anatomy includes the glenoid fossa, the articular eminence, and the condyles. The articular disk is not visualized on panoramic radiographs. However, the space occupied by the disk, the radiographic disk space, can be assessed.

(a) *Glenoid fossa.* The glenoid fossa is a convex depression in the floor of the cranial base. The fossa houses the articular disk when the jaws are in the closed position.
(b) *Articular eminence.* The articular eminence is a convex osseous projection from the cranial base and is anterior and inferior to the glenoid fossa. The articular eminence guides the rotation and translation of the mandible during opening of the jaws.
(c) *Condyle.* The condyle consists of the condylar neck and the condylar head. The condylar neck connects the ramus to the condylar head. The condylar head is the most superior portion of the mandible. The condylar head is a convex projection that is continuous with the condylar neck. On panoramic radiograph, the condylar head sits inferiorly to the glenoid fossa. The position of the condylar head is generally centered to slightly anteriorly placed within the glenoid fossa. Panoramic imaging of the condyles is relatively poor compared to CBCT imaging [7].
(d) *Radiographic disk space.* The radiographic disk space is a radiolucent space that is between the floor of the glenoid fossa and the superior surface of the condylar head.

3.5 Trigeminal Nerve (Cranial Nerve V)

The trigeminal nerve and its branches are the principle sensory nerves for the oral and maxillofacial region of the head and neck. The trigeminal nerve is also the motor nerve for the muscles of mastication. In this section, a brief review of the major branches of the trigeminal nerve exiting the cranium will be reviewed [8].

(a) *Trigeminal ganglion.* The trigeminal ganglion is the major sensory ganglion for the sensory nerves that innervate the oral and maxillofacial structures. The trigeminal ganglion sits within the anterior cranial base in a region called Meckel's cave (also known as the trigeminal cave) and gives rise to three major sensory nerves: the ophthalmic nerve (V1), the maxillary nerve (V2), and the mandibular nerve (V3) (Fig. 3.3a, b).
(b) *Ophthalmic nerve (V1).* The ophthalmic nerve is the most superior division of the trigeminal nerve. It leaves the trigeminal ganglion and courses through the lateral wall of the cavernous sinus and exits the skull through the superior orbital fissure. The ophthalmic nerve supplies sensory information to the scalp, forehead, and nose (Fig. 3.3b).
(c) *Maxillary nerve (V2).* The maxillary nerve is the middle division of the trigeminal nerve. It leaves the trigeminal ganglion and courses through the lateral wall of the cavernous sinus and exits the skull base through the foramen rotundum. The nerve continues horizontally in an anterior direction and first passes over the pterygopalatine fossa, where it gives off two small connecting branches that support the sphenopalatine ganglion. The nerve continues anteriorly and becomes the infraorbital nerve as it passes through the infraorbital groove, giving off branches of the posterior, middle, and anterior alveolar nerves. The infraorbital nerve then exits the skull through the infraorbital foramen and gives off sensory branches that innervate the midface (Fig. 3.3c).

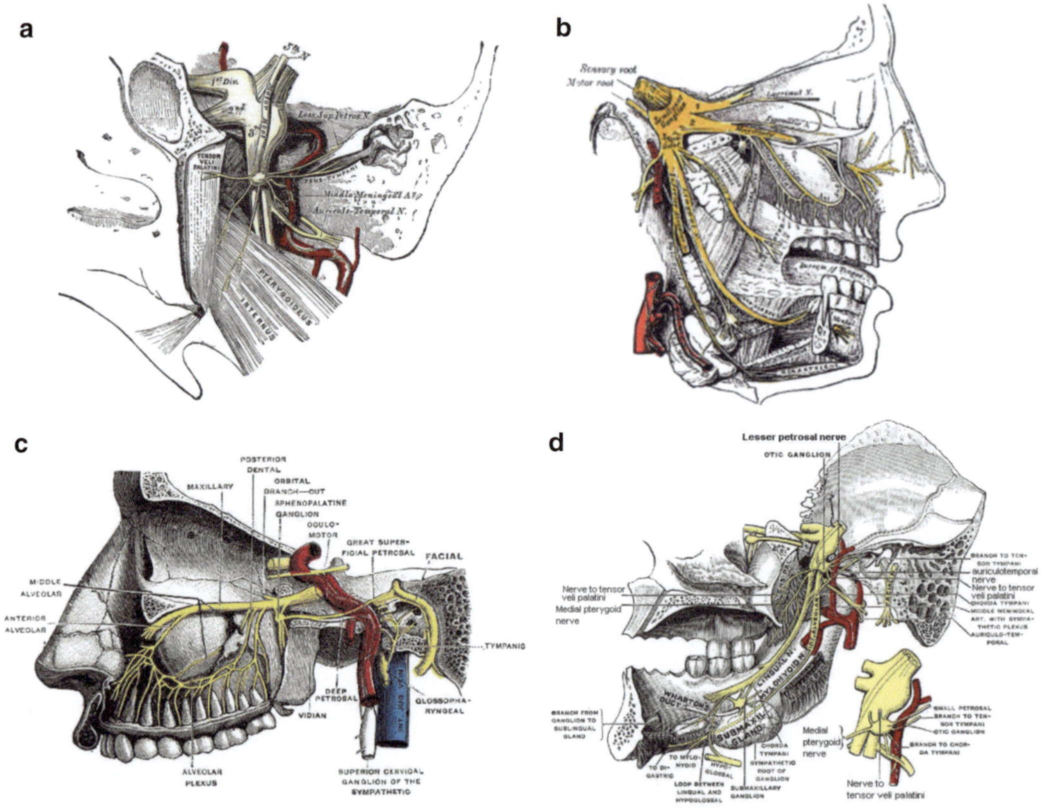

Fig. 3.3 (**a**, **b**) The trigeminal ganlion within the Meckel cave showing the three major sensory nerves V1, V2, and V3. (**c**) The maxillary nerve (V2) and its branches. (**d**) Major branches of the mandibular nerve (V3)

(d) *Mandibular nerve (V3).* The mandibular nerve is the inferior and largest branch of the trigeminal nerve. The mandibular nerve is a mixed nerve that has both sensory and motor functions. It leaves the trigeminal ganglion and exits the skull base through the foramen ovale. Upon exiting the foramen ovale, the maxillary nerve gives off a motor nerve to the medial pterygoid muscle and the sensory nerve, nervous spinosus. It branches into the anterior and posterior divisions. The anterior division gives off motor branches to the temporalis, lateral pterygoid, and masseter muscles and a sensory branch, the buccal nerve. The posterior division gives off sensory branches to the auriculotemporal, inferior alveolar, and lingual nerves. Its motor nerve innervates the mylohyoid muscle. The inferior alveolar nerve enters the mandible through the mandibular foramen and courses anteriorly to supply innervation to the mandibular teeth. The inferior alveolar nerve gives off one sensory branch, the mental nerve, which innervates the chin and lower lips (Fig. 3.3d).

3.6 Cone Beam Computed Tomography (CBCT)

Computed tomography (CT) was invented by electrical engineer Godfrey Hounsfield and physicist Allan Cormack, for which they were awarded the Nobel Prize in Physiology or Medicine in 1979 [9]. Though CT has many applications in medical imaging, its use in dentistry did not start until the early 2000s. The delay in dental applications was due to the many challenges in engineering and computer software design needed to make the CT machine smaller and faster for practical use in dental offices. One of the major challenges to overcome was in the delivery of X-rays for imaging. In medical CT, many passes of thinly sliced X-ray beams are needed to generate an image. To make CT acquisition faster for dental use, all the X-ray beams needed to generate multiple slices are emitted in one rotation of the X-ray source instead of multiple rotations of the X-ray source as in medical CT. Collectively, all of the X-ray beams form the shape of a cone, hence the name cone beam computed tomography (CBCT). CBCT has many advantages compared to intraoral and panoramic radiographs [10]. Advantages of CBCT include the following:

1. No superimposition of anatomy on image quality.
2. Anatomy can be viewed in a volume or in thin slices.
3. Anatomy can be viewed in any plane.
4. A pseudo-panoramic image can be generated.
5. There is no distortion or magnification of images.

Disadvantages of CBCT include the following:

1. More radiation dose to the patient
2. Image artifacts
3. Cost and availability of a CBCT machine

The viewing of CBCT images can be done in many different planes and orientations, but in general, for diagnostic interpretation, three standard planes oriented 90 degrees to each other are used. This standard viewing platform is called multiplanar cone beam computed tomography [11]. The three standard planes are the axial, sagittal, and coronal planes (Fig. 3.4). The axial plane slices the image from superior to inferior. The sagittal plane slices the image from medial to lateral. The coronal plane slices the image from anterior to posterior.

Each of the coplanar views gives unique visualization of anatomical structures and regions. Therefore, each anatomical structure and region should be evaluated in multiple planes before an interpretation is rendered. Only after a complete evaluation of an anatomical structure or region is

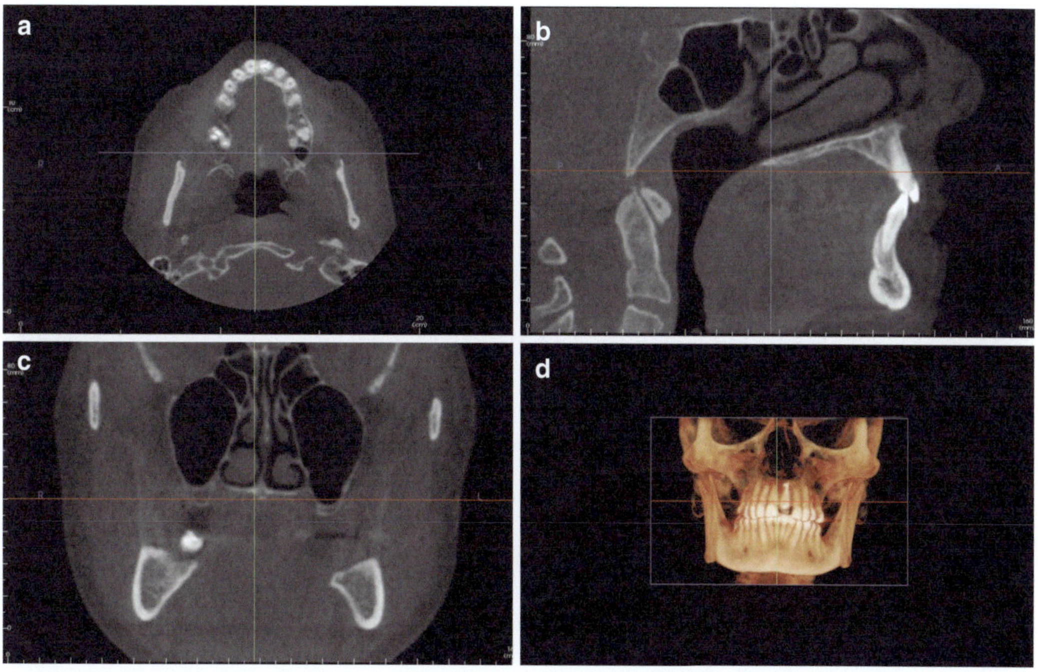

Fig. 3.4 (**a**) Axial section. (**b**) Sagittal section. (**c**) Coronal section. (**d**) Volume rendering

concluded should the clinician then move on to another anatomic structure or region. As for any evaluation of an image, a consistent systematic search is essential to ensure that the entire image has been visualized and evaluated.

It is important the reader acknowledges that CBCT is used for interpretation of the osseous structures. CBCTs are, in general, inadequate for capturing, with high fidelity, soft tissue anatomical structures. Although soft tissue anatomy is poorly visualized on CBCT, a proxy for gross evaluation is the osseous anatomical structures that the soft tissue passes through or attaches to. Changes to the osseous structures associated with soft tissue anatomical structures may directly or indirectly signal soft tissue changes.

The following is a review of common major anatomical structures visualized on CBCT images:

Paranasal Sinuses The paranasal sinuses consist of the frontal sinus, sphenoid sinus, ethmoid air cells, and maxillary sinuses. The paranasal sinuses are air-filled chambers that flank the nasal cavity. As the paranasal sinuses are air-filled structures, their normal anatomical presentation on CBCT is radiolucent.

(a) *Frontal sinus.* The frontal sinus is present in the anterior-inferior portion of the frontal bone. It has an irregularly shaped border and crosses the midline (Fig. 3.5b, d).
(b) *Sphenoid sinus.* The sphenoid sinus sits posterior and superior to the ethmoid air cells. The superior-posterior osseous structure of the sphenoid sinus forms the floor of the sella turcica, which houses the pituitary gland (Fig. 3.5c).
(c) *Ethmoid air cells.* The ethmoid air cells are paired structures that are superior to the nasal cavity. Each of the air cells are separated by delicate septa [12] (Fig. 3.5a, d).
(d) *Maxillary sinuses.* The maxillary sinuses are paired pyramid-shaped structures that lie lateral to the nasal cavity. The maxillary sinus shares walls with the floor of the orbit superiorly and the lateral wall of the nasal cavity medially.

Nasal Cavity The nasal cavity is an air-filled space in the midface that contains the nasal septum and the turbinates [13] (Fig. 3.6).

(a) *Nasal septum.* The nasal septum is a thin midline structure that separates the nasal cavity into two halves. Often, the nasal septum is deviated to one side or the other.
(b) *Middle and inferior turbinates.* The turbinates are J-shaped, paired structures with one-half of the pair on each side of the nasal cavity. The middle turbinates are extensions of the ethmoid bone and extend downward into the nasal cavity. The inferior turbinates are separate osseous structures that attach to the lateral wall of the nasal cavity.

Canals, Foramen, and Fossa The canals, foramen, and fossa are vital openings in the osseous structures that allow the passage of soft tissue structures. Knowledge of the location, normal anatomy, and soft tissue structures that utilize the openings is crucial for evaluation of possible pathosis contributing to orofacial pain.

Canals

(a) *Incisive canal.* The incisive canal is located in the anterior midline of the hard palate and contains the incisive nerve. On sagittal section, the canal projects inferiorly and anteriorly and is cylindrically shaped (Fig. 3.5c). On axial view, the incisive foramen is visualized as a circularly shaped, corticated radiolucency (Fig. 3.7a).
(b) *Greater palatine canal (pterygopalatine canal).* The greater palatine canal is a vertical canal that starts at the inferior end of the pterygopalatine fossa and ends in the posterolateral region of the horizontal plate of the palatine bone [14]. The canal transmits the greater and lesser palatine nerves and palatine vessels (Fig. 3.7a, b).
(c) *Vidian canal (pterygoid canal).* The vidian canal is a horizontal canal that communicates between the middle cranial fossa and ends in the pterygopalatine fossa [15]. The canal carries the vidian nerve (Figs. 3.9 and 3.10).

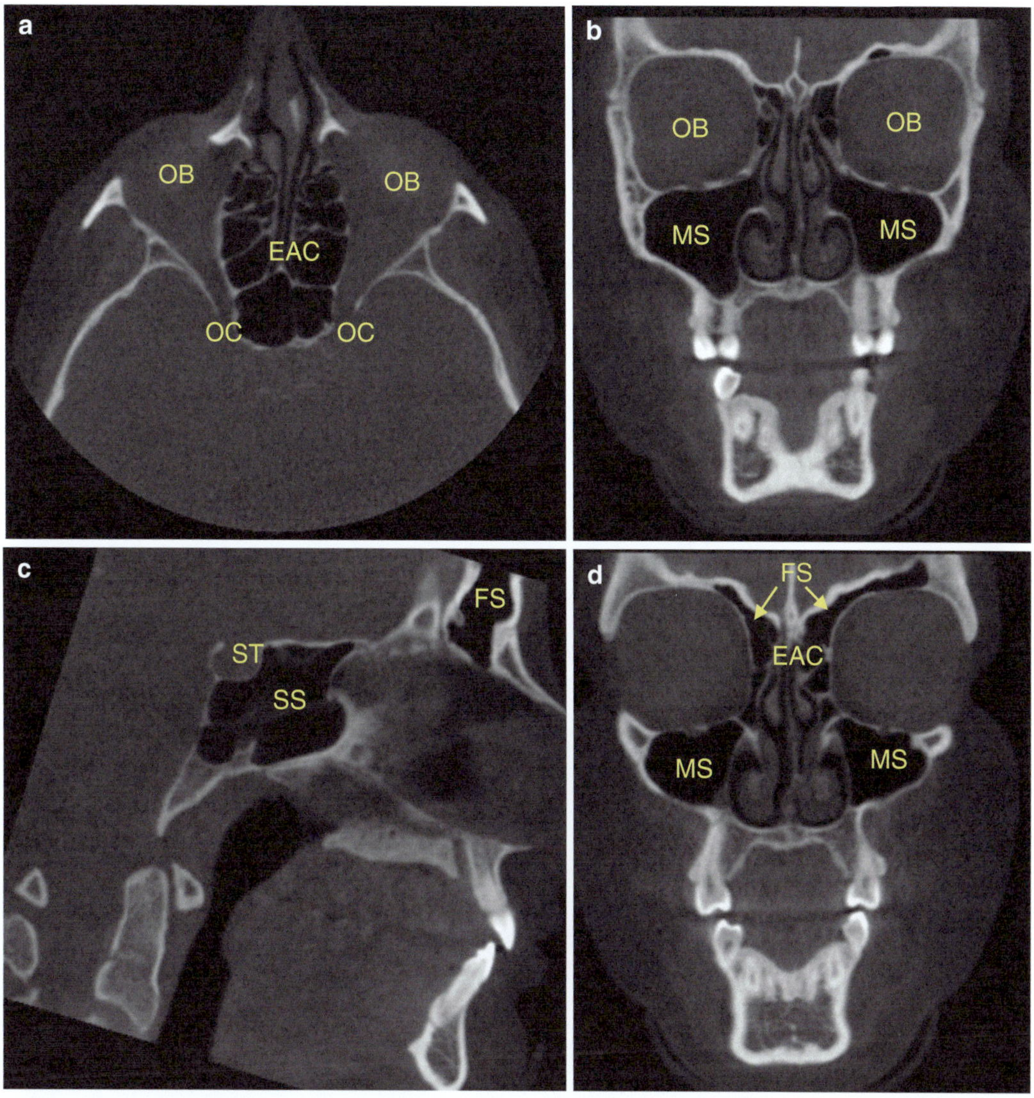

Fig. 3.5 (**a**) Axial view. (**b**, **d**) Coronal view. (**c**) Sagittal view. EAC ethmoid air cells, FS frontal sinus, MS maxillary sinus, OC optic canal, OB orbit, SS sphenoid sinus, ST sella turcica

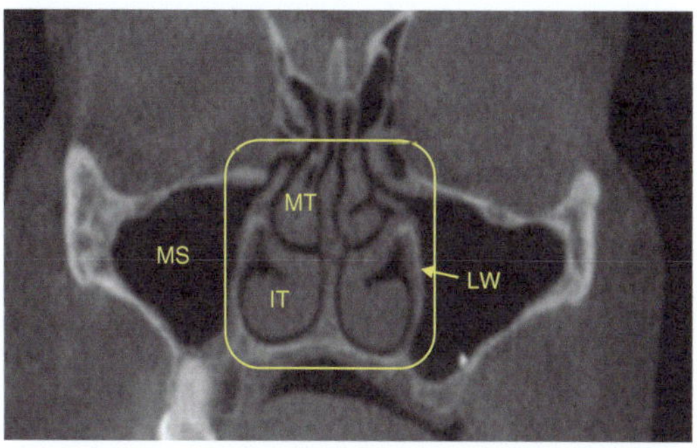

Fig. 3.6 Coronal view. Yellow rectangle: nasal cavity, IT inferior turbinate, LW lateral wall of the nasal cavity, MS maxillary sinus, MT middle turbinate

(d) *Infraorbital canal*. The infraorbital canal is a horizontal canal that starts at the infraorbital groove, traverses the maxilla, and ends at the infraorbital foramen. It transmits the infraorbital nerve, a branch of V2, and the infraorbital artery (Fig. 3.8).

(e) *Optic canal*. The optic canal is a communication between the middle cranial fossa and the orbit and transmits the optic nerve and the ophthalmic artery [12] (Fig. 3.5a).

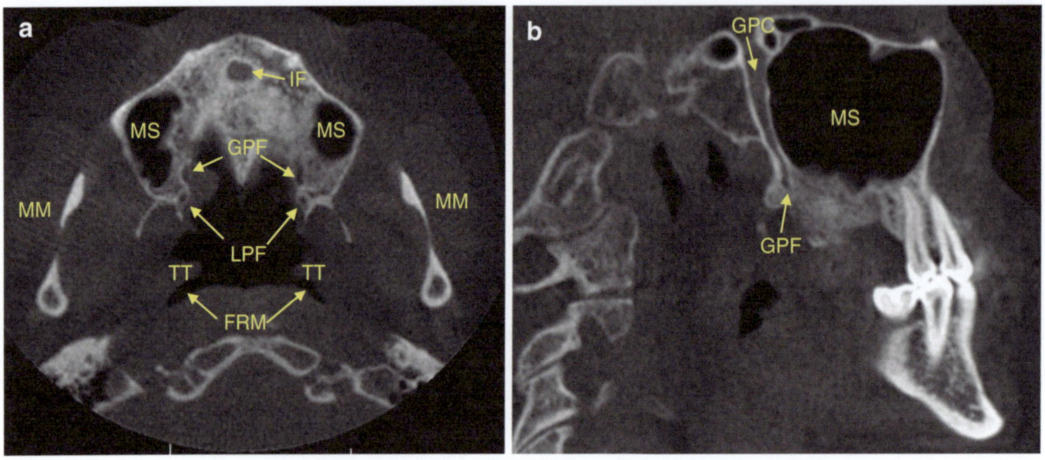

Fig. 3.7 (**a**) Axial section. (**b**) Sagital secton. FRM fossa of Rosenmuller, GPF greater palatine foramen, IF incisive foramen, LPF lesser palatine foramen, MM masseter muscle, MS maxillary sinus, TT torus tubarius

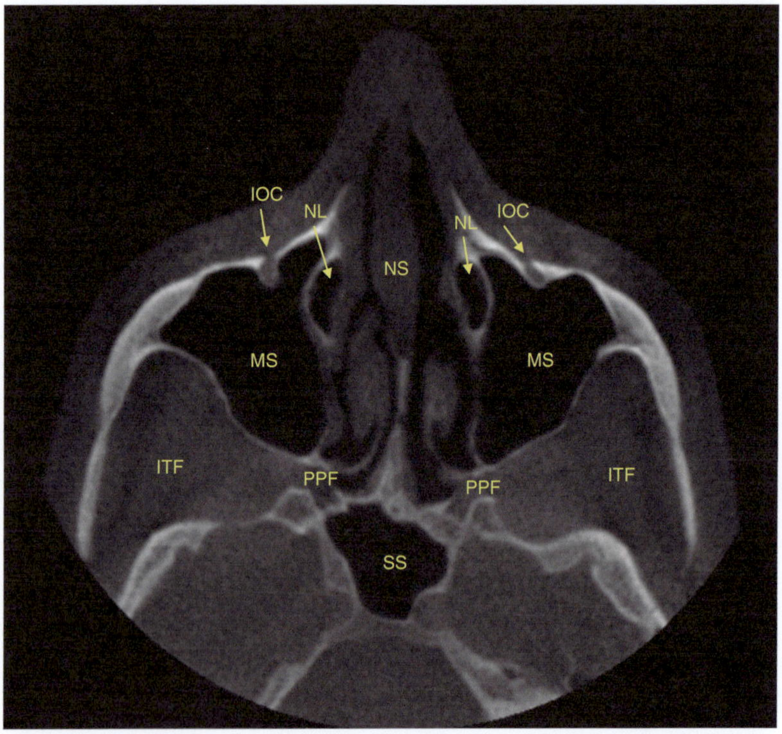

Fig. 3.8 CBCT axial section at the level of the sphenoid sinus. IOC infraorbital canal, ITF infratemporal fossa, MS maxillary sinus, NL nasolacrimal duct, NS nasal septum, PPF pterygopalatine fossa, SS sphenoid sinus

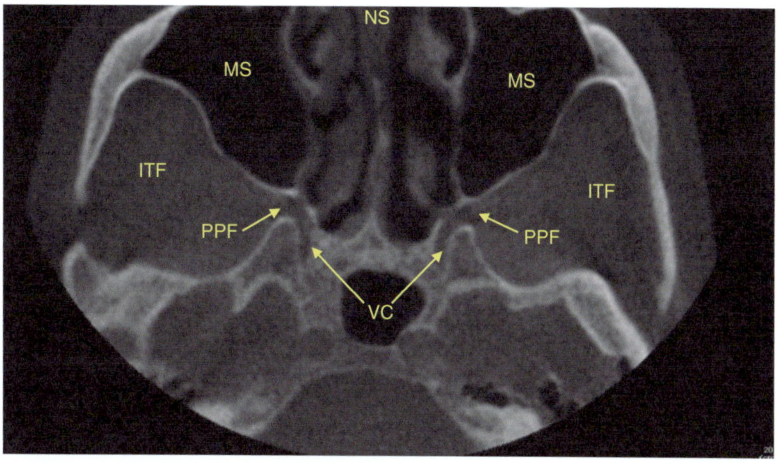

Fig. 3.9 Axial section. ITF infratemporal fossa, MS maxillary sinus, NS nasal septum, PPF pterygopalatine fossa, VC vidian canal

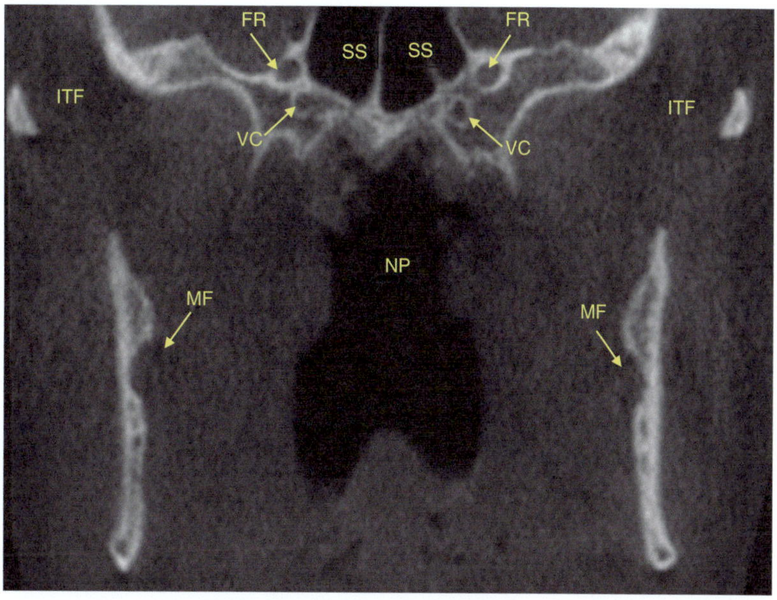

Fig. 3.10 CBCT coronal section through the sphenoid sinus. Yellow arrows: foramen rotundum, red arrows: vidian canal (pterygoid canal), white arrows: mandibular foramen, SS sphenoid sinus, NP nasopharynx

Foramen

(a) *Foramen ovale.* The foramen ovale is an oval-shaped opening in the sphenoid bone in the middle cranial fossa that transmits the mandibular branch of the trigeminal nerve V3 [16] (Fig. 3.11).

(b) *Foramen rotundum.* The foramen rotundum is a circular hole in the sphenoid bone in the middle cranial fossa that is located posterolateral to the foramen ovale. It allows passage of the maxillary branch of the trigeminal nerve V2 [16] (Figs. 3.10 and 3.11).

(c) *Infraorbital foramen.* The infraorbital foramen is the terminal portion of the infraorbital canal and is located in the maxilla inferior to the floor of the orbits. It transmits the infraorbital nerve (Fig. 3.12).

(d) *Greater palatine foramen.* The greater palatine foramen is located in the posterolateral region of the horizontal plate of the palatine bone. It transmits the greater palatine nerve (Fig. 3.7a, b).

(e) *Lesser palatine foramen.* The lesser palatine foramen is located in the horizontal plate of the palatine bone posterolateral to the greater palatine foramen. It transmits the lesser palatine nerve (Fig. 3.7a).

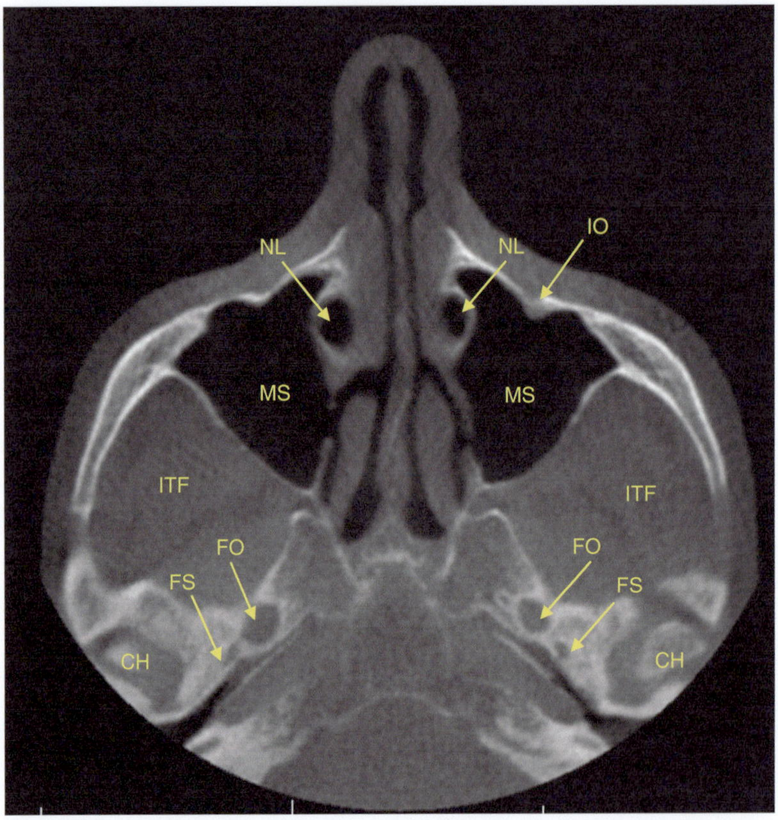

Fig. 3.11 CBCT axial section at the level of condyles. NL nasolacrimal ducts, IO infraorbital canal, MS maxillary sinus, FO foramen ovale, FS foramen spinosum, CH head of the condyle

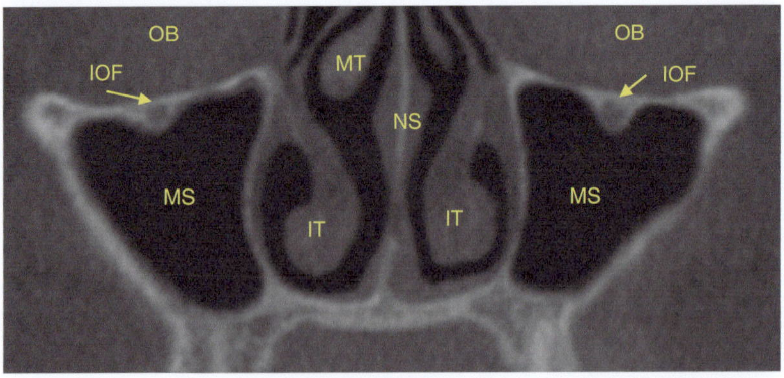

Fig. 3.12 The infraorbital foramen passing inferiorly to the floor of the orbits. IOF infraorbital foramen, IT inferior turbinate, MS maxillary sinus, MT middle turbinate, OB orbit

(f) *Mandibular foramen.* The mandibular foramen is an opening on the medial surface of the ramus. It is the entry point of the inferior alveolar nerve, which is a branch of the mandibular nerve V3 (Fig. 3.10).

Fossa

(a) *Pterygopalatine fossa.* The pterygopalatine fossa lies posterior to the posterior walls of the maxillary sinuses. It is bounded anteriorly by the perpendicular plate of the palatine bone and posteriorly by the pterygoid plate of the sphenoid bone. The pterygopalatine fossa connects anteriorly with the infraorbital canal, posteriorly with the vidian canal, and laterally with the infratemporal fossa. It contains the pterygopalatine ganglion, which transmits sensory, parasympathetic, and sympathetic nerve fibers to the face and nasal cavity [16] (Figs. 3.8 and 3.9).

(b) *Infratemporal fossa.* The infratemporal fossa is an irregularly shaped space that has anterior, posterior, medial, lateral, and superior walls but has no floor. It connects with the temporal fossa, the pterygopalatine fossa, and the orbit. The infratemporal fossa's contents include the medial and lateral pterygoid muscles and the temporalis muscle [17] (Figs. 3.8, 3.9, 3.10, and 3.11).

3.7 CBCT and the Imaging of the Temporomandibular Joints

Imaging of the temporomandibular joints (TMJs) can be done using a variety of imaging modalities (e.g., panoramic radiography, MRI, CT, and CBCT) [18]. Each of these modalities has its strengths and weaknesses. CBCT is a powerful imaging modality for interrogating the osseous structures of the TMJs and associated structures [19]. CBCT imaging does poorly when imaging the soft tissue structures associated with the TMJs, but it still can be used to evaluate, at least grossly, the outlines of the soft tissue structures and soft tissue spaces. The osseous structures that can be imaged with a CBCT scan include the glenoid fossae, the condyles, the articular eminences, and the medial and lateral pterygoid plates. Soft tissue structures and spaces that can be somewhat imaged are the lateral pterygoid and masseter muscles and the radiographic disk space. CBCT viewing software has developed several different viewing windows for evaluating the TMJs from multiplanar views (Fig. 3.13a, b) to a TMJ "Window" that allows for the viewing of both TMJs at once in two of the three viewing planes along with multiple slices through a single viewing plane (Fig. 3.13c).

3.7.1 Osseous Structures of the TMJs

(a) *Glenoid fossa.* The glenoid fossa is a bilateral oval depression in the temporal bone. The glenoid fossa houses the articular disk and the condylar head of the condyle. The roof of the fossa is a thin section of bone that separates the TMJ space from the middle cranial fossa. The anterior limit of the glenoid fossa coincides with the posterior slope of the articular eminence.

(b) *Condylar head.* The condylar heads are bilateral structures that extend superiorly from the condylar neck and are the most superior structure of the mandible. The condylar head's superior surface is generally smooth and convex. The mediolateral width is larger than the anteroposterior width. A thin layer of cortical bone covers the outer surface. The inner bone is cancellous bone. The condylar heads sit in the glenoid fossa with the jaws closed. On jaw opening, the condylar heads move inferiorly and anteriorly along the posterior slope of the articular eminence and come to rest approximately at the apex of the articular eminence. The articular disk sits in the space made by the superior surface of the condylar head and the glenoid fossa when the jaws are closed. This space is called the radiographic disk space (Fig. 3.13a, b).

(c) *Articular eminence.* The articular eminence is a bony protrusion on the inferior surface of

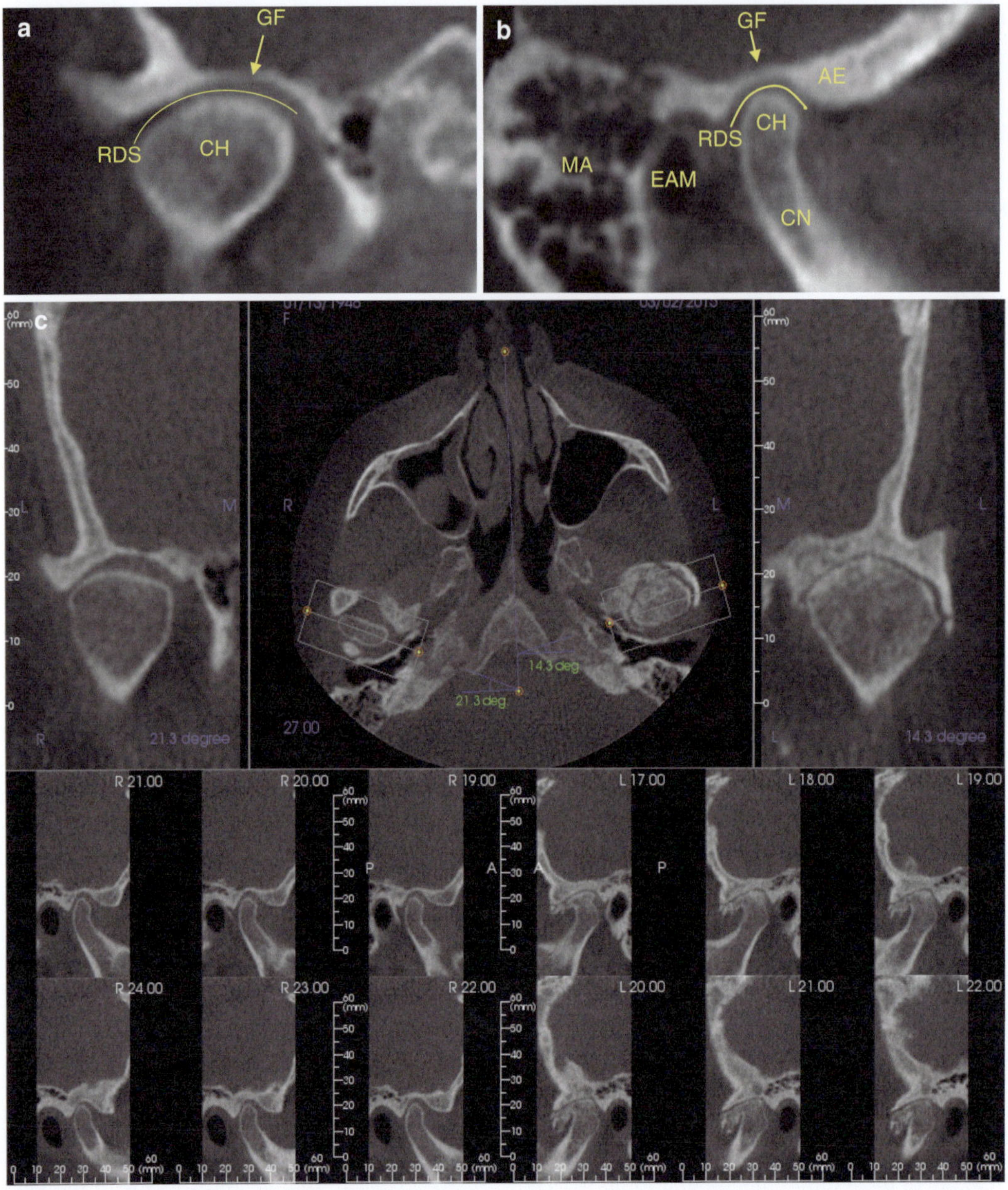

Fig. 3.13 (**a**) Coronal view of the TMJ. (**b**) Sagittal view of the TMJ. (**c**) TMJ window showing bilateral views of the TMJ with the coronal view in the upper left and right and serial sections through the TMJ in the bottom view. Notice the normal osseous structures in the right TMJ versus the severe degenerative joint changes in the left TMJ. AE articular eminence, CH condylar head, CN condylar neck, EAM external auditory meatus, GF glenoid fossa, MA mastoid air cells, RDS radiographic disk space

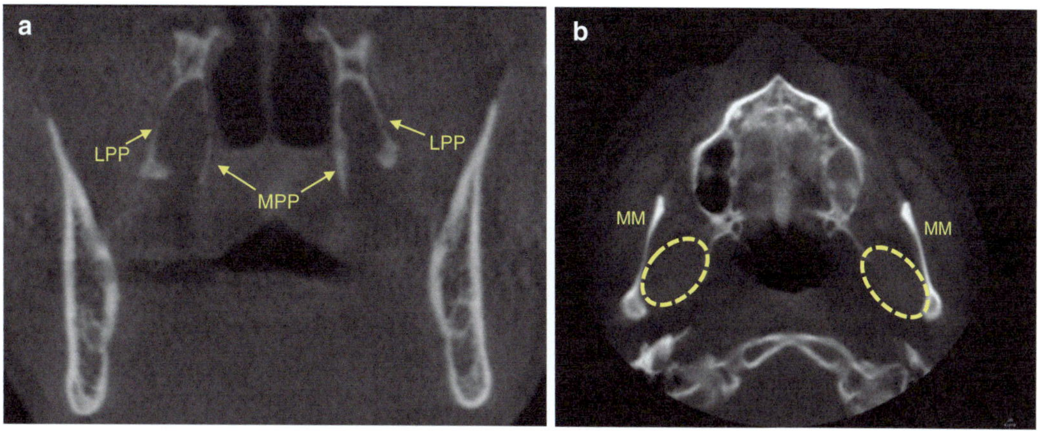

Fig. 3.14 (**a**) Coronal section. (**b**) Axial section. LPP lateral pterygoid plate, MM masseter muscle, MPP medial pterygoid plate. Yellow dashed line showing the outline of the lateral pterygoid muscle

the temporal bone. The posterior slope of the articular eminence is the anterior bony wall of the glenoid fossa. The articular eminence guides the condylar heads during mandibular rotation and translation (Fig. 3.13b).

(d) *Medial and lateral pterygoid plates.* The medial and lateral pterygoid plates are posteroinferior bony projections from the sphenoid bone. They are the bony support and origin of the medial and lateral pterygoid muscles, respectively [16, 20] (Fig. 3.14a).

3.7.2 Soft Tissue Structures and Soft Tissue Spaces

(a) *Lateral pterygoid muscle.* The lateral pterygoid muscle is a two-head muscle that inserts into the articular disk and fibrous capsule of the TMJ (superior or upper head) and inserts into the pterygoid fovea of the condylar neck (inferior or lower head). On CBCT axial sections, the faint soft tissue outline can be appreciated when the image contrast is manipulated (Fig. 3.14b).

(b) *Masseter muscle.* The masseter muscle is located on the lateral side of the ramus and mandible. The muscle's origin is the zygomatic arch, and its insertion is into the mandible. On CBCT axial sections, the soft tissue outline can be viewed when the image contrast is manipulated (Fig. 3.14b).

(c) *Radiographic disk space.* The radiographic disk space is the radiolucent space viewed on CBCT that houses the articular disk. The space is between the glenoid fossa superiorly and the head of the condyle inferiorly (Fig. 3.13a, b). Although the articular disk cannot be viewed on CBCT [21], narrowing of the space can be an indication of disk pathosis.

3.8 CBCT Pseudo-Panoramic Image

CBCT software has the capability to generate a pseudo-panoramic image. The pseudo-panoramic image has two advantages over a traditional panoramic radiograph: (1) There is no magnification or distortion of the image, and (2) superimposition is removed by the ability to slice through the image (Fig. 3.15a, b).

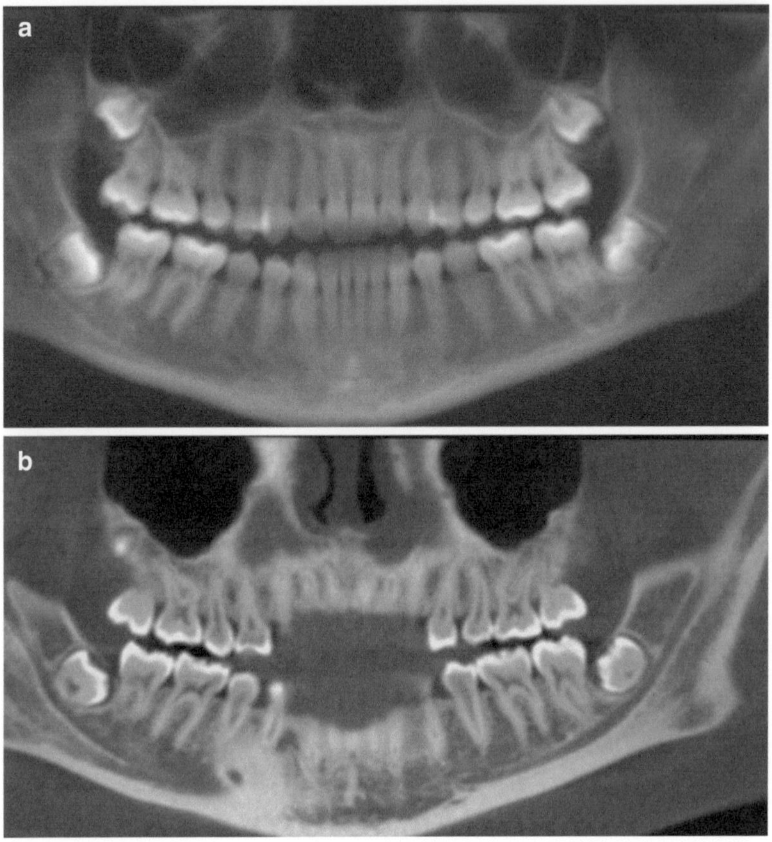

Fig. 3.15 (**a**) Pseudo-panoramic image. (**b**) A slice through the pseudo-panoramic image clearly showing the inferior alveolar canal by the removal of superimposition

3.9 Neck Structures

The neck connects the skull to the torso, and it extends from the base of the skull to the clavicles. There are many different (and vital) anatomical structures present in the neck. The preponderance of these structures is soft tissue. Of the imaging modalities generally available to the dentist or orofacial pain specialist, CBCT is the only imaging that frequently images neck structures usually limited to structures from the level of C1 to C3 or C4 when taking a large field of view. However, CBCTs have poor contrast resolution (i.e., they cannot differentiate between different soft tissues), and hence, all soft tissues whether normal or pathological have the same gray level. As is the case in general, if soft tissue pathosis is suspected, medical CT or MRI is the recommended imaging modality. In this section, the main anatomical structures imaged with CBCT are presented.

3.9.1 Structures in the Neck

(a) *Cervical spine.* The cervical spine is composed of eight vertebrae, and its primary function is to support and allow movement of the head. The first cervical vertebra is called C1 or atlas. The alanto-occipital joint located between the skull base and axis allows for extension and flexion of the head. The second vertebra is called C2 or axis. The axis has a bony prominence on its superior surface called the dens or odontoid process. The dens extends superiorly into the atlas and forms a joint that allows the head to rotate and swivel (Fig. 3.16a–c). The remaining cervical vertebrae are labeled C3–C8. Between adjacent cervical vertebrae is the intervertebral discs. The discs act as shock absorbers and allow for flexion of the spine. Imaging of the cervical spine, especially the

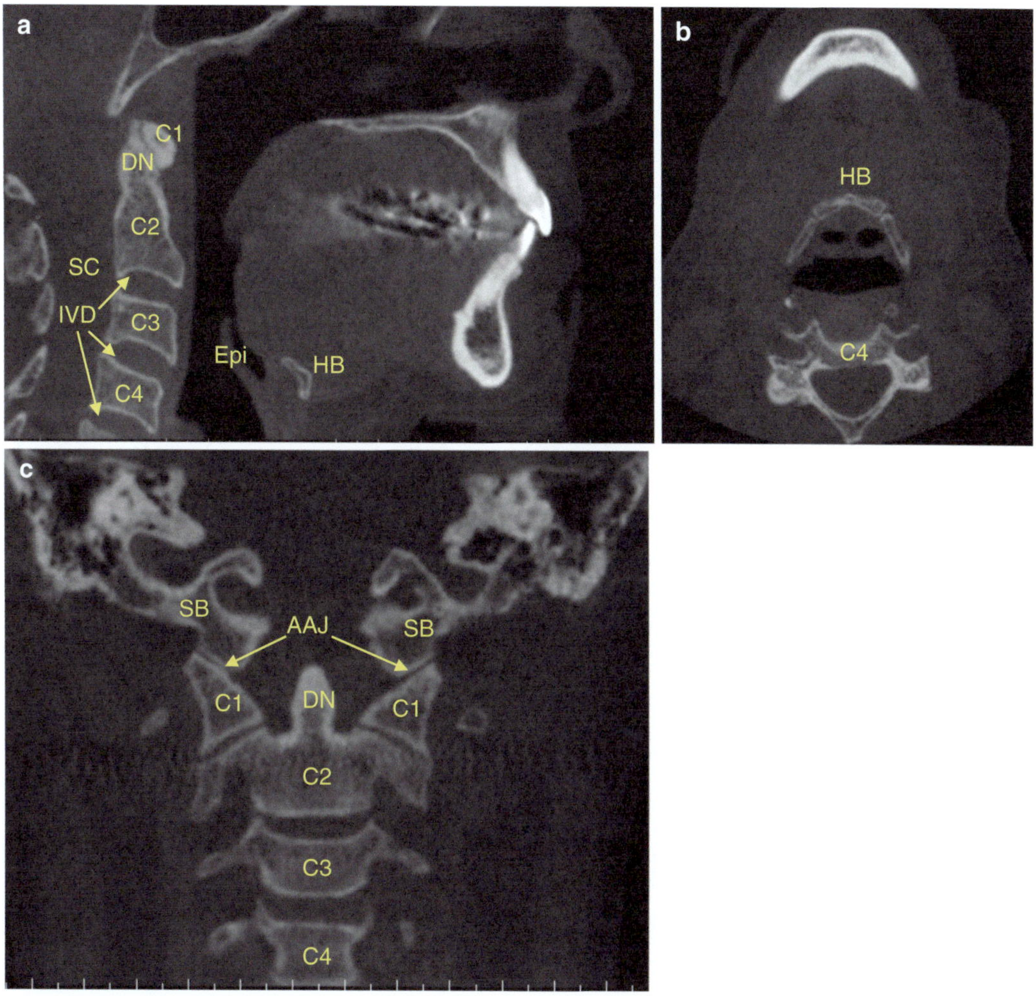

Fig. 3.16 (**a**) Sagittal section imaging structures in the midline. (**b**) Axial section at the level of C4. (**c**) Coronal section showing the base of the skull and cervical vertebrae. AAJ atlanto-occipital junction, C1 atlas, C2 axis, DN dens, Epi epiglottis, HB hyoid bone, IVD intervertebral disc, SB skull base, SC spinal canal

C1–C2, is important as this is a frequent site for osteoarthritis.

(b) *Hyoid bone.* The hyoid bone is a single, anterior, horseshoe-shaped, midline bony structure situated between the chin and the thyroid cartilage (Fig. 3.16a, b). It attaches to other osseous structures through muscles and ligaments as it does not articulate with any other bony anatomy. Muscle attachments include the suprahyoid and infrahyoid muscles. Ligament attachments include the stylohyoid, thyrohyoid, and hyoepiglottic ligaments. The hyoid bone functions in speech, swallowing, and breathing.

(c) *Epiglottis.* The epiglottis is a leaf-shaped flap of cartilage in the midline of the throat. Its base is below the tongue, and it extends superiorly and posteriorly in the pharynx to above the larynx. In its extended position, it allows air to pass into the trachea (Fig. 3.16a). During swallowing, the primary function of the epiglottis is to fold down and close off the trachea to prevent food, liquids, or other debris from being aspirated into the lungs.

3.10 Magnetic Resonance Imaging (MRI)

Magnetic resonance imaging or MRI is the gold standard for imaging cranial nerves [22] and soft tissue structures of the head and neck. MRI has another advantage over other imaging modalities such as panoramic radiography and CBCT in that MRI does not use ionizing radiation to acquire the image [23]. The use of MRI for imaging extracranial and intracranial structures has many applications in imaging the head and neck regions; however, they will not be reviewed in this chapter but will be introduced in other chapters of this book as needed. An example of MRI use in orofacial pain is provided here, as MRI may be used for evaluation of the TMJ [24]. This example will discuss internal displacement of the TMJ and introduce the reader to the visualization of the articular disk using MRI.

3.10.1 MRI Image Viewing

The acquisition of an MRI study allows many ways to manipulate the imaging parameters and change the monochromatic gray scale value of the anatomy. Unlike intraoral, panoramic, or CBCT imaging, where the contrast (radiolucency, radiopacity) of the anatomy is determined by the density of the tissues, MRI can change the contrast to make certain tissue brighter or darker depending on the needs of the study. Furthermore, MRI can suppress some tissues and make them dark (e.g., fat suppression) or enhance tissues (e.g., contrasting agents) and make them brighter. The critical point here is that the ability to interpret ionizing radiation imaging studies does not translate into the ability to read MRI studies. It would behoove any clinician without extensive training in reading and interpretation of head and neck MR images to consult with a neuroradiologist.

3.10.2 Internal Derangement of the TMJ

The articular disk is a bow tie-shaped fibrocartilaginous structure that sits between the glenoid fossa and articular eminence and the condylar head when the jaws are closed [25] (Fig. 3.17). Under normal physiological function, the articular disk remains between the greatest point of contact of the condylar head and the glenoid fossa and articular eminence as the mandible rotates and translates during jaw opening and closing.

Internal derangement of the TMJ occurs if the articular disk becomes displaced from its normal position with the condylar head. The two most common types of internal derangement of the TMJ are (1) disk displacement with reduction and (2) disk displacement without reduction [26]. The techniques for imaging the TMJ using MRI are many and have been reviewed elsewhere [27]. The most common displacement of the articular disk in internal derangement is an anterior displacement of the disk relative to the condylar head (Figs. 3.18a and 3.19a). Posterior displacement of the articular disk is rare, with a reported prevalence of 0.7–2.2% of cases [26].

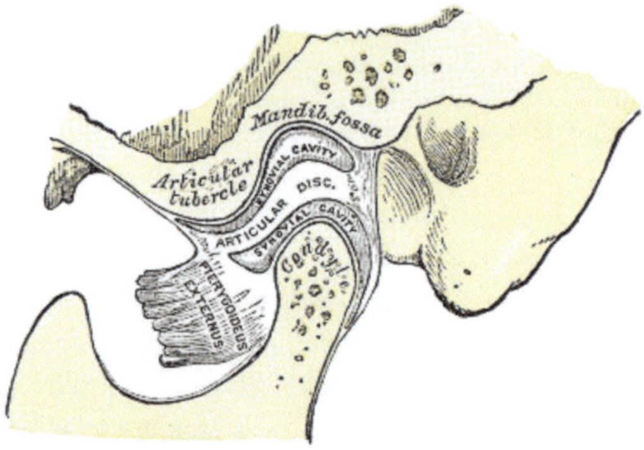

Fig. 3.17 The articular disk interposed between the condylar head and the glenoid fossa and articular eminence with the jaws closed

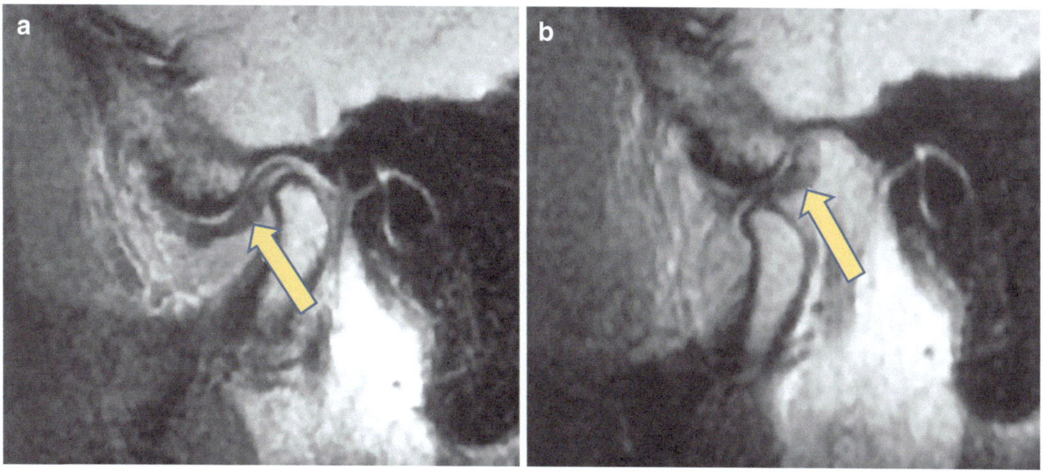

Fig. 3.18 Disk displacement with reduction. (**a**) Anterior displacement of the articular disk. (**b**) The articular disk returning to its normal position upon opening and closing of the jaws

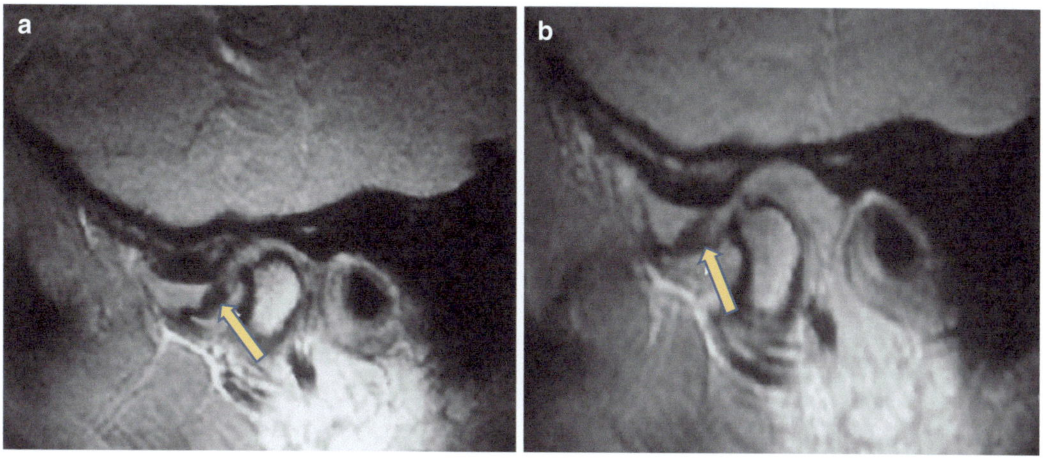

Fig. 3.19 Disk displacement without reduction. (**a**) Anterior displacement of the articular disk. (**b**) The articular disk does not return to its normal position upon opening and closing of the jaws

3.10.3 Disk Displacement with Reduction

In disk displacement with reduction, the articular disk becomes displaced at some time during the opening and closing of the jaws (Fig. 3.18a). Upon a variable number of cycles of jaw opening and closing, the articular disk will return to its normal position in relation to the condylar head (Fig. 3.18b). Further cycles of jaw opening and closing will again displace the articular disk, and the cycle of disk displacement and reduction will continue.

3.10.4 Disk Displacement Without Reduction

In disk displacement without reduction, the articular disk becomes displaced at some time during the opening and closing of the jaws (Fig. 3.19a). Unlike disk displacement with reduction, however, on any number of cycles of opening and closing of the jaws, the articular disk stays displaced and does not return to its normal relationship with the condylar head (Fig. 3.19b).

3.11 Conclusion

In this chapter, normal imaging structures imaged with periapical radiographs, panoramic radiographs, and CBCT scans were reviewed. A brief introduction to MRI was also presented. For the clinician, the importance of knowing normal imaging anatomy cannot be overstated. A clinician must know what normal looks like before abnormal can be identified. In addition, a clinician must choose the most appropriate imaging modality. The choice of which imaging modality, if any, must be guided by the clinical history and examination and clinical judgment. As presented in this chapter, multiple imaging modalities can image the same anatomy. However, each modality has its strengths and weaknesses. The choice of imaging modality that will best answer the clinical question should be selected.

References

1. Shintaku W, Enciso R, Broussard J, Clark GT. Diagnostic imaging for chronic orofacial pain, maxillofacial osseous and soft tissue pathology and temporomandibular disorders. J Calif Dent Assoc. 2006;34(8):633–44.
2. Whyte A, Matias M. Imaging of orofacial pain. J Oral Pathol Med. 2020;49(6):490–8.
3. Gupta A, Devi P, Srivastava R, Jyoti B. Intra oral periapical radiography - basics yet intrigue: a review. Bangladesh J Dent Res Educ. 2014;4:83.
4. Suomalainen A, Pakbaznejad Esmaeili E, Robinson S. Dentomaxillofacial imaging with panoramic views and cone beam CT. Insights Imaging. 2015;6(1):1–16.
5. Schiffman E, Ohrbach R, Truelove E, Look J, Anderson G, Goulet JP, et al. Diagnostic Criteria for Temporomandibular Disorders (DC/TMD) for clinical and research applications: recommendations of the International RDC/TMD Consortium Network* and Orofacial Pain Special Interest Group†. J Oral Facial Pain Headache. 2014;28(1):6–27.
6. Epstein JB, Caldwell J, Black G. The utility of panoramic imaging of the temporomandibular joint in patients with temporomandibular disorders. Oral Surg Oral Med Oral Pathol Oral Radiol Endod. 2001;92(2):236–9.
7. Winocur E, Reiter S, Krichmer M, Kaffe I. Classifying degenerative joint disease by the RDC/TMD and by panoramic imaging: a retrospective analysis. J Oral Rehabil. 2010;37(3):171–7.
8. A pictorial review of cranial nerves imaging anatomy and pathology: part 1—anatomy. Contemp Neurosurg 2022;44(14):8.
9. Schulz RA, Stein JA, Pelc NJ. How CT happened: the early development of medical computed tomography. J Med Imaging (Bellingham, Wash). 2021;8(5):052110.
10. Liang H. Imaging in orofacial pain. Dent Clin N Am. 2018;62(4):533–51.
11. Elmorsy K, Elsayed L, Elkhateeb S. Case report: ectopic third molar in the maxillary sinus with infected dentigerous cyst assessed by cone beam CT. F1000Res. 2020;9:209.
12. von Arx T, Lozanoff S, Bornstein MM. Extraoral anatomy in CBCT – a literature review. Part 2: Zygomatico-orbital region. Swiss Dent J. 2020;130(2):126–38.
13. von Arx T, Lozanoff S, Bornstein MM. Extraoral anatomy in CBCT – a literature review. Part 1: Nasoethmoidal region. Swiss Dent J. 2019;129(10):804–15.
14. Tomaszewska IM, Kmiotek EK, Pena IZ, Środniawa M, Czyżowska K, Chrzan R, et al. Computed tomography morphometric analysis of the greater palatine canal: a study of 1,500 head CT scans and a systematic review of literature. Anat Sci Int. 2015;90(4):287–97.
15. Gong W, Cao W, Zhang W, Xiang R, Xu Y. Imaging anatomy of the vidian canal and its clinical significance. Quant Imaging Med Surg. 2023;13(12):8704–28.
16. von Arx T, Lozanoff S, Bornstein MM. Extraoral anatomy in CBCT – a literature review. Part 3: Retromaxillary region. Swiss Dent J. 2020;130(3):216–28.
17. Arya S, Rane P, D'cruz A, Hathiram BT, Khattar VS. Infratemporal fossa, masticator space and Parapharyngeal space: can the radiologist and surgeon speak the same language? Otorhinolaryngol Clin Int J. 2012;4:125–35.
18. Mallya SM, Ahmad M, Cohen JR, Kaspo G, Ramesh A. Recommendations for imaging of the temporomandibular joint. Position statement from the American Academy of Oral and Maxillofacial Radiology and the American Academy of Orofacial Pain. J Oral Facial Pain Headache. 2023;37(1):7–15.
19. Brooks SL, Brand JW, Gibbs SJ, Hollender L, Lurie AG, Omnell K-Å, et al. Imaging of the temporomandibular joint: a position paper of the American

Academy of Oral and Maxillofacial Radiology. Oral Surg Oral Med Oral Pathol Oral Radiol Endod. 1997;83(5):609–18.
20. Guerrero ME, Beltran J, de Laat A, Jacobs R. Can pterygoid plate asymmetry be linked to temporomandibular joint disorders? Imaging Sci Dentist. 2015;45(2):89–94.
21. Barghan S, Tetradis S, Mallya S. Application of cone beam computed tomography for assessment of the temporomandibular joints. Aust Dent J. 2012;57(Suppl 1):109–18.
22. Romano N, Federici M, Castaldi A. Imaging of cranial nerves: a pictorial overview. Insights Imaging. 2019;10(1):33.
23. Algarín JM, Díaz-Caballero E, Borreguero J, Galve F, Grau-Ruiz D, Rigla JP, et al. Simultaneous imaging of hard and soft biological tissues in a low-field dental MRI scanner. Sci Rep. 2020;10(1):21470.
24. Bag AK, Gaddikeri S, Singhal A, Hardin S, Tran BD, Medina JA, et al. Imaging of the temporomandibular joint: an update. World J Radiol. 2014;6(8):567–82.
25. Runci Anastasi M, Cascone P, Anastasi GP, Santoro G, Nicita F, Picciolo G, et al. Articular disc of a human temporomandibular joint: evaluation through light microscopy, immunofluorescence and scanning electron microscopy. J Funct Morphol Kinesiol. 2021;6(1):22.
26. Young AL. Internal derangements of the temporomandibular joint: a review of the anatomy, diagnosis, and management. J Indian Prosthodont Soc. 2015;15(1):2–7.
27. Mehndiratta A, Kumar J, Manchanda A, Singh I, Mohanty S, Seth N, et al. Painful clicking jaw: a pictorial review of internal derangement of the temporomandibular joint. Pol J Radiol. 2019;84:e598–615.

4 Radiation Physics and Health Safety Concerns

Mel Mupparapu, Brad M. Hong, and Irene H. Kim

4.1 Introduction

Knowledge of radiation physics, radiation biology, and radiation protection is paramount to the dental practitioner including the orofacial pain specialist, especially the understanding of the principles of imaging and the rationale for ordering either the radiograph or a study involving a radiopharmaceutical agent. This chapter also outlines a brief history of radiology, from the discovery of X-ray by William Roentgen and his contemporaries to the discovery and application of the X-ray for imaging. The understanding of the effects of radiation took years, and unfortunately, the lives of many health care practitioners were affected before human effects of radiation were completely understood. This chapter also outlines both traditional and advanced imaging principles used in image production.

4.2 History of Dental Radiography

Within weeks of the publication of Roentgen's discovery of X-rays in 1895, Dr. Otto Walkhoff of Germany obtained possibly the first dental radiograph on himself in 1896. About the same period, Dr. Frank Harrison of Sheffield, England, took a dental radiograph of a 7-year-old girl, carefully recorded his work, and published it in the *Journal of British Dental Association* in 1896. The credit of introducing radiographs to dentistry goes to four pioneers who worked independently on imaging of the teeth and oral cavity: Drs. Walkhoff and Koenig in Germany, Dr. Edmund Kells in the United States, and Dr. Harrison in England [1].

In the early years of the twentieth century, rapid developments took place in the design of medical and dental X-ray-generating equipment. After Roentgen's discovery, several scientists independently developed a "focus tube" which is essentially made by moving the parallelly placed anode to an angled one, leading to smaller source of X-rays and hence sharper images and longer tube life. The X-ray tubes during this period had air which was considered a source of electrons (Fig. 4.1). Constant depletion of air led to the hit or miss X-ray production. The X-ray tubes then were made with small projections within the glass tube with a small opening closed by a screw cap to let the air in upon depletion to a vacuum. This process was very cumbersome, and the operator was forced to test upon themselves or an assistant before using on a patient. This was well before the effects of radiation were largely known to the scientific world. The development and introduction of alternating current (AC) and transformers

M. Mupparapu (✉) · B. M. Hong · I. H. Kim
Division of Oral and Maxillofacial Radiology, University of Pennsylvania School of Dental Medicine, Philadelphia, USA
e-mail: mmd@upenn.edu

G. A. Kaspo, G. D. Klasser (eds.), *Orofacial and Head Pain*,
https://doi.org/10.1007/978-3-032-08275-6_4

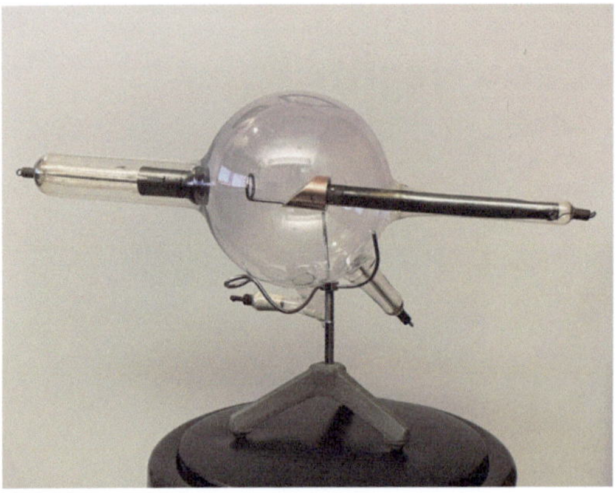

Fig. 4.1 Crookes tube dated circa 1910–1919 approximately after the discovery of X-rays and early experimentation with the air-filled cathode tubes. This Crookes tube was created with hand-blown techniques and is not a vacuum tube

improved this situation greatly, but it was not until Dr. William Coolidge patented his "hot cathode" technology in 1913 that there was a significant improvement in the production of X-rays. The Coolidge tube used tungsten filament as cathode in a vacuum X-ray tube. The X-ray machines manufactured from 1905 to 1913 had exposed high-voltage wires and had the risk of electrocution. Victor CDX, a shock-proof X-ray machine was introduced in the United States in 1918 that used an oil-filled container to house the X-ray tube and electrical wires. This was a method of insulation, modifications of which are still being used in today's modern X-ray machines [2, 3].

A major development in oral and maxillofacial radiography came in the twentieth century with the introduction of panoramic radiography. Panoramic radiography, with an intraoral source of radiation, was initially developed in the 1940s and 1950s, but it was not until Dr. Yrjo Veli Paatero, a Finnish scientist who built on the previous ideas of researchers, invented a panoramic X-ray machine that had an extraoral source of radiation with a "slit-beam collimator" [4, 5].

Panoramic radiographic machines today offer a wide variety of options including selective radiography of areas within the jaws, extraoral bitewing radiography, tomography for the temporomandibular joint (TMJ) and sinuses, and an added option of converting these machines to cone beam CT machines.

The introduction of *F-speed film/Insight film* toward the end of the century reduced the radiation doses to essentially half of what was used for D-speed films that were used until then. This reduced the time of exposure drastically to fractions of seconds. All the films were processed chemically using the chemicals developer and fixer. Automated processors were introduced to the dental profession, transporting exposed films on a roller in the machine through the developer, water, fixer, and water, and then drying them within the processor before they were collected for viewing and interpretation. About the same time, a French dentist named Francis Mouyen developed the RadioVisioGraphy (RVG), which was the beginning of digital radiography. This development was the start of the migration away from the age-old film radiography as a recording medium while reducing the radiation dose to the patient even further. This was followed by introduction of CCD and CMOS-based digital radiographic sensors that eliminated the need for chemical processing and storage of X-ray films. Digital images are captured electronically, stored on a computer, and viewed upon demand, making capturing, storing, and viewing a seamless process while also keeping the radiation doses as low as possible. This added to the concept of *As Low As Reasonably Achievable* (ALARA), making the use of radiation safe for all dental patients [6, 7, 8, 9].

4.3 Physics of Radiation

Radiation is the transmission of energy through space and matter and occurs in two forms, electromagnetic and particulate. X-rays are part of the electromagnetic radiation. In electromagnetic radiation, the movement of energy is a combination of magnetic and electric fields, and radiation is generated when the electrically charged particle's velocity is changed. Other examples of electromagnetic radiation include gamma rays, ultraviolet rays, visible light, infrared radiation (heat), microwaves, and radio waves. On the electromagnetic spectrum, the higher-energy types of radiation are ultraviolet rays, X-rays, and gamma rays. These types of energies are capable of ionizing matter. Higher-energy gamma rays originate in the nuclei of radioactive atoms, whereas X-rays are produced outside of the nucleus as a result of the interaction of electrons with large atomic nuclei [9].

4.3.1 X-Ray Machine

The X-ray machine consists of a power supply, control panel, and head or tube head which contains the X-ray tube. An image receptor is the material on which the latent image is created. The receptor may be a film, fluoroscope, or digital receptor and is processed either chemically or digitally to produce a radiograph. The X-ray tube is positioned within the tube head with components of the power supply, and the tube is often recessed within the tube head to improve the quality of the radiographic image [8].

The basic design of a Coolidge tube was introduced in 1913. It consisted of a cathode as a source of electrons, an anode, and an evacuated glass tube. The electrons from the cathode strike the anode to produce X-ray photons (Fig. 4.2). Coolidge tubes require a power supply to heat a filament to generate electrons and establish a high-voltage potential between the anode and cathode to accelerate the electrons. The filament in the cathode is the source of electrons and is a coil of tungsten wire 1 cm long and 0.2 cm in diameter mounted on two stiff wires for support to carry the electric current. The wires are connected to high- and low-voltage electric sources, and the incandescence of the wire causes the release of electrons. Tungsten has a high atomic number of 74 and is most efficient at producing X-rays. Its high melting point of 3370°C can withstand the high temperatures generated when photons are produced, and the low vapor pressure helps maintain the vacuum in the tube at those high operating temperatures. It also has a high thermal conductivity that dissipates the heat into the copper stem. The cathode also features a focusing cup which is a negatively charged concave reflector that repels electrons. The focusing cup is made of nickel or molybdenum and directs the electrons from the filament to a focal spot on the anode. Electrons travel from the cathode to the anode by repellant forces on the negatively charged cathode and the attractive forces on the positively charged anode [8].

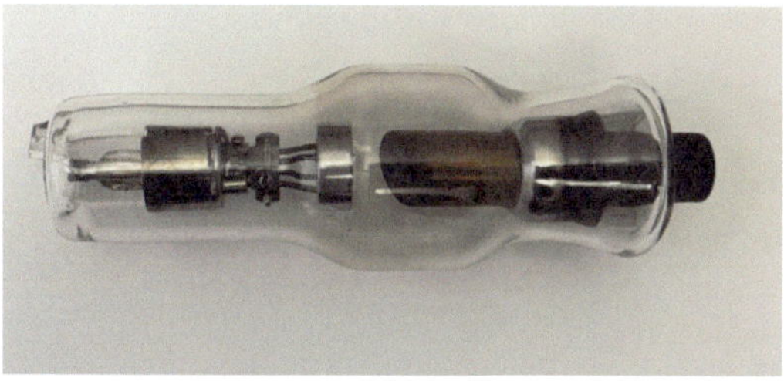

Fig. 4.2 This smaller version of the X-ray tube, known as the "Coolidge tube" was a vacuum X-ray tube that is now known as the "modern X-ray tube" due to its small size and vacuum sealing

The anode contains a tungsten target embedded in a copper stem that converts the kinetic energy of the electrons from the filament into photon energy or X-rays. This is an inefficient process where 99% of the energy is lost as heat. The tungsten is embedded in a large block of copper which is a good thermal conductor that can dissipate the heat from the tungsten, thereby reducing the risk of target melting. Oil surrounds the X-ray tube for insulation [9].

Handheld X-ray machines Portable or handheld X-ray machines have made their way into dental practices since the introduction of the first of its kind, the Nomad®, in the early 2000s. The Nomad® (Fig. 4.3), a battery-operated and handheld dental X-ray machine, was tested for radiation safety, backscatter radiation, and overall effectiveness. Although there are distinct differences in the indications and techniques of using such devices compared with the wall-mounted traditional X-ray machines, these machines are considered radiation-emitting

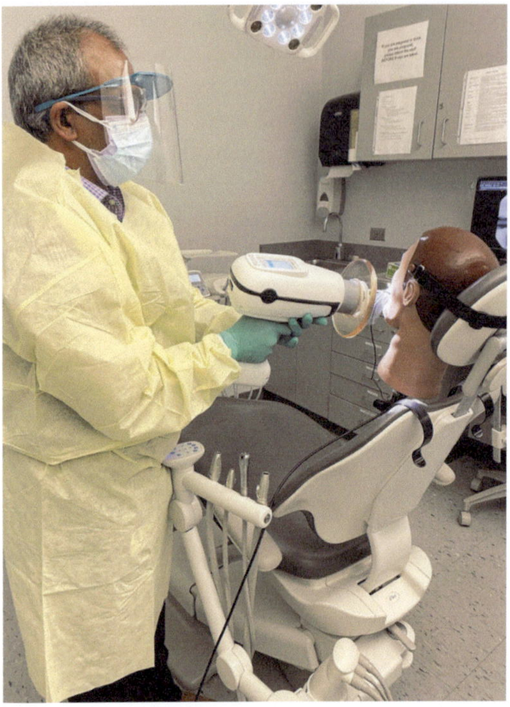

Fig. 4.3 Here the operator is seen holding the handheld, battery-operated X-ray machine simulating the exposure on a DXTTR mannequin. In real-life situations, both the operator and the patient should have a protective apron. (Image courtesy: Dr. Mel Mupparapu)

devices that present no greater risk than the standard X-ray machines, and the measured doses were well below the recommended levels of radiation [10, 11].

4.3.2 Image Quality

Voltage is the potential difference between two electric charges, and in an X-ray tube, the voltage is measured between the negative cathode and positive anode. When the voltage is increased, the speed of the electrons is increased, causing the electrons to strike the target with a greater force resulting in a radiograph beam with a shorter wavelength. Voltage is measured in volts or kilovolts (1 kV = 1000 V). A polychromatic beam is the result of varying kilovoltage in an AC tube. The two most important parameters regarding radiographic exposure are density and contrast in a film-based detector. In a digital detector, other factors such as bit depth come into play, but the kilovoltage peak (kVp) is a key factor. An adjustment in kVp changes the contrast of a dental radiograph. A low kilovoltage setting (<70 kVp) results in an image with high contrast. A high kilovoltage setting (>80 kVp) results in an image with low contrast. Radiographic exposure parameters are typically between 60 kVp and 70 kVp, and between 5 mA and 8 mA using direct current (DC) radiographic machines. The AC radiographic machines are no longer recommended for digital sensors [12].

The resolution of an image in intraoral digital radiography is limited by the thickness of the layer, not pixel size. Resolution is measured in line pairs resolved per millimeter (lp/mm or lppm) and is also limited by what can be detected by the human eye. Normally, the film resolution is greater than 20 lppm. Intraoral photostimulable phosphor (PSP) detector resolution is between 7 lppm to 14 lppm, and charge-coupled device/complementary metal oxide semiconductor (CCD/CMOS) sensor resolution is between 10 lppm and 24 lppm. While digital imaging systems can capture up to 256 different densities, monitors may or may not display all of the densities captured in one screen. If the resolution of the monitor is higher than the captured densities, there will not be an issue displaying those images. However, the human eye can only distinguish approximately 32 different densities, which is a limiting factor in the diagnostic process [13].

Studies have shown that the ability to recognize incipient dental carious lesions is not dependent on the image sensor (film or digital), the system used, or how it is displayed [13].

4.3.3 Kilovoltage Peak (kVp), Milliamperage (mA), and Exposure Times

The general recommendation when the kVp is increased by 15 for AC machines is to decrease the exposure time by half when the milliampere (mA) is fixed or cannot be altered. When the kVp is decreased by 15, the exposure time should be doubled. Radiation output is proportional to the square of kVp. Increasing the kVp results in an increased density and hence lower contrast. Decreasing the kVp results in lighter density and hence higher contrast, which is recommended for all dental radiographic examinations. When the kVp is increased, the mA seconds must be decreased in order to maintain the previous radiographic density. Radiation output is proportional to mA. Radiation output is also proportional to exposure time [14].

Radiographic images are either stored within a practice management software independently or in a picture archiving and communication system that is connected to practice management software. This method is especially true when the volume of the radiographic data is high and needs networking for large group practice situations, or a dental school environment [9].

4.3.4 Radiation Sources

Radiation comes from both natural and artificial sources. In the United States, the average annual radiation exposure is approximately 3.6–7.2 mSv, or 0.36–0.72 rem. A large proportion of annual exposure to background radiation (80–82%) comes from natural sources, such as radon (2 mSv, 55% of radiation exposure), internal sources (0.39 mSv, 11% of radiation exposure), terrestrial sources (0.28 mSv, 8% of radiation exposure), and cosmic sources (0.27 mSv, 8% of radiation exposure). A smaller proportion (18%) of annual exposure to background radiation comes from artificial sources, such as X-ray diagnosis (0.39 mSv, 11% radiation exposure), nuclear medicine (0.14 mSv, 4% of radiation exposure), and consumer products (0.10 mSv, 3% of radiation exposure). Less than 2% of annual radiation exposure comes from other sources. These include occupational sources, nuclear fuel, and fallout, each of which carries <0.01 mSv and comprises <0.03% of background radiation exposure [15, 16].

Internal sources are the second largest source of natural radiation, resulting from the ingestion of food and water that contain radionuclides. The average annual *E* due to the presence of uranium and thorium and their decay products (primarily potassium-40, but also rubidium-87, carbon-14, tritium, and a dozen or more extraterrestrially produced radionuclides) is estimated at 0.40 mSv (400 μSv) per year in the United States.

In the United States, the average annual exposure to terrestrial radiation is estimated at 0.28 milliSv (280 μSv since 1 milliSv = 1000 μSv), which is 8% of the average annual *E* (Fig. 4.4). This quantity of radiation exposure is minimal compared to the quantity received by people living in other regions [17].

At sea level, the annual exposure to cosmic radiation is about 240 μSv. Cosmic radiation doubles with each 2000-meter increase in elevation. At an elevation of 1600 meters (about 1 mile, or the elevation of Denver, CO), it is approximately 500 μSv per year. At an elevation of 3200 meters (about 2 miles, or the elevation of Leadville, CO), it is approximately 1250 μSv per year. Given the altitude and latitude distribution of the US population, and a 20% reduction in radiation exposure due to structural shielding during time spent indoors, the average cosmic radiation exposure is about 240–260 μSv per year. A single, 5-h airline flight in the middle latitudes at an altitude of 12 kilometers results in about 25 μSv of cosmic radiation exposure [15, 18].

4.3.5 Comparative Effective Doses

The effective dose of background radiation is approximately 3600 μSv per year. When this is compared to diagnostic radiographs, the effective doses from dental radiographs are quite low. A set of four bitewing films approximately equals 2–3 microSv, a full mouth series of radiographs equals about 10–15 μSv, and a TMJ tomogram is approximately 2 μSv. Both a cephalometric radiograph and a panoramic radiograph equal approximately 6–11 μSv. In comparison to medical diagnostic radiographs, posteroanterior (PA) and lateral chest planar films are approximately 170 μSv [11, 19].

Computed tomography (CT) is now often used in medicine and dentistry. In medicine, a chest CT is about 7800 microSv, and a spiral/

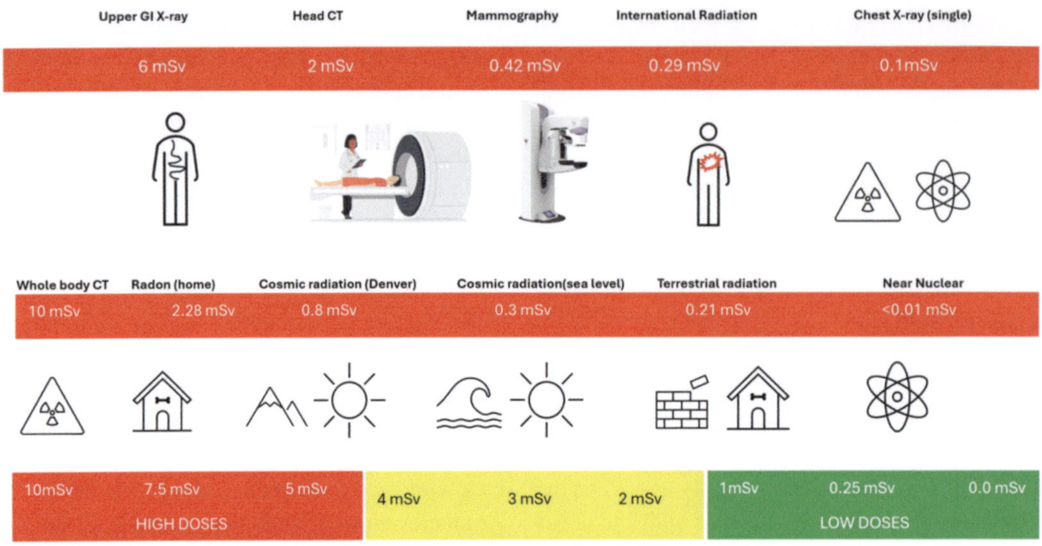

Fig. 4.4 A cartoon depicting the average background radiation doses to US population and equivalent doses from both natural background and additional doses from common medical and dental X-ray procedures. It is color-coded to depict the low and high ends of the dose spectrum

helical CT is approximately 30,000 microSv. In contrast, in dentistry, a CT of the mandible and maxilla equals approximately 2100 microSv. A mandibular CT is about 150–700 microSv, and the maxillary CT is about 1400 microSv. Most recently, cone beam CT (CBCT) is used to examine the oral maxillofacial structures. The effective dose of CBCT equals approximately 52–57 microSv [11, 19].

4.3.6 Effects of Radiation on Cells and Body

Changes in cellular organelles occur and manifest many hours after moderate doses of radiation. The nucleus of the cell, particularly the DNA within the chromosomes, is more sensitive to radiation than the cytoplasm. If a cell is irradiated after DNA synthesis, it may result in a single-arm aberration, also known as a *chromatid aberration*. If the same cell is irradiated before DNA synthesis, it results in a double-arm aberration, also known as a *chromosome aberration*. These changes are not seen at diagnostic radiation levels but more from therapeutic doses [20, 21].

Radiosensitivity varies according to cell type. As early as 1906, French radiobiologists Bergonié and Tribondeau observed that cells from various organs of the same individual may respond differently to irradiation. They recognized that the most radiosensitive cells possess a high mitotic rate, long mitotic future, and primitive differentiation [20]. Like cell types, the organs of the body exhibit varying radiosensitivity. The lymphoid organs, intestines, kidneys, liver, bone marrow, and mucous membranes are examples of organs with high radiosensitivity. The salivary glands, lungs, growing bone, growing cartilage, and fine vasculature exhibit intermediate radiosensitivity. The optic lens, muscle cells, mature erythrocytes, and neurons have low radiosensitivity [21].

4.3.7 Radiation Protection

Carcinogenesis from dental radiographs is relatively low. The risk of cancer from dental radiographs is 11 per million dental radiographic examinations. This is low in comparison to other risks such as hospital accidents and choking deaths which are 13 per million and boating accidents which is 4.6 per million. In medicine, CT scans are commonly performed on patients. The effective dose (E) from a CT of the chest and abdomen is equivalent to 1000 chest films. Although dental radiography is a weak carcinogen, the risk is increased due to the large number of people exposed. However, if everyone were exposed to dental radiographs, the number of new cancer cases would only increase by 0.2%. In dentistry, practitioners practice ALARA (As Low As Reasonably Achievable) to protect their patients. The techniques to reduce radiation exposure include patient selection, choice of equipment, choice of technique, and protection of personnel [11, 19, 22].

In terms of patient selection, dentists should exercise professional judgment when prescribing diagnostic radiographs. They should take into consideration the patient's history and consider both the dental and medical health needs of the patient. There are published selection criteria guidelines for symptomatic and asymptomatic patients available, and the administrative use of radiation should not be used solely for the purpose of education, documentation, or licensure [22].

The source-to-image receptor distance for intraoral radiography is recommended to be between 20 and 40 cm but shall not be less than 20 cm (8 inches) [23], and rectangular collimation of the X-ray beam should always be used. Filters should be used to remove low-energy X-ray photons selectively from the X-ray beam. This filtration decreases the patient exposure to radiation without loss of radiographic information. Patients should be protected with lead aprons and thyroid collars, provided these do not interfere with the examination. Greater than 90% of scatter is absorbed by lead aprons and shields. The current data shows that the mean exposure at skin entrance of a single dental periapical film is 217 mR. If the gonadal dose is equal to 1/10,000 of the total beam exposure, the dose from one dental periapical film would be 0.02 mR which is 50 times less than the negligible dose of 1 mR.

Dental X-ray machines should be operating at greater than 60 kVp, and there is no practical usage at greater than 80 kVp. Constant kilovoltage (kVc) machines should operate in the range of 60–80 kVc. The recommended mA for E speed film at 70 kVp is around 3.6–4.2 mA. If the practitioner still uses film as a recording medium, films should be processed following the manufacturer-recommended conditions with proper processing equipment in a dark room with safelights. An automatic processor with an appropriate safelight hood may also be used. Quality control of the darkroom should be routinely performed with sensitometry, dosimetry, step wedge, reference film, chemical monitoring, and daylight processor maintenance [22].

The personnel of the dental clinic should also be protected by taking into consideration the shielding design, barriers, distance, position, and use of personal dosimeters. The public should be protected with a total E of less than 1 milli Sievert (mSv) per year. Shielding design involves increasing the thickness of building material by adding lead, gypsum, drywall, concrete, and steel. The operator should stand at least 6 feet from the tube head during exposure, and barriers should be designed to allow for visual contact and communication with the patient during the procedure. When using the handheld intraoral machines, both the operator and the patient should be protected with personal protective shielding. Lead thickness of 2 mm is used in leaded aprons, or non-leaded aprons (with lead equivalent material) can be used for patient and operator shielding. In digital imaging, radiographic techniques should be adjusted for the minimum patient dose required to produce an appropriate signal-noise ratio to provide the best image quality. Underexposure results in a decreased signal-noise ratio with a loss of diagnostic information with a grainy image. Although the dental radiographic guidelines recommend obtaining panoramic radiographs on edentulous patients as their first image during a dental visit, these radiographs are also obtained instead of full mouth series in teeth and jaws that appear healthy on history and physical examination visits [24].

4.4 Types of Radiographic Images

4.4.1 Intraoral Radiographs

The three common intraoral radiographs used to assess the patient's dentition and its supporting anatomy are periapical, bitewing, and occlusal radiographs. Periapical views are best for evaluating orofacial pain related to the pulp or periodontal structures. Bitewing views are best for the diagnosis of interproximal dental caries, height of the interproximal bone, and the condition of existing restorations. Occlusal radiographs offer a larger view of the dentition and the supporting structures in the buccal/lingual dimension and can be used on patients with a limited ability to open their mouth [25].

4.4.2 Extraoral Radiographs: Skull Views and Panoramic Radiographs

Skull views are needed when the area of examination exceeds the detector size used to capture the dental images, i.e., periapical or bitewing radiographs. To obtain skull views, the X-ray machine needs to be equipped with a cephalostat or a positioning device for the skull. The patient is typically standing or sitting in a chair while the head is adjusted within the cephalostat and the Frankfurt horizontal plane is adjusted depending on the type of skull image needed. The common skull views are postero-anterior skull (PA skull), antero-posterior skull (AP skull), reverse Townes, Waters view, submento-vertex (SMV), and lateral oblique views of the body of the mandible or ramus. All have specific indications for viewing the facial bones, orbits, mandible including the TMJ, and sinuses. The most useful skull view by far is the Waters view as it shows the craniofacial bones as well as the cervical vertebrae and dens when the patient opens the mouth during the positioning.

Dubbed in the clinical world as the "poor man's CT," the Waters view shows most facial bony structures and the cranium, although it is considered the gold standard for the evaluation of paranasal sinuses. The advent of computed tomography made this technique less useful.

Dental panoramic radiographs (DPR) have a complex magnification pattern as a direct result of the image production mechanisms. To obtain an ideal image, the operator must make sure that the patient is positioned within the machine's "focal trough" or the center of the image plane. There are several aiding guides to make sure this happens including the bite block, chin rest, positioning lights, and lateral side guides. Within the focal trough, both vertical and horizontal image magnifications are equally matched. If the patient is not positioned well within these confines, magnifications are not only pronounced but also differ based on the anatomic location. For example, the inaccuracies are more marked in the anterior region of the jaws as opposed to the posterior region since the focal trough is narrow anteriorly and has less tolerance to errors. Panoramic radiographs, although used for the detection of large carious lesions, generalized periodontal disease, large apical lesions, evaluation of impacted teeth and jaw fractures, identification of systemic disease, and the assessment of TMJ pathology, are limited in use due to the technique being a tomography and the resolutions being low, unless used as an initial exam in partially or completely edentulous patients. This cannot be used as a substitute for intraoral radiography for evaluation of proximal caries and apical inflammatory disease. The limitations of panoramic radiography in the evaluation of TMJ pathology must be considered. Changes in the bony structures are identified only on the lateral slopes or central parts of the condyle, given the oblique orientation of the beam relative to the long axis of the condyle. Only gross changes involving the articular eminence and glenoid fossa are evident due to the superimposition of the base of the skull and zygomatic arches [9, 26, 27].

4.4.3 Cone Beam Computed Tomography

Cone beam computed tomography (CBCT) is a three-dimensional imaging modality that was introduced to dentistry in 1998, with commercially available scanners in the new millennium. CBCT has been used in multiple applications for the diagnosis of dental and maxillofacial disorders, trauma, and treatment planning purposes. In terms of orofacial pain, CBCT can evaluate maxillofacial trauma and pathology involving the salivary glands, nasal cavity, paranasal sinuses, maxilla, mandible, alveolar bone, and dentition (Figs. 4.5 and 4.6). It can also evaluate orofacial pain associated with implant placement, third molar proximity to the inferior alveolar nerve, external/internal resorption of teeth related to impactions, and overall root morphology and anatomy of the teeth and their surrounding structures [9, 25].

Large CBCT fields of view (FOV) are acquired with resolutions ranging from 200 to 400 μm (microns). In many dental specialties that require the visualization of details like the lamina dura or the periodontal ligament space, furcation defects, root anatomy, fractures, and complex pathways of pulp in high resolution, small-volume CBCT imaging is used with pixel sizes as small as 60–70 μm.

Children and adolescents need CT with lowered dose, and therefore, CBCT would be their choice of imaging modality compared to the medical CT (MDCT/MSCT). The FOVs can be tailored to suit the imaging needs in pediatric dental patients, thereby reducing the effective doses [E], as collectively there is an obligation to our patients to achieve maximum diagnostic ability using minimum dose as noted in the principle of ALARA (As Low as Reasonably Achievable) [9, 22].

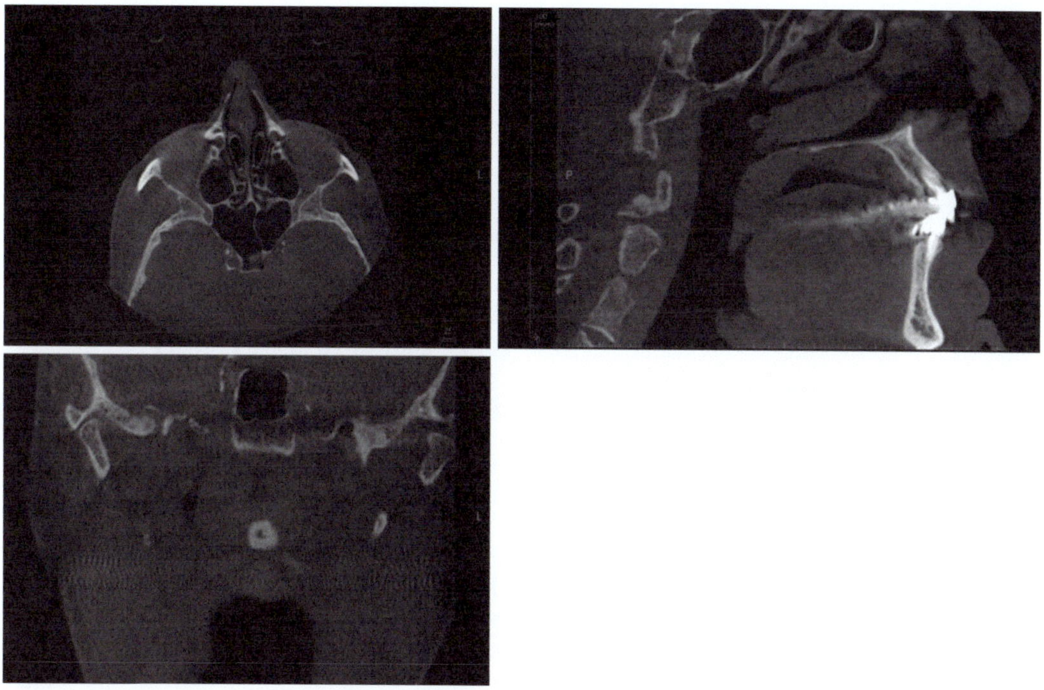

Fig. 4.5 A cone beam CT (CBCT) axial, sagittal, and coronal reconstructions (clockwise) depicting calcifications within the cavernous sinus area intracranially. Typically, CBCT volumes are obtained to rule out the maxillofacial disease as part of investigation for orofacial pain and headache

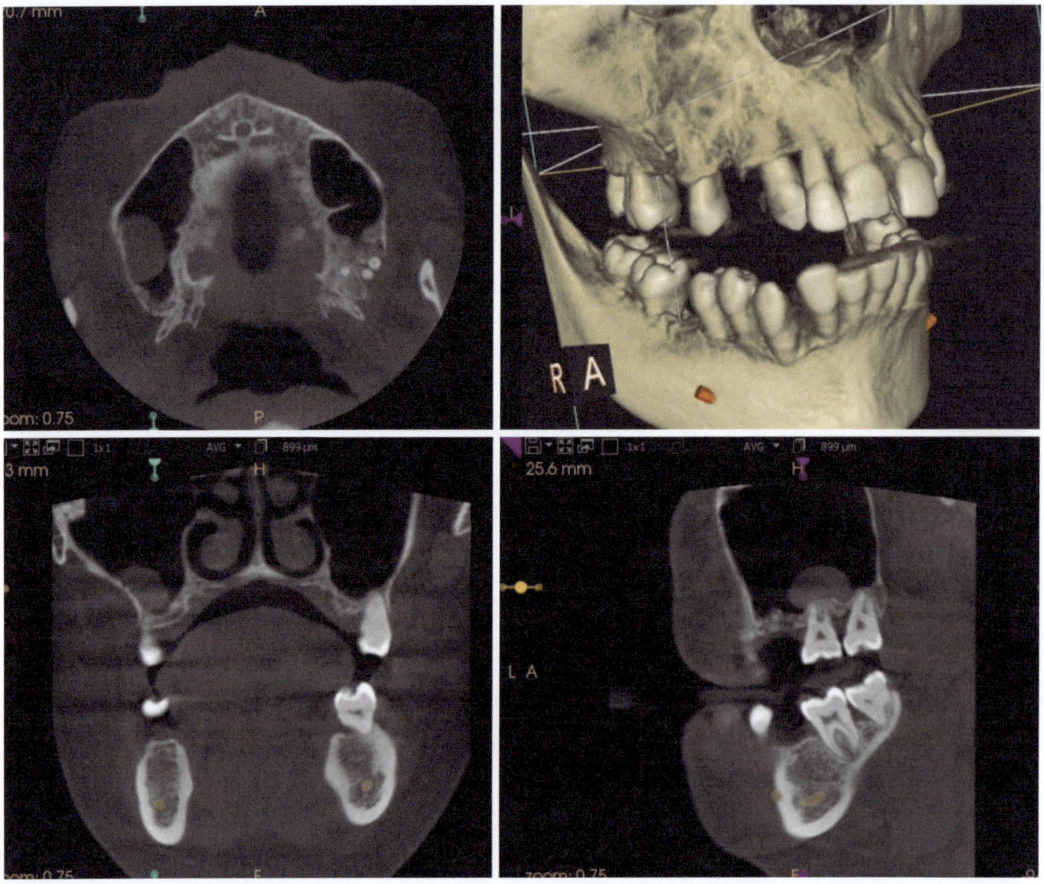

Fig. 4.6 A CBCT axial, 3D, sagittal, and coronal constructions showing a large mucous retention cyst within the right maxillary sinus. Patient has AAP stage 4 periodontal disease

4.4.4 Computed Tomography

The CT scan-derived image is in the digital format. It consists of a square matrix of pixels (picture elements), the three-dimensionality of each pixel represents a voxel (volume element) of the given section of a patient. Voxel can be calculated by multiplying pixel area and slice thickness. A CT section has a finite thickness. The size of this voxel depends on the matrix size, the selected field of view (FOV), and the section thickness. The average linear attenuation coefficients of the patient's anatomy correspond to the spatial locations of these pixels. The numerical pixel matrix corresponding to a spatial location in the image is converted into an image based on the allocation/transformation of the pixel values to a corresponding gray scale value.

CT numbers (Hounsfield units (HU)) are defined as the attenuation values of the imaged tissues normalized to that of water.

According to the definition of CT number (HU), the CT numbers of air and water range from −1000 to 0, respectively. The conventional (traditional) CT scanner uses a fan-shaped X-ray beam, which takes a single slice image per scan and continues to the next slice scan position. The spiral or helical CT scanner uses a continuous acquisition mode in which the fan-shaped X-ray beam and detector (or multidetector) move along a helical or spiral path relative to the object acquiring the data. Multidetector CT (MDCT) is equipped with a 2D array of detector elements which replaced the linear array of detector elements (in a single-slice CT) used in conventional and spiral CT scanners. The 2D detector array allows CT scanning to acquire multiple slices (or sections) of large volume simultaneously, and greatly increases the speed of CT image acquisition.

The advantage of MDCT is faster scanning, as more parts of the body are contained in each turn of the gantry. For MDCT, multiple slices are reconstructed per projection by the multiple rows of detectors. In MDCT, the pitch is calculated by dividing the table movement by the entire beam width. This yields numbers like the single-slice version: a pitch of 1 corresponds to contiguous helices [28].

4.4.4.1 Dual-Energy CT (DECT) and Detector-Based Spectral CT

DECT, also known as spectral CT, uses two different X-ray energy tubes (most frequently rated at 80 kVp and 140 kVp) compared with the general single-energy helical CT, thus allowing the image enhancement of substances with the use of subtraction imaging techniques, which have separate attenuation behaviors at different energies. DECT can already facilitate better discrimination of tissues, thus making it easier to differentiate between materials, such as tissues containing calcium and iodine that can appear similar on traditional, monochromatic CT techniques. It can also potentially increase diagnostic accuracy in a wide range of clinical applications [9, 25, 29].

4.4.5 Bone Scintigraphy

Bone scintigraphy or radionuclide scans are examples of radioisotope imaging. In contrast to other imaging techniques, the radiation source is positioned within the body. Radiographic isotopes that emit gamma rays from within the body can be imaged, and the isotope selection is based on its affinity to the tissue of interest that is being investigated. The short-lived tracer isotopes can be delivered via injection, inhalation, or by mouth, and a gamma camera detects and builds an image from the areas where the radiation is emitted [30].

Technetium (^{99m}Tc) is the most commonly used isotope and has played a significant role in the diagnosis of oral maxillofacial disorders. In patients with idiopathic facial pain (IFP), a positive ^{99m}Tc scan was strongly correlated with the location of the pain in IFP and IFP patients demonstrated significantly more hot spots than control patients [31]. Bone scintigraphy has also been used in the diagnosis of osteoarthritis of the TMJ, chronic obstructive parotitis, sialolithiasis, and Sjogren syndrome [32].

4.4.6 Positron Emission Tomography

Positron emission tomography (PET) is a procedure used in radiology to create images for evaluating the function of the organ or tissue for disease or other conditions. Predominantly used for evaluation of the heart and brain, it is also used for detection of cancer and evaluation of cancer treatment. Radiopharmaceuticals are used to tag substances that are used naturally by the particular organ or tissue. Functioning or hyperfunctioning cells accumulate the radionuclide substance, which is measured by its emission outside of the patient's body. For example, in PET scans of the brain, a radioactive atom is applied to glucose (blood sugar) to create a radionuclide called fluorodeoxyglucose (FDG), because the brain uses glucose for its metabolism. FDG is widely used in PET scanning. Other substances may be used for PET scanning, based on the purpose of the scan. If blood flow and perfusion of an organ or tissue are of interest, the radionuclide may be a type of radioactive oxygen, carbon, nitrogen, or gallium.

The radionuclide is administered intravenously to the patient. The scanner moves slowly over the parts of the body being investigated. The positrons emitted by the breakdown of the radionuclide collide with electrons near the decay event, creating gamma rays (annihilation photons). These gamma rays are captured by the detector, and the information is fed to the computer that creates an image map of the organ or tissue. The quantity of radionuclide collected in the tissue or organ indicates the level of the function that can be used to assess the clinical

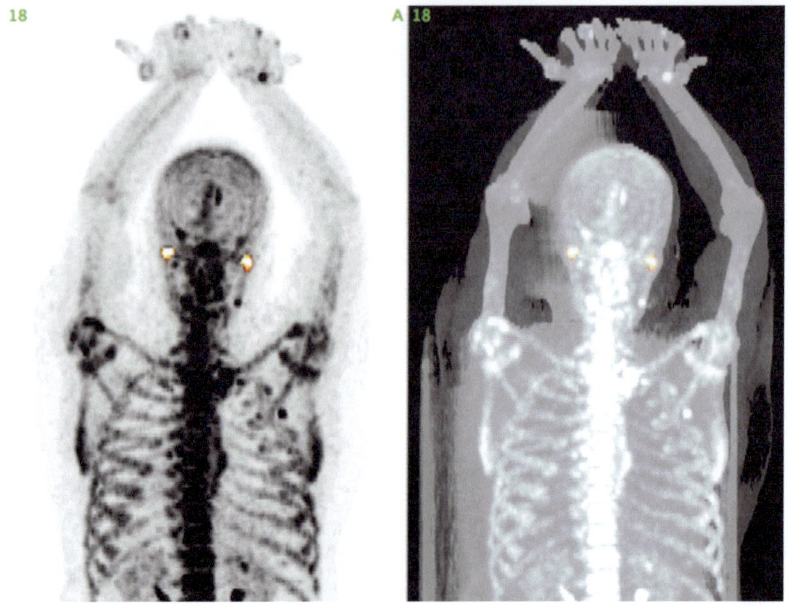

Fig. 4.7 PET/CT fusion images showing the active uptake of FDG in the region of temporomandibular joints bilaterally using a special software called ROVER® which detects and quantifies the uptake of FDG

status of the organ or tissue. Fusion techniques are developed that can combine PET with CT and PET with MRI called PET-CT and PET-MR techniques.

Positron emission tomography (PET) and positron emission tomography/CT (PET/CT) are novel technologies that have shown increasing relevance in the detection and management of TMJ RA. One such example is shown in Fig. 4.7, which not only evaluated the presence of rheumatoid arthritis but also enabled quantification using a software called "ROVER." Similarly, PET-MR techniques are becoming popular in the world of nuclear medicine [33].

4.5 Conclusion

Imaging of craniofacial structures both using radiation and non-radiation sources has its value in not only identifying structures within the head and neck that are abnormal but also differentiating various densities within the head and neck region that show the anatomic detail. This is useful in evaluating a patient who presents with orofacial pain and complex head and neck abnormalities that first manifest as pain. Odontogenic pathology must be ruled out before investigating further for neurogenic causes and intracranial pathology. Starting from intraoral radiography and utilizing various imaging modalities including ultrasound, CBCT, MDCT, MRI, and PET scans, all have a role to play in the identification and isolation of pathology causing orofacial pain. This chapter detailed the role of imaging modalities, quality of imaging, the potential detriment of radiation, and information on the ways to protect the patient and the operator from radiation hazards.

References

1. Horner K, Drage N, Brettle D. Twenty-first century imaging. 1st ed. London: Quintessence Publishing Company; 2007. p. 1–12.
2. Jacobsohn PH, Fedran RJ. Making darkness visible: the discovery of X-ray and its introduction to dentistry. J Am Dent Assoc. 1995;126:1359–67.
3. Tubiana M. Wilhelm Conrad Röntgen and the discovery of X-rays. Bull Acad Natl Med. 1996;180(1):97–108.
4. Hallikainen D. History of panoramic radiography. Acta Radiol. 1996;37:441–5.
5. Graber TM. Panoramic radiography. Angle Orthod. 1966;36:293–311.
6. Molteni R. The way we were (and how we got here): fifty years of technology changes in dental and

maxillofacial radiology. Dentomaxillofac Radiol. 2021;50:20200133.
7. Ruprecht A. Oral and maxillofacial radiology: then and now. J Am Dent Assoc. 2008;139(Suppl):5S–6S.
8. Horner K, Drage N, Brettle D. Quint-essentials imaging 3: 21st century imaging. London: Quintessence Publishing co. Ltd; 2008. p. 1–165.
9. Mupparapu M, Nadeau C. Oral and maxillofacial imaging. Dent Clin N Am. 2016;60:1–37.
10. Goren AD, Bonvento M, Biernacki J, Colosi DC. Radiation exposure with the NOMAD portable X-ray system. Dentomaxillofac Radiol. 2008;37(2):109–12.
11. Gray JE, Bailey ED, Ludlow JB. Dental staff doses with handheld dental intraoral X-ray units. Health Phys. 2012;102:137–42.
12. Fosbinder R, Orth D. Essentials of radiologic science. Philadelphia: Lippincott Williams & Wilkins; 2011.
13. Cederberg RA, Frederiksen NL, Benson BW, Schulman JD. Influence of the digital image display monitor on observer performance. Dentomaxillofac Radiol. 1999;28:203–7.
14. Basics of radiation physics. Available at: https://hps.org/publicinformation/ate/faqs/radiation.html NCRP Report No. 160. In: Ionizing radiation exposure of the population of the United States, 2009. https://ncrponline.org/publications/reports/ncrp-report-160-2. Accessed 30 March 2025.
15. Natural background radiation. Government of Canada In: Natural background radiation, 2020. https://www.cnsc-ccsn.gc.ca/eng/resources/fact-sheets/natural-background-radiation. Accessed 21 Nov 2024.
16. United States Environmental Protection Agency. In: Radiation sources and doses, 2024. https://www.epa.gov/radiation/radiation-sources-and-doses. Accessed 21 Nov 2024.
17. United States Environmental Protection Agency. In: Calculate your radiation dose, 2024. https://www.epa.gov/radiation/calculate-your-radiation-dose. Accessed 21 Nov 2024.
18. Shatskiy I. Effective doses and radiation risks from common dental radiographic, panoramic and CBCT examinations. Radiat Prot Dosim. 2021;195:296–305.
19. Hall EJ. Scientific view of low-level radiation risks. Radiographics. 1991;11(3):509–18.
20. Hall EJ. Radiation biology for pediatric radiologists. Pediatr Radiol. 2009;39(Suppl 1):S57–64.
21. Kim IH, Singer SR, Hong DJ, Mupparapu M. Fundamentals of radiographic interpretation for the dentist. Dent Clin N Am. 2021;65:409–25.
22. Radiation Protection in Dentistry. Recommendations of the National Council on radiation protection and measurements [NCRP report 145, 2003]. Bethesda, MD: National Council for Radiation Protection and Measurements; 2003.
23. Kim IH, Mupparapu M. Dental radiographic guidelines: a review. Quintessence Int. 2009;40:389–98.
24. Liang H. Imaging in orofacial pain. Dent Clin N Am. 2018;62:533–1.
25. Hallikainen D. History of panoramic radiography. Acta Radiol. 1996;37(3):441–5.
26. Epstein JB, Caldwell J, Black G. The utility of panoramic imaging of the temporomandibular joint in patients with temporomandibular disorders. Oral Surg Oral Med Oral Pathol Oral Radiol Endod. 2001;92(2):236–9.
27. Kopp AF, Heuschmid M, Kuettner A, et al. Multislice computed tomography: basic principles and clinical applications. Electromedica. 2000;68(2):94–105.
28. Jung H. Basic physical principles and clinical applications of computed tomography. Prog Med Phys. 2021;32:1–17.
29. Whaites E, Drage N. Essentials of dental radiography and radiology. 6th ed. Philadelphia: Elsevier Health Sciences; 2013.
30. Bouquot JE, Spolnik K, Adams W, et al. Technetium-99mTc MDP imaging of 293 quadrants of idiopathic facial pain: 79% show increased radioisotope uptake. Oral Surg Oral Med Oral Pathol Oral Radiol. 2012;114:83–92.
31. DEXA Scan. In: Radiation Health. https://www.cdc.gov/radiation-health/data-research/facts-stats/dexa-scan.html#:~:text=At%20a%20glance,conditions%2C%20such%20as%20bone%20thinning. Accessed on 26 Dec 2024.
32. Mupparapu M, Oak S, Chang YC, et al. Conventional and functional imaging in the evaluation of temporomandibular joint rheumatoid arthritis: a systematic review. Quintessence Int. 2019;50(9):742–53.
33. Greiser A, Christensen J, Fuglsig JMCS, et al. Dental-dedicated MRI, a novel approach for dentomaxillofacial diagnostic imaging: technical specifications and feasibility. Dentomaxillofac Radiol. 2024;53(1):74–85.

Imaging of Odontogenic Pain—Homotopic/Primary

5

Carla Y. Falcon and Bassam M. Kinaia

5.1 Introduction

Odontogenic pain is a category of complex disorders that include the soft tissue and the bony structures in the head and neck areas [1]. Odontogenic pain can be caused by pathological conditions related to dental, somatic, or neurologic origins [1]. Dental treatments (non-surgical and surgical therapies) may also result in postoperative odontogenic pain. Generally, odontogenic pain can be temporarily relieved using pharmacological agents such as anesthetics, anti-inflammatory medications, and analgesic medications [2, 3]. Despite the origin, correct clinical diagnosis and radiographic image selection are critical in determining the appropriate treatment for odontogenic pain. Diagnosis requires a comprehensive review of the patient's medical history, dental history, and clinical examination, combined with appropriate imaging techniques. The selection of the imaging technique is closely dependent on the information obtained during the examination. Imaging techniques generally include two-dimensional (2D) and/or three-dimensional (3D) imaging and ought to show soft tissue and bony structures to examine for the presence and extent of disease and/or absence of disease [4].

C. Y. Falcon (✉)
Diplomate, American Board of Endodontics, Department of Endodontics, Rutgers School of Dental Medicine, Newark, NJ, USA
e-mail: falconcy@sdm.rutgers.edu

B. M. Kinaia
Diplomate, American Board of Periodontology, Diplomate, International Congress of Oral Implantology, Graduate Periodontics Program, University of Detroit Mercy, Detroit, MI, USA

Intraoral imaging is the most common 2D radiography technique to assess the teeth and supporting structures and includes periapical, bitewing, and occlusal radiographs. Extraoral imaging includes 2D and 3D radiography such as panoramic, cone beam computed tomography (CBCT), and magnetic resonance imaging (MRI) [4]. Odontogenic pain therapies often include dentists and/or physicians selecting appropriate treatment for pain relief. This chapter focuses on the usefulness of imaging techniques to determine sources of odontogenic pain and select appropriate therapeutic methods.

5.2 Dental Caries

Dental caries is the most common noncommunicable disease worldwide (WHO). Untreated dental caries can result in pain and infection, resulting in the need for costly dental treatment or tooth loss [5]. Periodic exams by dentists are recommended to evaluate for the clinical and radiographic presence of dental caries [6]. Visual-tactile detection has limited accuracy for the detection of non-carious lesions, particularly on interproximal surfaces [7]. Bitewing radiography is the most common and most efficient radiographic modality used to assess for inter-

G. A. Kaspo, G. D. Klasser (eds.), *Orofacial and Head Pain*,
https://doi.org/10.1007/978-3-032-08275-6_5

proximal dental caries [7–10]. Radiographic caries detection has been found to be highly accurate for interproximal lesions and for lesions that extend into dentin [11]. It is relatively insensitive for radiographic caries detection for initial carious lesions [11]. The frequency of radiographic evaluation for dental caries varies based on the patient's caries risk factors. Increased risk factors for dental caries include poor oral hygiene, high frequency of exposure to sucrose-containing foods, and deficient fluoride intake [6]. The American Dental Association generally recommends a posterior bitewing examination for children at 6- to 12-month intervals and at 6- to 18-month intervals for adults with a high caries risk level. For children with a low caries risk assessment, a radiographic examination is recommended at intervals of 12–24 months, and 18–36 months for adults [6]. A patient's risk for caries can change over time, and the frequency of radiographic assessment should change accordingly [6].

5.3 Pulpal Diseases

Pulpal issues are generally categorized through clinical evaluation of the pulpal and periradicular status and are frequently associated with pain. Pulpal pain is often described as "sharp," "sharp and lancinating," "slow," "dull," or "crawling," depending on the pain pathway, with A-delta nerve fibers evoking the former and c-fibers evoking the latter [12]. Dental caries, fractures, cracks, dental trauma, and periodontal disease can result in pulpal changes as well as pain.

Pulpitis is inflammation of the dental pulp and is clinically categorized as reversible or irreversible. If pulpitis is untreated, pulp necrosis can occur. Pulpitis and pulp necrosis can cause apical periodontitis, which is inflammation and/or destruction of the apical periodontium of pulpal origin. It can also trigger an inflammatory reaction, resulting in an abscess. Pain levels can vary based on the diagnosis and patient factors [13, 14].

Clinical evaluation of the pulpal and periradicular status includes an evaluation of the patient's medical and dental history, the patient's report of the chief complaint(s), and clinical tests, most commonly, thermal, electrical, percussion, palpation, and circumferential periodontal probing [15]. Depending on the patient's reported symptoms and results to initial testing, some additional tests may be indicated, such as bite test, transillumination, test cavity, anesthesia, additional periodontal examination/evaluation, and observation of occlusal discrepancies [15]. The American Association of Endodontists provides a diagnostic nomenclature (Table 5.1) which is useful in the diagnosis of pulpal issues [16, 17].

- Intraoral radiographs are considered the imaging modality of choice in the initial radiographic assessment of pulpal issues and for immediate postoperative assessment of endodontic treatment [18]. This includes a periapical radiograph, preferably using the paralleling technique, with complete view of all roots, root apices, and associated periarticular structures [19]. The periapical radiograph allows for assessment of any periradicular changes, as well as anticipated anatomy and case complexity in the event endodontic treatment or extraction is recommended [15]. The horizontal and vertical angulation of the radiographic beam is helpful in separating structures, such as multiple roots, that may be superimposed on a 2D image [20, 21]. A loss of mineral content and bone changes are needed to visualize periapical changes such as apical periodontitis radiographically [19]. The periapical index is a scoring system for registration of apical periodontitis in radiographs [22] (Table 5.2).

CBCT is a supplemental diagnostic aid which can further allow for the evaluation of the tooth and periradicular structures. It is important to note that CBCT is not recommended to be used routinely for endodontic diagnosis or for screening purposes in the absence of clinical signs and symptoms [18]. Careful consideration of field of view and dose is incumbent upon the clinician when considering the adjunctive use of CBCT, as

Table 5.1 A summary of American Association of Endodontists Diagnostic Nomenclature [16, 17]

Normal Pulp
In normal pulp, the pulp is symptom-free and normally responsive to pulp testing. Although the pulp may not be histologically normal, a "clinically" normal pulp results in a mild or transient response to thermal cold testing, lasting no more than 1–2 seconds after the stimulus is removed, and a similar response to adjacent and contralateral teeth.
Reversible Pulpitis
In reversible pulpitis, subjective and objective findings indicate that the inflammation should resolve and the pulp return to normal following appropriate management of the etiology. The patient often reports discomfort when a stimulus such as cold or sweet is applied. The patient reports resolution within a couple of seconds following the removal of the stimulus. Typical etiologies may include exposed dentin (dentinal sensitivity), caries, or deep restorations. There are no significant radiographic changes in the periapical region of the suspect tooth, and the pain experienced is not spontaneous. Following management of the cause, the tooth requires further evaluation to determine whether the "reversible pulpitis" has returned to a normal status.
Symptomatic Irreversible Pulpitis
In symptomatic irreversible pulpitis, subjective and objective findings indicate that the vital inflamed pulp is incapable of healing. The patient often reports a sharp pain upon thermal stimulus, lingering pain (often 30 seconds or longer after stimulus removal), spontaneous pain, and referred pain. Common causes include deep caries, extensive restorations, or fractures affecting the pulpal tissues. Treatment usually includes endodontic treatment or extraction.
Asymptomatic Irreversible Pulpitis
In asymptomatic irreversible pulpitis, subjective and objective findings indicate that the vital inflamed pulp is incapable of healing. The patient often does not report any clinical symptoms and usually respond normally to thermal testing but may have had trauma or deep caries that would likely result in, or has already resulted in, pulp exposure following removal. Treatment usually includes endodontic treatment or extraction.
Pulp Necrosis
Pulp necrosis indicates the death of the dental pulp. The patient does not report symptoms of pulpal origin, and the pulp is non-responsive to pulp testing. Treatment usually includes endodontic treatment or extraction.
Previously Treated
Previously treated indicates that the tooth has been endodontically treated, and the canals are obturated with an obturating material.
Previously Initiated Therapy
Previously initiated therapy indicated that the tooth has received partial endodontic therapy such as pulpotomy or pulpectomy. Depending on the level of therapy, the tooth may or may not respond to pulp testing modalities.
Normal Apical Tissues
Teeth with normal periradicular tissues that are not sensitive to percussion or palpation testing. The lamina dura surrounding the root is intact, and the periodontal ligament space is uniform.
Symptomatic Apical Periodontitis
Symptomatic apical periodontitis indicates the presence of inflammation, usually of the apical periodontium, producing clinical symptoms including a painful response to biting and/or percussion or palpation. In radiographic assessment, it might or might not be associated with an apical radiolucent area. Treatment may include occlusal adjustment, endodontic treatment, or extraction.
Asymptomatic Apical Periodontitis
Asymptomatic apical periodontitis indicates the presence of inflammation and destruction of apical periodontium that is of pulpal origin. In radiographic assessment, it appears as an apical radiolucent area and does not produce clinical symptoms upon testing (no pain on percussion or palpation). Treatment may include endodontic treatment, extraction, and/or biopsy.
Acute Apical Abscess
Acute apical abscess is an inflammatory reaction to pulpal infection and necrosis characterized by rapid onset, spontaneous pain, extreme tenderness of the tooth to pressure, pus formation, and swelling of associated tissues. There may be no radiographic signs of destruction and the patient often experiences malaise, fever, and lymphadenopathy. Treatment may include endodontic treatment or extraction in addition to emergency treatment such incision and drainage and/or antibiotic therapy.
Chronic Apical Abscess
Chronic apical abscess is an inflammatory reaction to pulpal infection and necrosis characterized by gradual onset, little or no discomfort, and an intermittent discharge of pus through an associated sinus tract. Radiographically, there are typically signs of osseous destruction such as a radiolucency. To identify the source of a draining sinus tract when present, a gutta-percha cone is carefully placed through the stoma or opening until it stops and a radiograph is taken.
Condensing Osteitis
Condensing osteitis is a diffuse radiopaque lesion representing a localized bony reaction to a low-grade inflammatory stimulus usually seen at the apex of the tooth. Treatment may include endodontic treatment or extraction.

Table 5.2 A summary of the Periapical Index used to evaluate radiographic changes of the periarticular area [79, 80]

Score 1: Normal periapical structures
Score 2: Small changes in bone structure
Score 3: Changes in bone structure with some mineral loss
Score 4: Apical periodontitis with well-defined radiolucent area
Score 5: Severe apical periodontitis with exacerbating features

Table 5.3 Summary of recommendations of the AAE and AAOMR Joint Position Statement "Use of Cone Beam Computed Tomography in Endodontics—2015/2016 Update" [18]

Recommendation 1: Intraoral radiographs should be considered the imaging modality of choice in the evaluation of the endodontic patient.
Recommendation 2: Limited FOV CBCT should be considered the imaging modality of choice for diagnosis in patients who present with contradictory or nonspecific clinical signs and symptoms associated with untreated or previously endodontically treated teeth.
Recommendation 3: Limited FOV CBCT should be considered the imaging modality of choice for initial treatment of teeth with the potential for extra canals and suspected complex morphology, such as mandibular anterior teeth, maxillary and mandibular premolars and molars, and dental anomalies.
Recommendation 4: If a preoperative CBCT has not been taken, limited FOV CBCT should be considered as the imaging modality of choice for intra-appointment identification and localization of calcified canals.
Recommendation 5: Intraoral radiographs should be considered the imaging modality of choice for immediate postoperative imaging.
Recommendation 6: Limited FOV CBCT should be considered the imaging modality of choice if clinical examination and 2-D intraoral radiography are inconclusive in the detection of vertical root fracture.
Recommendation 7: Limited FOV CBCT should be the imaging modality of choice when evaluating the nonhealing of previous endodontic treatment to help determine the need for further treatment, such as nonsurgical, surgical, or extraction.
Recommendation 8: Limited FOV CBCT should be the imaging modality of choice for nonsurgical retreatment to assess endodontic treatment complications, such as overextended root canal obturation material, separated endodontic instruments, and localization of perforations.
Recommendation 9: Limited FOV CBCT should be considered as the imaging modality of choice for presurgical treatment planning to localize root apex/apices and to evaluate the proximity to adjacent anatomical structures.
Recommendation 10: Limited FOV CBCT should be considered as the imaging modality of choice for surgical placement of implants.
Recommendation 11: Limited FOV CBCT should be considered the imaging modality of choice for diagnosis and management of limited dento-alveolar trauma, root fractures, luxation, and/or displacement of teeth and localized alveolar fractures, in the absence of other maxillofacial or soft tissue injury that may require other advanced imaging modalities.
Recommendation 12: Limited FOV CBCT is the imaging modality of choice in the localization and differentiation of external and internal resorptive defects and the determination of appropriate treatment and prognosis.
Recommendation 13: In the absence of clinical signs or symptoms, intraoral radiographs should be considered the imaging modality of choice for the evaluation of healing following nonsurgical and surgical endodontic treatment.
Recommendation 14: In the absence of signs and symptoms, if limited FOV CBCT was the imaging modality of choice at the time of evaluation and treatment, it may be the modality of choice for follow-up evaluation. In the presence of signs and symptoms, refer to Recommendation #7.

CBCT has a higher radiation exposure to the patient than intraoral imaging. The American Association of Endodontists and the American Academy of Oral and Maxillofacial Radiology published a joint position statement on the use of cone beam computed tomography in endodontics (Table 5.3).

5.4 Periodontal Diseases

Periodontal health is important to maintain good overall dental and medical health, and if not maintained, it may result in pain and negatively impact the patient's health and quality of life

[23]. For the most part, periodontal pain is a relatively low-grade, localized pain associated with chronic low-grade infection such as gingivitis and periodontitis. Sometimes, the pain may present as acute severe pain associated with high infection such as abscesses of the gingiva or periodontium, necrotizing periodontal disease, herpetic lesions, peri-implantitis, or endodontic-periodontal involvement [24, 25].

Generally, orofacial pain associated with periodontal diseases may not be easily diagnosed. Therefore, correct imaging techniques combined with clinical examination are necessary for appropriate diagnosis and treatment selection. Each imaging technique has advantages and disadvantages as well as technical limitations, making it imperative to select the appropriate imaging based on the clinical scenario [26].

5.4.1 Chronic Periodontitis

The American Academy and European Federation of Periodontology consensus reports support clinical examination combined with two-dimensional (2D) full mouth series (FMS) as the gold standard for periodontal evaluation (Fig. 5.1) [27, 28]. The 2D FMS radiographs normally include bitewings, periapical, and panoramic. For periodontitis patients, vertical bite-

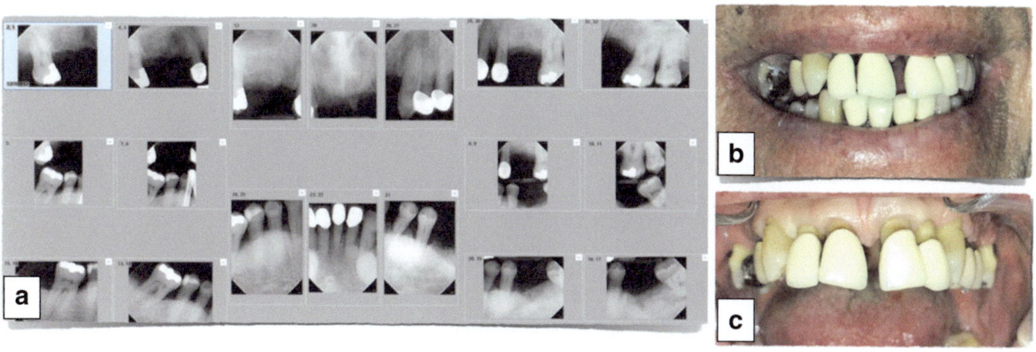

Fig. 5.1 (**a**) Full mouth radiographs of a 72-year-old male with generalized periodontitis showing moderate to severe bone loss. (**b**) Smile picture showing black triangles and diastema anteriorly. (**c**) Facial clinical view showing gingival recession

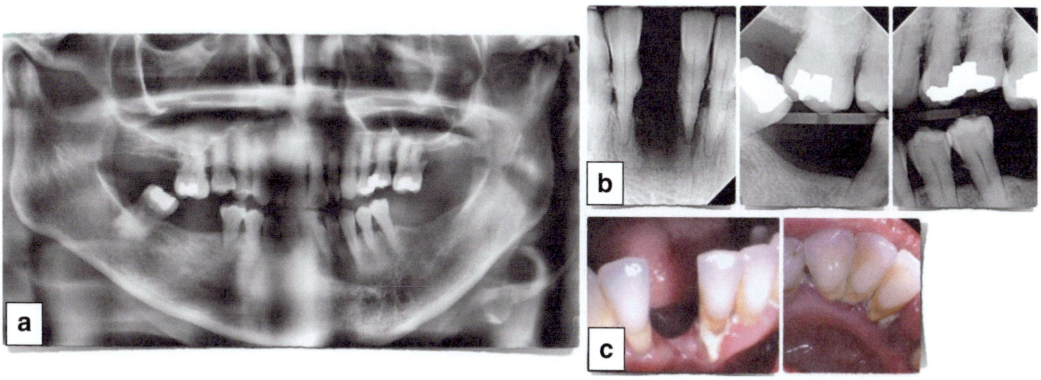

Fig. 5.2 (**a**) Panoramic radiograph of a 68-year-old male with generalized periodontitis showing moderate to severe bone loss with partial edentulism. (**b**) Periapical and vertical bitewing radiographs showing crestal bone loss and calculus presence. (**c**) Facial and lingual clinical views showing calculus presence with gingival recession

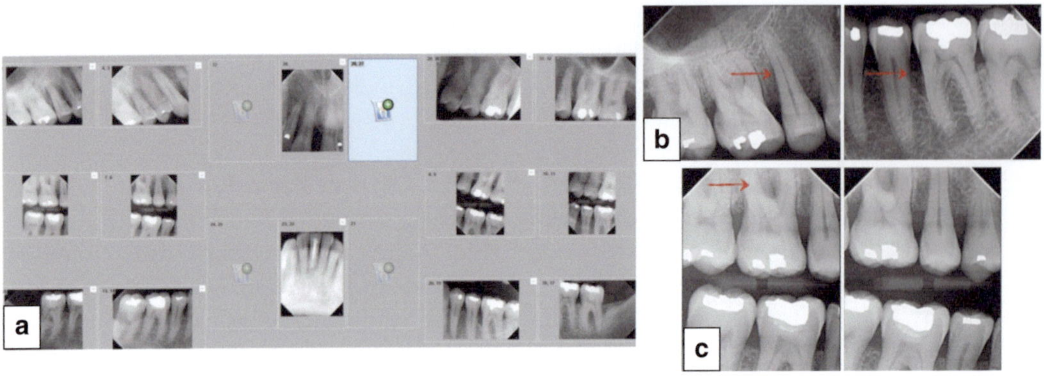

Fig. 5.3 (**a**) Full mouth radiographs of a 57-year-old male with generalized periodontitis showing moderate to severe bone loss. (**b**) Periapical radiographs showing vertical bone loss around #4 and #19 (red arrows). (**c**) Vertical bitewing radiographs showing furcation bone loss #3 (red arrow)

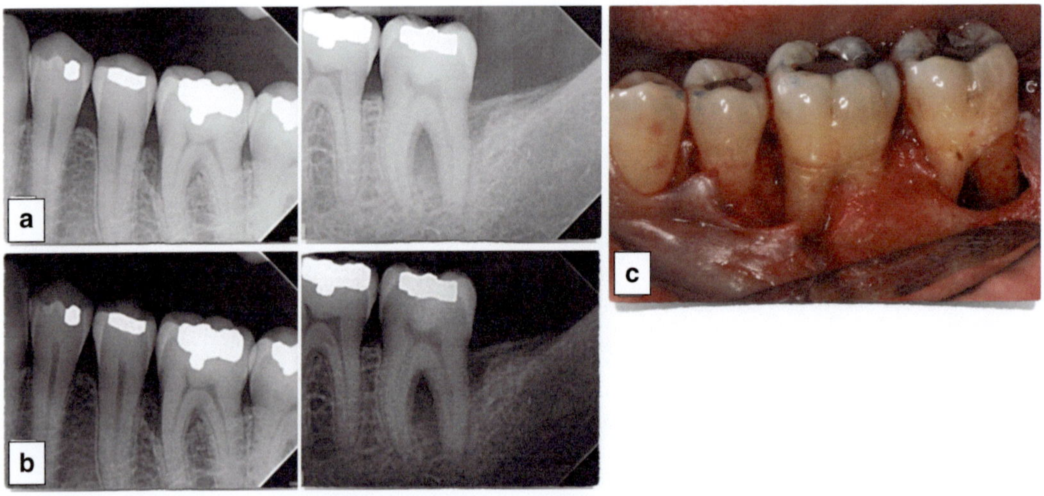

Fig. 5.4 (**a**) Digital periapical radiographs showing bone loss #18, 19. (**b**) Increasing radiolucency of the digital periapical radiographs shows more clearly the vertical and furcation bone loss #18, 19. (**c**) Clinical facial view confirming the presence of vertical and furcation bone loss #18, 19

wings combined with periapical and panoramic radiographs are required to visualize the bone levels (Fig. 5.2). This allows appropriate assessment of the bone levels, calculus presence, bone loss pattern, and identification of pathologies (Fig. 5.3) [29]. Compared to conventional 2D radiographs, digital imaging improves the efficiency of radiographs detecting subtle bony density changes with lower radiation dose. The use of 2D digital subtraction imaging, measuring the difference in bone level changes at two different time points, increases diagnostic accuracy and periodontal disease progression (Fig. 5.4) [30]. Despite the usefulness of 2D radiographs, clinicians may encounter overlapping of anatomic structures and mis-estimation of caries (Fig. 5.5) [31]. Furthermore, 2D radiographs are sufficient to detect interproximal bony changes but are not accurate in detecting buccal and lingual bone loss [32]. Three-dimensional (3D) imaging such as CBCT is a useful tool for periodontal disease diagnosis and management. CBCT offers higher resolution allowing accurate detection of vertical and furcation bone loss, and fenestration and

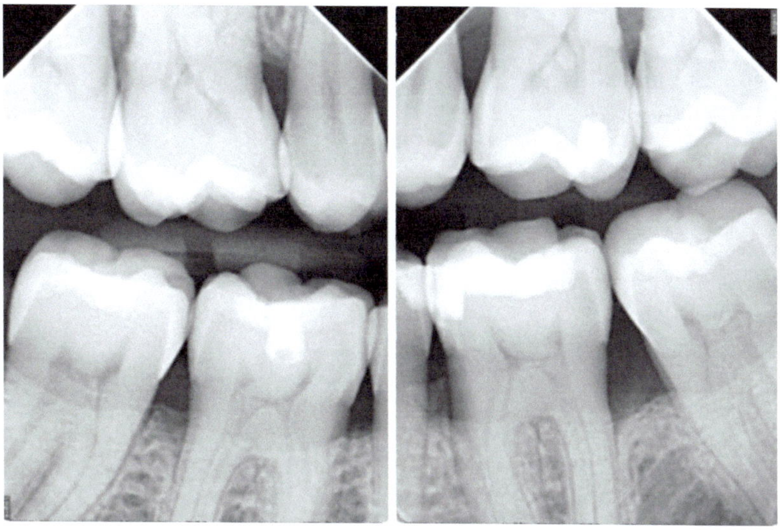

Fig. 5.5 Vertical bitewing radiographs showing overlap interproximally

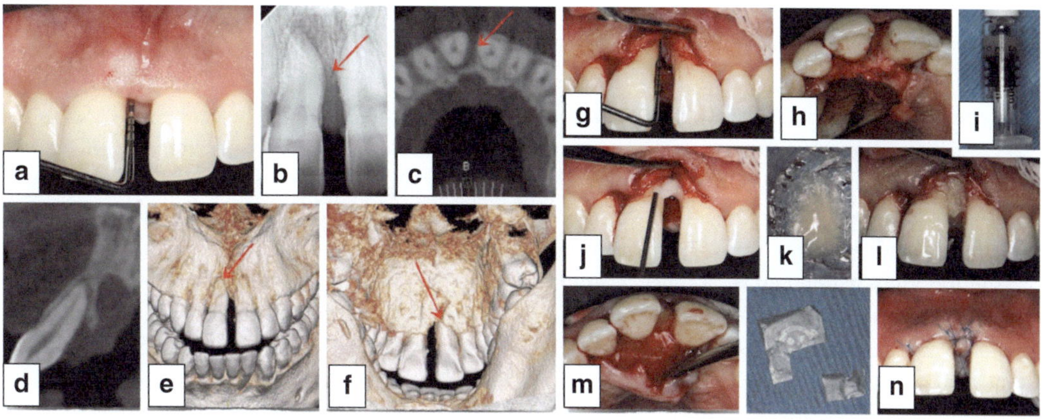

Fig. 5.6 (**a**) Initial clinical facial view showing deep probing depth #8. (**b**) Initial periapical radiograph showing vertical bone loss #8 (red arrow). (**c**) Initial CBCT occlusal view showing circumferential bone loss #8 (red arrow). (**d**) Initial CBCT cross-sectional view showing palatal bone loss #8. (**e, f**) CBCT facial and palatal views showing severe bone loss #8 (red arrows). (**g, h**) Surgical clinical facial and occlusal views showing circumferential bone loss #8. (**i**) Growth factor. (**j**) Detoxifying root surface with EDTA. (**k**) Bone allograft placement mixed with growth factor. (**l**) Graft and growth factor added to fill the bony defect #8. (**m**) Amnion-chorion membrane adapted. (**n**) Primary closure obtained with non-resorbable sutures. (**o**) CBCT occlusal view at 9 months showing bone fill #8 (red arrow). (**p**) A 9-month periapical radiograph showing vertical bone fill #8 (red arrow). (**q**) CBCT cross-sectional view showing palatal bone fill #8 (red arrow). (**r**) CBCT palatal view showing proper bone fill #8 (red arrow). (**s**) Clinical facial view showing healthy periodontium with diastema closed #8–9. (**t**) Clinical palatal view during orthodontic treatment showing healthy periodontium

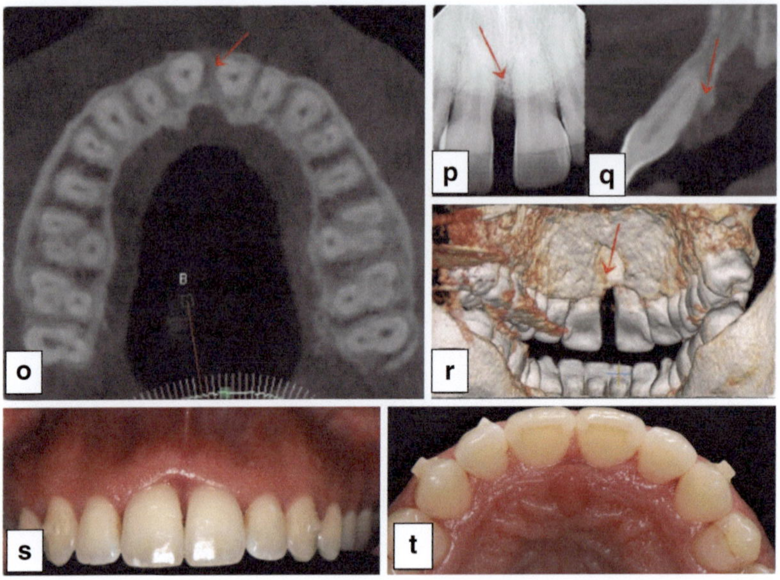

Fig. 5.6 (continued)

dehiscence bony defects (Fig. 5.6a–f). Based on the CBCT and bone loss assessment, regenerative periodontal therapy is employed to restore the damaged periodontium (Fig. 5.6g–n). Clinical and radiographic follow-ups with rigorous periodontal maintenance are necessary to monitor the periodontium and ensure periodontal stability (Fig. 5.6o–t) [33, 34]. Walter et al. examined the use of CBCT in detecting furcation invasions (FI) in patients with generalized chronic periodontitis (FI = 22). They assessed the accuracy in detecting grade I, II, and III FI and concluded that CBCT is a reliable imaging technique for FI detection and treatment selection [35]. CBCT is also superior to 2D imaging in detecting fenestration and dehiscence bony defects, which is important in assessing the extent of bone loss [36]. When dehiscence defects extend 50% or more of the root length with a thin periodontal phenotype, regenerative periodontal therapy combined with soft tissue grafting is recommended to stabilize the periodontium (Fig. 5.7a–k). Braun et al. investigated the use of CBCT to detect vertical, fenestration, and dehiscence bony defects. The study results showed better diagnosis of bony defects using CBCT (vertical 21%, dehiscence 25%, fenestration 33%) compared to periapical radiographs [36]. In addition to CBCT, MRI can detect soft and hard tissue changes within the periodontium. A recent study evaluated the use of MR imaging in assessing periodontal disease severity and extent. Probst et al. compared clinical findings, panoramic, and MRI in 42 periodontitis and 34 periodontally healthy patients. The study showed that the MRI results were consistent with clinical findings and able to detect bony changes before a bony defect occurs [37]. Recently, artificial intelligence (AI) models are being investigated in diagnosis and treatment of periodontal diseases. A systematic review by Revilla-León et al. reported on AI findings from 24 publications. AI models using intraoral photographs and radiographic images showed accuracy in detecting dental plaque (73.6–99%) and alveolar bone loss (73.4–99%) as well as diagnosing gingivitis (67.7–78.20%) and periodontitis (47–81%) [38]. Once the diagnosis is made based on the correct imaging technique, management often involves non-surgical and surgical periodontal therapies to stabilize the periodontium.

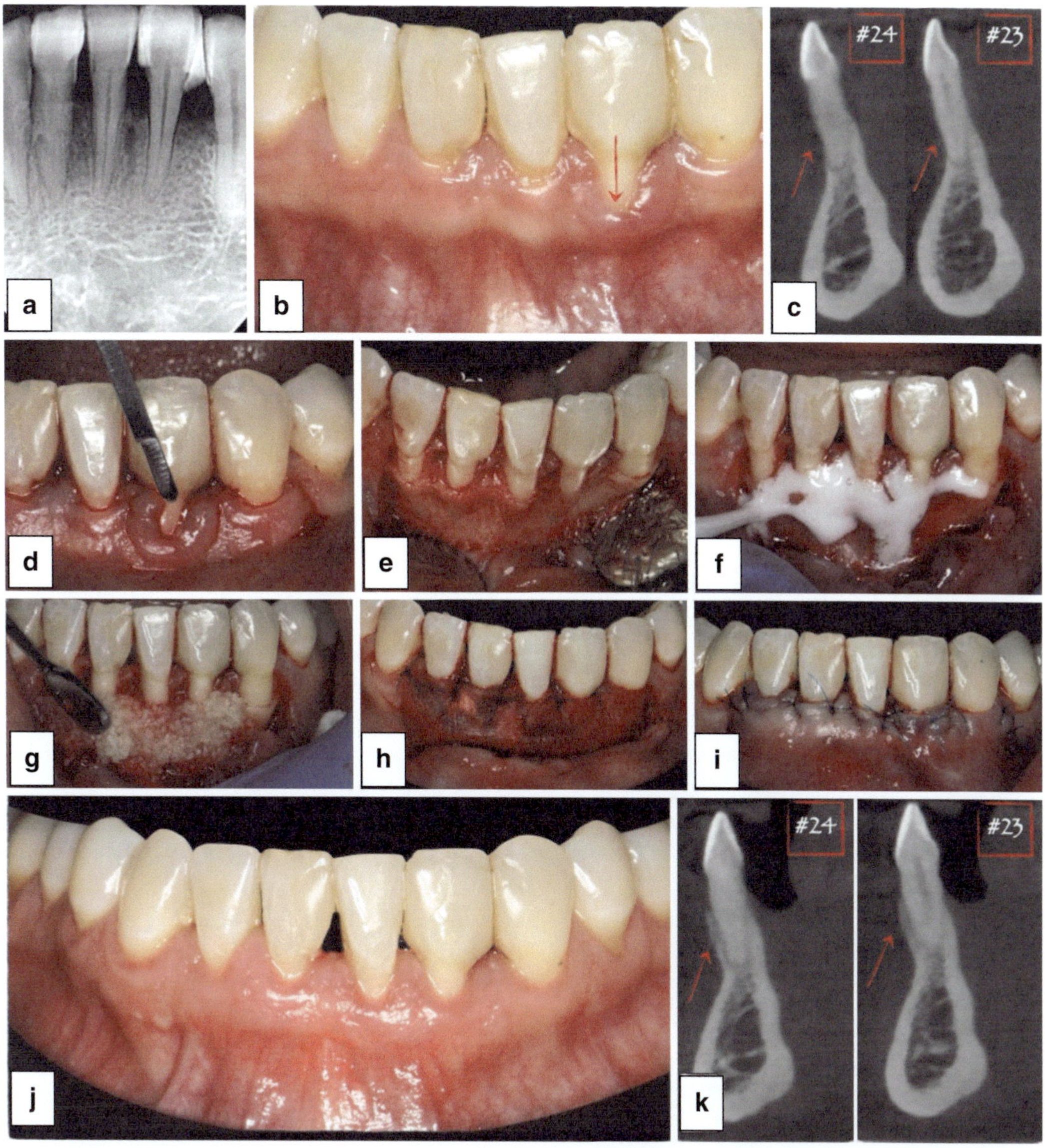

Fig. 5.7 (**a**) Initial periapical radiograph showing horizontal bone loss #23–26. (**b**) Initial clinical facial view showing gingival recession with thin periodontal phenotype #23 (red arrow). (**c**) CBCT cross-sectional view showing dehiscence bone loss facially #23, 24 (red arrows). (**d**) Surgical clinical facial view showing sulcular incision with microsurgical blade. (**e**) Full-thickness flap reflection showing fenestration and dehiscence. (**f**) Detoxifying root surfaces with EDTA. (**g**) Bone allograft placement. (**h**) Soft tissue xenograft placement. (**i**) Primary closure obtained with non-resorbable sutures. (**j**) Final clinical facial view showing thick periodontal phenotype with reduction in gingival recession at 12-month follow-up. (**k**) CBCT cross-sectional view showing proper bone fill facially #23, 24 (red arrows)

5.4.2 Acute Periodontal Diseases

Although periodontal pain is generally chronic, low-grade, localized dull pain, acute periodontal disease is often associated with more severe pain [24, 25]. The most common acute periodontal diseases include periodontal abscesses, necrotizing periodontal diseases, and endodontic-periodontal lesions. They often lead to painful and rapid destruction of the connective tissue and alveolar bone. They present as dental emergencies where early diagnosis and management are necessary [39].

5.4.2.1 Periodontal Abscesses and Necrotizing Periodontal Diseases

Periodontal abscesses include gingival or periodontal abscesses, endodontic abscesses, those resulting from surgery/trauma, peri-coronal abscess, or foreign body impaction. Periodontal abscesses are the third most common dental emergency (7.7–14.0%) after endodontic abscesses and peri-coronal abscesses [39]. Patients' symptoms generally include pain, swelling, tenderness, or suppuration. They are often associated with deep periodontal probing (7.3–9.3 mm) and tooth mobility (56.4–100%) [39]. Periodontal abscesses often cause rapid periodontal tissue destruction, negatively affecting the tooth prognosis and possibly leading to systemic dissemination of the dental infection [39, 40]. Clinically, visual examination and a periodontal probe is used to identify the periodontal pocket and bony defect. The extent of the bone loss is confirmed with 2D and 3D radiographic imaging. The treatment aims to drain the abscess either through non-surgical periodontal therapy (scaling and root planning) or surgical periodontal therapy using incision and drainage combined with antibiotic and analgesic medications (Fig. 5.8) [23, 24].

Necrotizing periodontal diseases (NPD) include necrotizing gingivitis, necrotizing periodontitis, and necrotizing stomatitis. Factors that may predispose patients to NPD include stress,

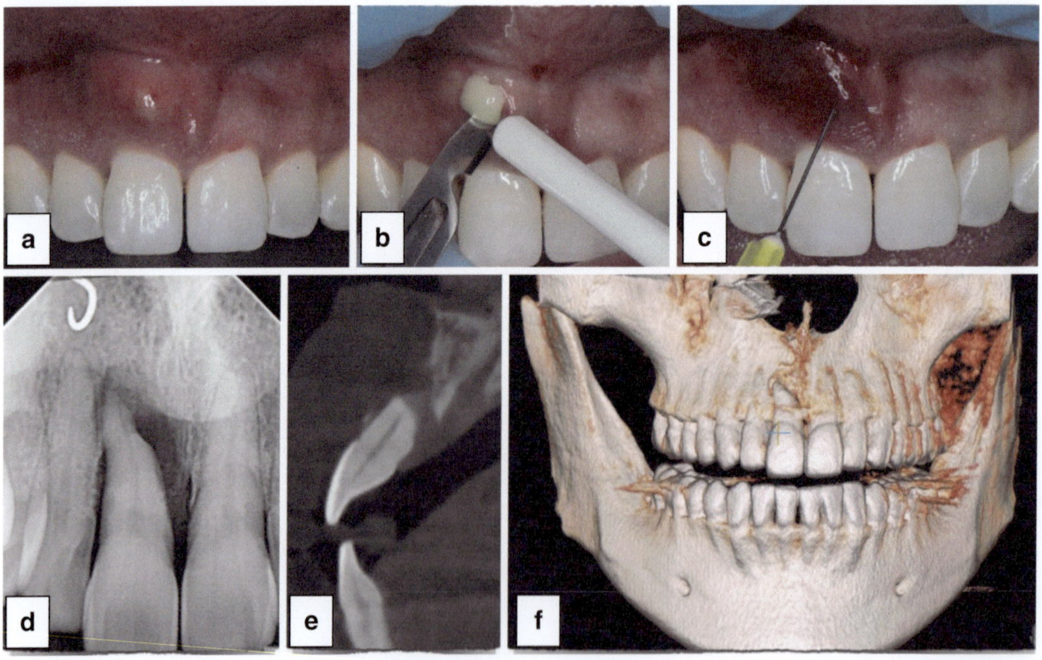

Fig. 5.8 (**a**) Clinical facial view showing fluctuant painful swelling #8. (**b**) Facial view showing drainage of periodontal abscess #8. (**c**) Facial view showing non-surgical therapy and irrigation with antibacterial solution. (**d**) Periapical radiograph showing large radiolucency and bone loss #8. (**e**) CBCT cross-sectional view showing fenestration #8 facially and dehiscence palatally. (**f**) CBCT facial view showing severe bone loss

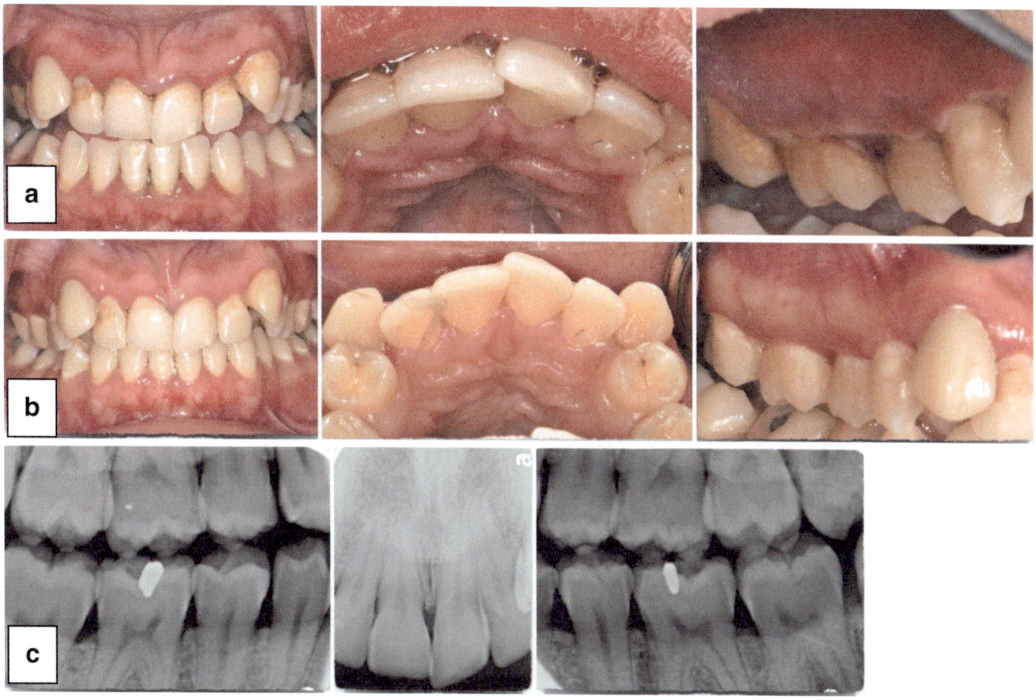

Fig. 5.9 (**a**) Pretreatment clinical facial and occlusal views showing necrotizing periodontitis. (**b**) Post-treatment clinical facial and occlusal views showing reduction in inflammation. (**c**) Periapical and bitewing radiographs showing minimal bone loss

tobacco, alcohol, age, poor diet, and lack of oral hygiene, as well as HIV infection [41, 42]. NPD diagnosis is primarily based on clinical findings, and imaging techniques are complementary (Fig. 5.9) [39]. NPD are painful and may cause rapid destruction of periodontal soft and hard tissues. The use of 2D or 3D imaging outlines the bone loss severity and extent [23]. Thus, similar to chronic periodontitis, 2D and 3D imaging are used to select a proper treatment option. This includes the use of vertical bitewings, periapical, panoramic, and CBCT [29]. CBCT imaging is advantageous to 2D imaging, but it may have some limitations associated with beam-hardening artifacts, especially in the presence of dental implants, restorations, and metal posts, which can cause image distortion (Fig. 5.10). Despite such limitations, CBCT provides accurate diagnosis of the bony defect topography compared to 2D imaging and is therefore more appropriate for selecting appropriate treatment options (Fig. 5.11) [26]. Prompt periodontal treatment with improvement in oral hygiene combined with antibiotics is necessary to control the supra- and subgingival biofilm for predictable outcomes.

5.4.2.2 Endodontic-Periodontal Lesions (EPL)

Endodontic-periodontal lesions (EPL) are inflammatory responses to microorganisms, leading to pulpal tissue and periodontal damage and loss. Both periodontal and endodontic lesions may affect the same tooth simultaneously and/or may be present as a single lesion. What appears to be a periodontal lesion may be symptoms of an endodontic lesion and vice versa, often making the diagnosis and treatment planning a challenge for clinicians (Fig. 5.12) [43, 44].

An interdisciplinary approach is necessary to understand etiology and symptoms based on clinical and radiographic examinations as discussed above. Radiographic imaging is a critical part in EPL diagnosis, treatment, and follow-up [19]. Traditionally, 2D periapical radiographs

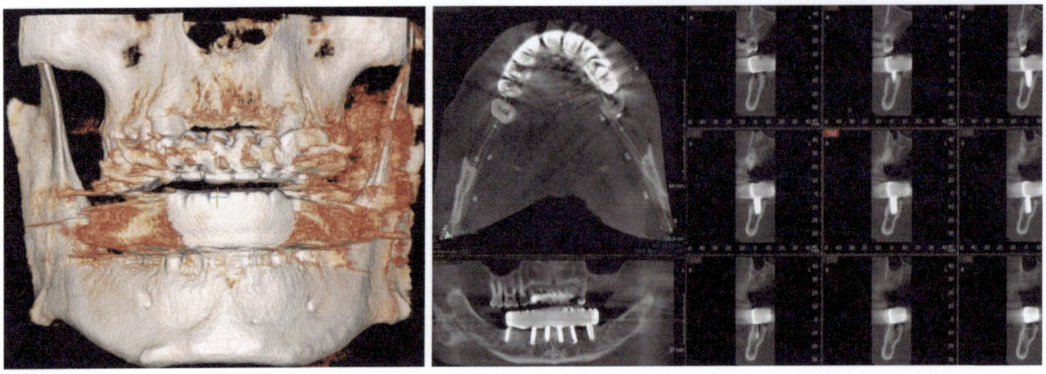

Fig. 5.10 CBCT showing beam-hardening artifacts in the presence of dental implants with image distortion

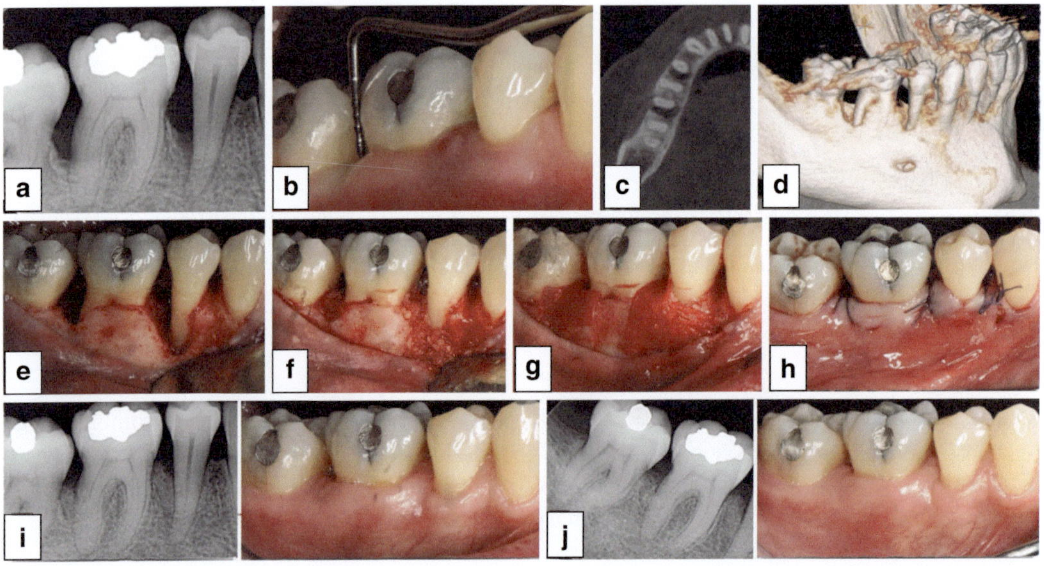

Fig. 5.11 (**a**) Periapical radiograph showing vertical bone loss #29, 30. (**b**) Clinical facial view showing deep probing depth #30. (**c**) CBCT occlusal view showing circumferential bone loss #29, 30. (**d**) CBCT facial view showing vertical bone loss. (**e**) Facial view showing bone loss extent. (**f**) Bone allograft placement #29, 30. (**g**) Collagen membrane adaptation #29, 30. (**h**) Primary closure with resorbable sutures. (**i**) A 9-month follow-up showing proper bone fill radiographically with stable periodontium clinically. (**j**) An 18-month follow-up showing proper bone fill radiographically and healthy periodontium

are the most common imaging technique used to identify odontogenic pain associated with EPL (Fig. 5.13) [4]. CBCT is a three-dimensional imaging that provides greater accuracy in assessing EPL as well as tooth-related anatomical factors (Fig. 5.14) [19]. CBCT enhances the endodontic pre-surgical planning, diagnosis, and treatment, thereby reducing postoperative complications [45, 46]. A study by Chogle et al. evaluated 45 patients in need of endodontic treatment (30 with CBCT, 15 without CBCT). The use of CBCT showed 19% more accurate pulpal diagnosis and 30% better apical diagnosis, concluding that CBCT imaging has a significant advantage in determining the etiology of endodontic pathoses and in treatment recommendation [46]. Another study by Gurusamy et al. evaluated endodontic therapy outcome (pain and swelling) in 52 patients (88 teeth). Patients were randomly assigned to CBCT or periapical (PA)

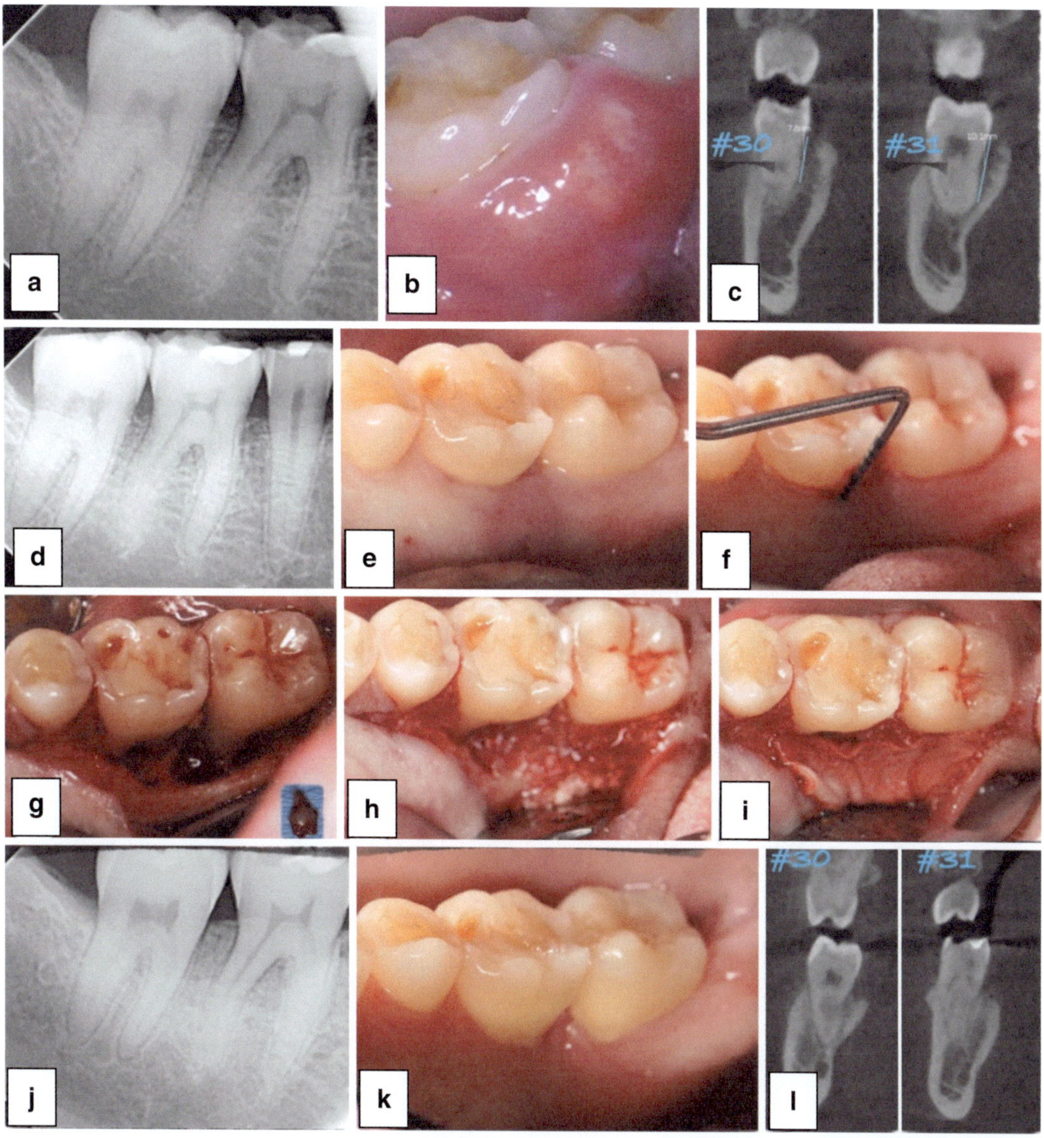

Fig. 5.12 (**a**) Initial periapical radiograph showing radiolucency and furcation bone loss #30–31. (**b**) Initial clinical lingual view showing fluctuant swelling #30, 31. (**c**) Initial CBCT cross-sectional view showing lingual bone loss #30, 31 but not fully extending to the root apices. (**d**) Post-antibiotic treatment periapical radiograph showing loss of bone mineralization crestally #30–31. (**e**, **f**) Post-antibiotic treatment clinical lingual views showing reduction in swelling #30, 31 but persistent deep probing depth. (**g**) Full-thickness flap reflection showing circumferential bone loss with bone fragment removed #30–31. (**h**) Bone allograft placement. (**i**) Collagen membrane adaptation. (**j**) A 12-month follow-up radiograph showing proper bone fill #30–31. (**k**) A 12-month follow-up lingual view showing gingival recession with stable periodontium #30, 31. (**l**) A 12-month follow-up CBCT cross-section view showing proper bone fill #30, 31 lingually

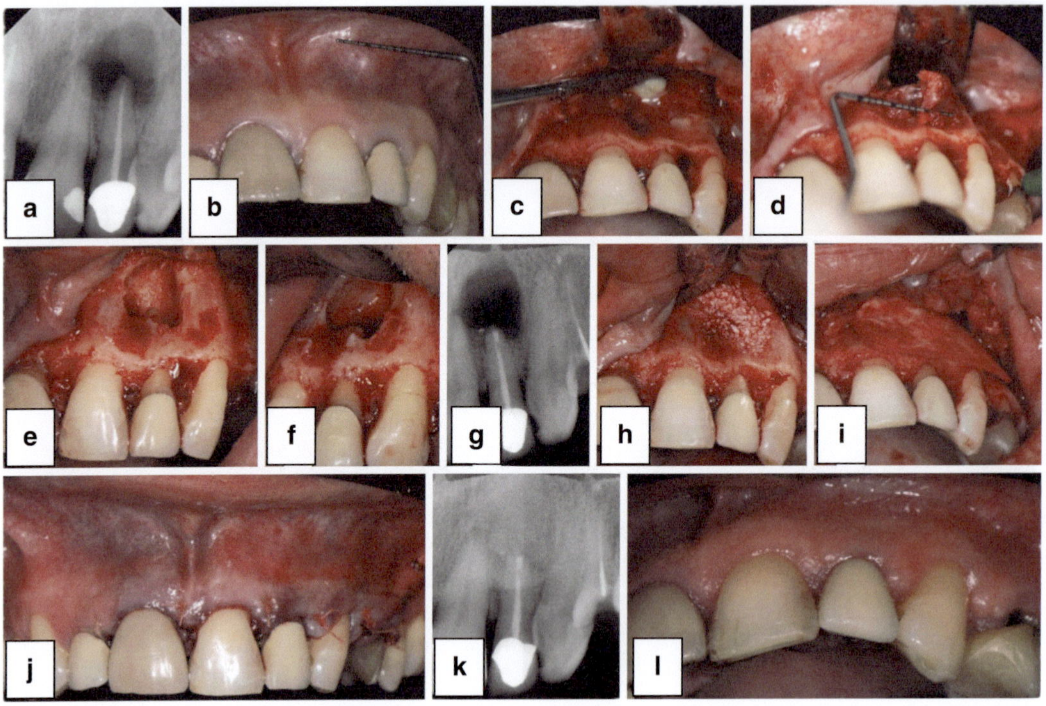

Fig. 5.13 (**a**) Initial periapical radiograph showing large radiolucency #10. (**b**) Clinical facial view showing fluctuant swelling #10 apically. (**c**) Clinical facial view showing exudate #10. (**d**) Facial view showing large granulation tissue. (**e**) Facial view showing defect #10 completely degranulated. (**f**) Facial view showing apicocectomy #10. (**g**) Periapical radiograph showing retrograde filling #10. (**h**) Bone allograft placement. (**i**) Collagen membrane adaptation. (**j**) Primary closure with resorbable sutures. (**k**) A 6-month periapical radiograph showing proper bone fill #10. (**l**) A 6-month facial view showing healthy periodontium and stable #10

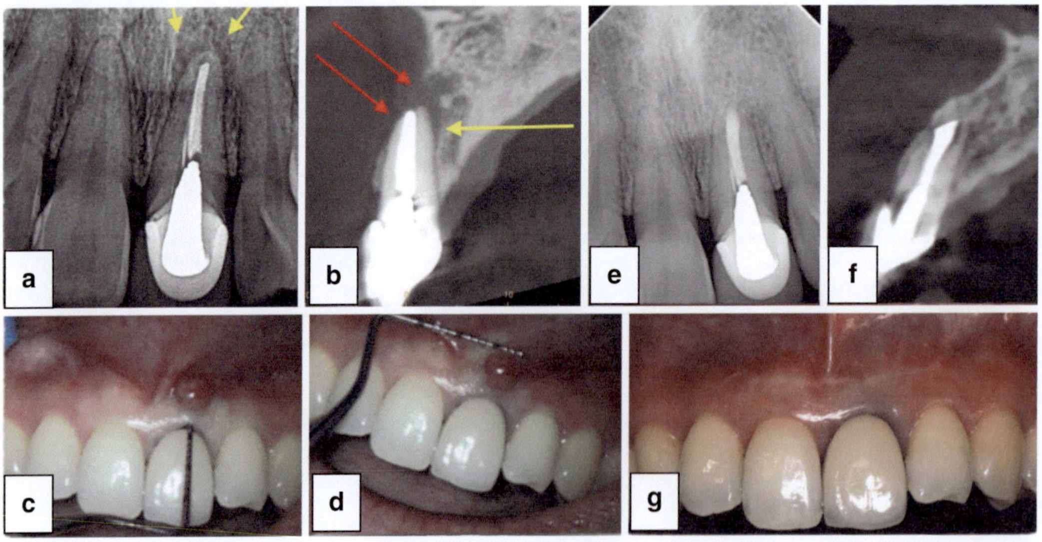

Fig. 5.14 (**a**) Initial periapical radiograph showing radiolucency #9 (yellow arrows). (**b**) CBCT cross-section showing fenestration and apical bone loss #9 (yellow and red arrows). (**c, d**) Clinical facial view showing fistula drainage apically with 2–3 mm probing depth. (**e**) A 6-month periapical radiograph post apicocectomy and guided tissue regeneration showing proper bone fill #9. (**f**) Clinical facial view showing stable periodontium #9. (**g**) A 6-month CBCT cross-section view showing proper bone fill #9

groups. The CBCT group experienced significantly less post-endodontic treatment pain and swelling compared to the PA group [45]. Recent studies are examining the use AI models in diagnosis and treatment planning. AI combined with CBCT can be a valuable tool to aid the clinician [47]. Furthermore, recent studies looked into the use of MRI for dento-maxillofacial radiology. Dental-dedicated MRI (ddMRI) is a new method that may have dento-maxillofacial applications, but it is relatively new and more studies are needed to validate its efficacy in the dental field [48].

5.5 Cracked and/or Tooth Fractures

Cracked tooth syndrome (CTS) is a condition where the patient reports a "sharp" pain during mastication, particularly pain on release of biting, and pain upon temperature stimulation. Symptoms can change as the crack progresses (Fig. 5.15) [49]. It affects approximately 5% of adults annually, with 45% of cracked teeth having one or more symptoms [50, 51]. The most common patient-reported symptoms are pain to cold (37%), followed by pain upon biting (16%), and the least was spontaneous pain (11%) [51].

There are five types of longitudinal tooth fractures: craze lines, fractured cusps, cracked teeth, split teeth, and vertical root fractures (VRF) [52]. There are multiple diagnostic imaging techniques to detect a cracked tooth including periapical, panoramic, CBCT, mirco-CBCT radiography, light transillumination, ultrasound wave, optical coherence tomography (OCT), and MRI [49, 53]. In a clinical setting, a periapical radiograph and bitewing radiograph are the initial imaging modalities of choice. A crack is unlikely to be frankly visualized, as visualization is strongly influenced by the angle of the beam rays (Fig. 5.16) [54]. Limited field-of-view CBCT can assist in the diagnosis of a suspected crack. As in periapical radiographs, the frank crack is unlikely to be directly visualized, but patterns of bone loss associated with cracks or vertical root fractures can be visualized [55].

Micro-CBCT offers higher resolution and sensitivity compared to conventional CBCT in detecting CTS and VRF. Micro-CBCT combined with flap reflection and microscope is the "gold standard" to visualize fractures, but it is not in general clinical use (Fig. 5.17) [49, 56]. Discernment between a crack and vertical root fracture is important, as vertical root fractures have a poor treatment prognosis, but teeth with cracks can be maintained with endodontic treatment and full cuspal restoration [55]. Alaugaily et al. evaluated clinical and radiographic parameters to differentiate between cracked teeth (Fig. 5.15) and vertical root fractured (Fig. 5.18) teeth using 2D and 3D imaging [55]. Cracked teeth were found to be associated with probing depths of <6 mm, the presence of an angular defect on the CBCT scan, and an intact cortical

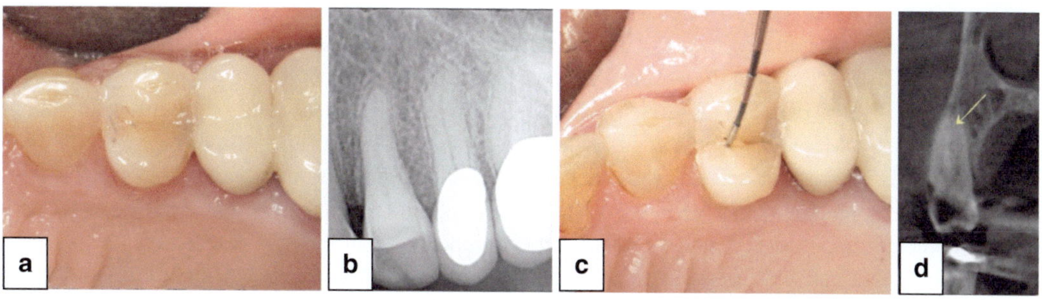

Fig. 5.15 (**a**) Initial occlusal view of a 61-year-old female complaining of cold sensitivity and pain upon biting #12. (**b**) Periapical radiograph showing normal bone pattern. (**c**) Occlusal view of #12 with periodontal probe showing separation in the central groove area "cracked tooth." (**d**) CBCT cross-section view showing thin radiolucent line in the center of #12 (yellow arrow)

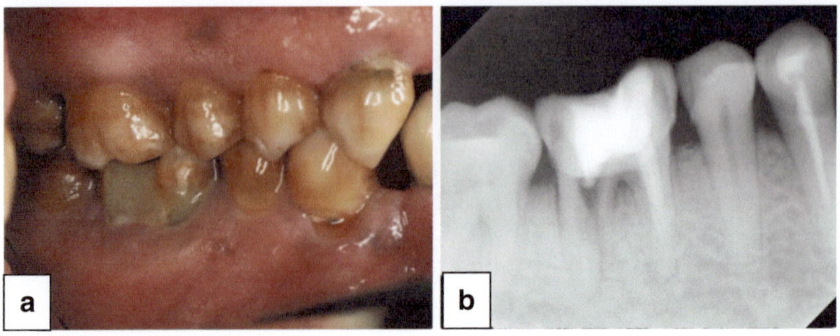

Fig. 5.16 (**a**) Initial facial view of a 73-year-old male complaining of pain upon biting on a heavily restored #30. (**b**) Periapical radiograph showing vertical root fracture #30

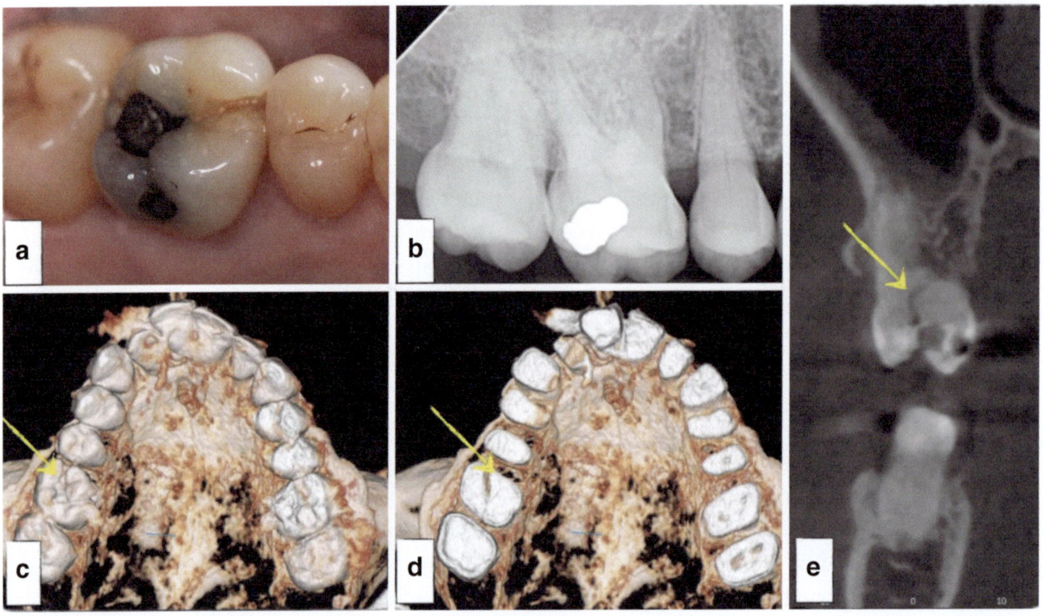

Fig. 5.17 (**a**) Initial occlusal view of a 58-year-old male complaining of thermal sensitivity #3. (**b**) Periapical radiograph showing normal bone pattern. (**c**, **d**) Occlusal view of #3 moving the scan from occlusal to root area to show the cracked tooth position (yellow arrows). (**e**) CBCT cross-section view showing thin radiolucent line through the occlusal to root area #3 (yellow arrow)

plate, whereas vertical root fractures are associated with a probing depth of ≥6 mm, a J-shaped defect on the CBCT scan, and the absence of the cortical plate (Fig. 5.19) [55]. Similar findings were reported by Mareque-Bueno et al., when comparing CBCT to periapical in detecting cracked teeth, split teeth, and VRF teeth. The CBCT detected bone loss patterns associated with cracked teeth and VRF (71%) compared to lower detection with preapical radiographs (42%) [57].

Ultrasound wave is based on mechanical vibration of structures, generally the upper limit of human hearing (>20 kHz) [58]. Currently, ultrasonic imaging is not used due to the complex geometry of the tooth and the unclear mechanism of ultrasound on dentin and enamel [49]. Optical coherence tomography (OCT) is a 2D or 3D imaging that detects backward reflection of biologic tissues. OCT can be used as a diagnostic method to detect enamel surface demineralization, early caries, and tooth fracture [59–61]. OCT has high sensitivity to detect cracks, microcracks, and VRF [62, 63]. Although MRI is generally not used to detect cracked teeth, it still has a high diagnostic value.

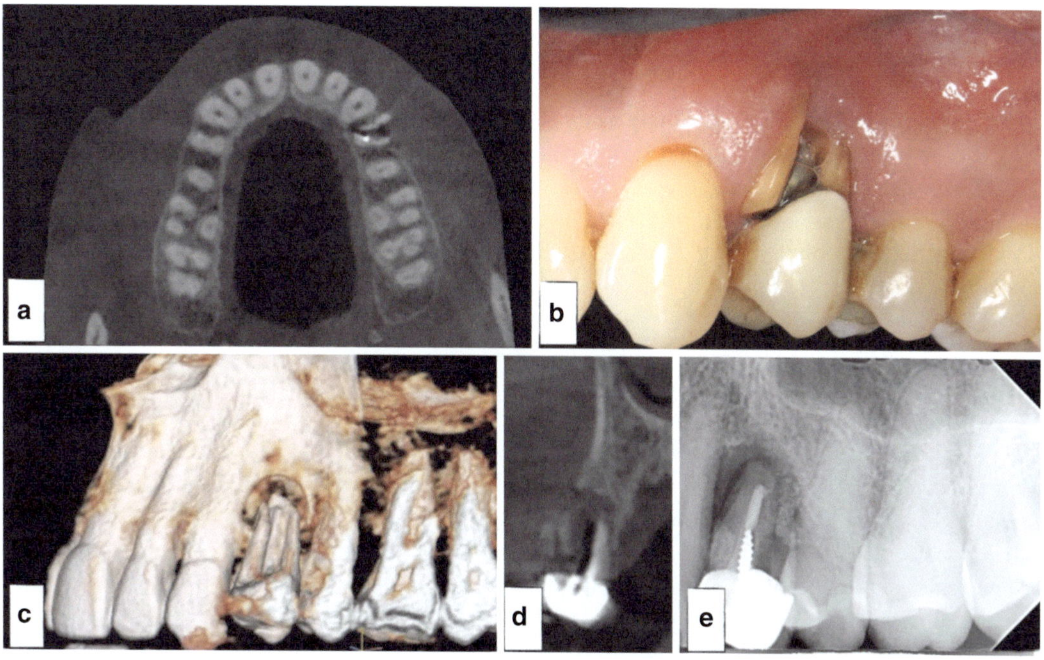

Fig. 5.18 (**a**) CBCT occlusal view showing vertical root fracture #12. (**b**) Facial view of a 66-year-old male complaining of pain upon biting #12. (**c**) CBCT facial view showing complete bone loss #12. (**d**) CBCT cross-section view showing VRF with complete bone loss #12. (**e**) Periapical radiograph showing J-shaped radiolucency #12

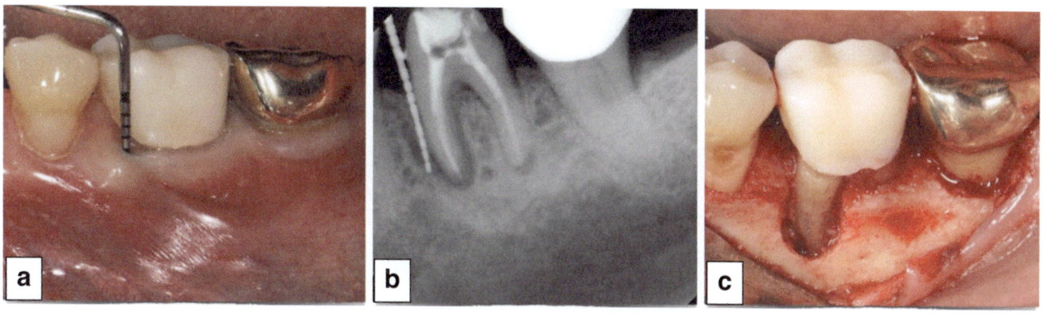

Fig. 5.19 (**a**) Initial facial view showing isolated deep probing depth #19. (**b**) Periapical radiograph showing J-shaped radiolucency around mesial root #19. (**c**) Clinical facial view showing vertical root fracture with bone loss confound to #19 mesial root

Idiyatullin et al. evaluated the diagnostic capability of MRI to detect cracked teeth and showed great ability to detect subtle microcracks in dental structures [64, 65].

Once the diagnosis is made based on the clinical and radiographic/imaging examinations, treatment options can be discussed. Generally, all cracked teeth will require a crown but may not need a root canal treatment. For VRF teeth, extraction and dental implant replacement is often recommended [66].

5.6 Tooth Impactions

Tooth impactions can cause pressure and pain and can be diagnosed through clinical examination, noting the absence of the tooth in its normal position combined with the radiographic assessment showing the position of the unerupted tooth [67]. Third molars are the most commonly impacted tooth, followed by maxillary canines [68]. Systematic reviews have found that CBCT is indicated when conventional radiography such as periapical and panoramic radiographs does not provide sufficient information for impacted teeth [69, 70].

5.7 Failed Dental Procedures (Overextended Root Canal Fillings, Root Perforations)

In endodontic treatment, underfilling of the root canal space or untreated canals can result in persistent bacterial presence which can result in apical periodontitis or abscess, with the clinical and radiographic signs and symptoms as described above [71]. Overfilling of the root canal space, which presents radiographically as root filling material beyond the apex of the tooth, can result in tissue damage and inflammation [71]. Radiographically, it will present with filling material beyond the anatomic apex. Apical surgery may be necessary to remove the overextended material. Extrusion into vital structures, such as the inferior alveolar nerve canal, is an emergency condition, as it can cause permanent damage to the nerve via trauma, pressure, or neurotoxicity [72]. Extrusion into the inferior alveolar nerve canal can result in pain in the location as well as radiating pain [73]. Early surgical exploration and debridement may reverse the side effects of endodontic treatment on the inferior alveolar nerve [72].

Root perforations are another iatrogenic event which can present with pain. Radiographically, a perforation can present as misalignment between the root canal filling or restorative material (post/dowel) and the root or root canal space [74]. Multiple angled radiographs assist in the diagnosis and location of a suspected perforation [20, 21]. CBCT is also helpful in diagnosing and assessing treatment options of a suspected perforation. However, beam hardening and artifacts secondary to radio-opaque materials can negatively impact the interpretation of the CBCT [18, 75, 76].

Perforations may present with associated periodontal defects such as epithelial downgrowth and bone loss, which may require periodontal treatment in addition to any endodontic perforation repair procedures [77]. Prognosis depends on root size, location relative to epithelial attachment, and accessibility for repair [78].

5.8 Conclusion

Proper selection and prescription of two-dimensional and three-dimensional assessment via periapical radiographs and CBCT are essential in the diagnosis of endodontic and periodontal issues to correctly manage odontogenic pain.

References

1. Renton T. Dental (Odontogenic) pain. Rev Pain. 2011;5(1):2–7.
2. Santos EC, Huller D, Brigola S, Ferreira MD, Pochapski MT, Dos Santos FA. Pain management in periodontal therapy using local anesthetics and other drugs: an integrative review. J Dent Anesth Pain Med. 2023;23(5):245–56.
3. Romero-Reyes M, Arman S, Teruel A, Kumar S, Hawkins J, Akerman S. Pharmacological Management of Orofacial Pain. Drugs. 2023;83(14):1269–92.
4. Liang H. Imaging in orofacial pain. Dent Clin N Am. 2018;62(4):533–51.
5. Sugars and dental caries [updated 9 November 2017]. Available from: https://www.who.int/news-room/fact-sheets/detail/sugars-and-dental-caries.
6. Administration ADACoSAaUSFaD. Dental radiographic examinations: recommendations for patient selection and limiting radiation exposure, 2012.
7. Rindal DB, Gordan VV, Litaker MS, Bader JD, Fellows JL, Qvist V, et al. Methods dentists use to diagnose primary caries lesions prior to restorative treatment: findings from The Dental PBRN. J Dent. 2010;38(12):1027–32.
8. Newman B, Seow WK, Kazoullis S, Ford D, Holcombe T. Clinical detection of caries in the primary dentition with and without bitewing radiography. Aust Dent J. 2009;54(1):23–30.
9. Hopcraft MS, Morgan MV. Comparison of radiographic and clinical diagnosis of approximal and occlusal dental caries in a young adult population. Community Dent Oral Epidemiol. 2005;33(3):212–8.

10. da Silva RP, Assaf AV, Pereira SM, Mialhe FL, Ambrosano GM, Meneghim Mde C, et al. Validity of caries-detection methods under epidemiological setting. Am J Dent. 2011;24(6):363–6.
11. Schwendicke F, Tzschoppe M, Paris S. Radiographic caries detection: a systematic review and meta-analysis. J Dent. 2015;43(8):924–33.
12. Bender IB. Pulpal pain diagnosis—a review. J Endodont. 2000;26(3):175–9.
13. Pak JG, White SN. Pain prevalence and severity before, during, and after root canal treatment: a systematic review. J Endodont. 2011;37(4):429–38.
14. Rechenberg DK, Munir A, Zehnder M. Correlation between the clinically diagnosed inflammatory process and periapical index scores in severely painful endodontically involved teeth. Int Endod J. 2021;54(2):172–80.
15. Endodontics AAo. Guide to clinical endodontics, 2019.
16. Glickman GN. AAE Consensus Conference on Diagnostic Terminology: background and perspectives. J Endodont. 2009;35(12):1619–20.
17. Endodontics AAo. Endodontic diagnosis Fall, 2013.
18. Special Committee to Revise the Joint AAEAPSouoCiE. AAE and AAOMR joint position statement: use of cone beam computed tomography in endodontics 2015 update. Oral Surg Oral Med Oral Pathol Oral Radiol. 2015;120(4):508–12.
19. Setzer FC, Lee SM. Radiology in endodontics. Dent Clin N Am. 2021;65(3):475–86.
20. Walton RE. Endodontic radiographic technics. Dent Radiogr Photogr. 1973;46(3):51–9.
21. Fava LR, Dummer PM. Periapical radiographic techniques during endodontic diagnosis and treatment. Int Endod J. 1997;30(4):250–61.
22. Endodontics AAo. Glossary of endodontic terms, 2020.
23. Miranda-Rius J, Brunet-Llobet L, Lahor-Soler E. The periodontium as a potential cause of orofacial pain: a comprehensive review. Open Dent J. 2018;12:520–8.
24. Edens MH, Khaled Y, Napenas JJ. Intraoral pain disorders. Oral Maxillofac Surg Clin North Am. 2016;28(3):275–88.
25. Gaurilcikaite E, Renton T, Grant AD. The paradox of painless periodontal disease. Oral Dis. 2017;23(4):451–63.
26. Jacobs R, Fontenele RC, Lahoud P, Shujaat S, Bornstein MM. Radiographic diagnosis of periodontal diseases - current evidence versus innovations. Periodontol 2000. 2024;95(1):51–69.
27. Chapple ILC, Mealey BL, Van Dyke TE, Bartold PM, Dommisch H, Eickholz P, et al. Periodontal health and gingival diseases and conditions on an intact and a reduced periodontium: Consensus report of workgroup 1 of the 2017 World Workshop on the classification of periodontal and peri-implant diseases and conditions. J Clin Periodontol. 2018;45(Suppl 20):S68–77.
28. Papapanou PN, Sanz M, Buduneli N, Dietrich T, Feres M, Fine DH, et al. Periodontitis: Consensus report of workgroup 2 of the 2017 World Workshop on the classification of periodontal and peri-implant diseases and conditions. J Clin Periodontol. 2018;45(Suppl 20):S162–S70.
29. Ismail A, Al YF. The role of radiographic imaging in the diagnosis and management of periodontal and peri-implant diseases. Dent Clin N Am. 2024;68(2):247–58.
30. Bragger U. Digital imaging in periodontal radiography. A review. J Clin Periodontol. 1988;15(9):551–7.
31. Eickholz P, Kim TS, Benn DK, Staehle HJ. Validity of radiographic measurement of interproximal bone loss. Oral Surg Oral Med Oral Pathol Oral Radiol Endod. 1998;85(1):99–106.
32. Lang NP, Hill RW. Radiographs in periodontics. J Clin Periodontol. 1977;4(1):16–28.
33. du Bois AH, Kardachi B, Bartold PM. Is there a role for the use of volumetric cone beam computed tomography in periodontics? Aust Dent J. 2012;57(Suppl 1):103–8.
34. Acar B, Kamburoglu K. Use of cone beam computed tomography in periodontology. World J Radiol. 2014;6(5):139–47.
35. Walter C, Kaner D, Berndt DC, Weiger R, Zitzmann NU. Three-dimensional imaging as a pre-operative tool in decision making for furcation surgery. J Clin Periodontol. 2009;36(3):250–7.
36. Braun X, Ritter L, Jervoe-Storm PM, Frentzen M. Diagnostic accuracy of CBCT for periodontal lesions. Clin Oral Investig. 2014;18(4):1229–36.
37. Probst M, Burian E, Robl T, Weidlich D, Karampinos D, Brunner T, et al. Magnetic resonance imaging as a diagnostic tool for periodontal disease: a prospective study with correlation to standard clinical findings-is there added value? J Clin Periodontol. 2021;48(7):929–48.
38. Revilla-Leon M, Gomez-Polo M, Barmak AB, Inam W, Kan JYK, Kois JC, et al. Artificial intelligence models for diagnosing gingivitis and periodontal disease: a systematic review. J Prosthet Dent. 2023;130(6):816–24.
39. Herrera D, Retamal-Valdes B, Alonso B, Feres M. Acute periodontal lesions (periodontal abscesses and necrotizing periodontal diseases) and endo-periodontal lesions. J Periodontol. 2018;89(Suppl 1):S85–S102.
40. Silva GL, Soares RV, Zenobio EG. Periodontal abscess during supportive periodontal therapy: a review of the literature. J Contemp Dent Pract. 2008;9(6):82–91.
41. Miranda-Rius J, Brunet-Llobet L, Lahor-Soler E. Ecstasy (3, 4-methylenedioxymethamphetamine, MDMA) related necrotising ulcerative gingivitis. BMJ Case Rep. 2009;2009:2009:bcr06.2008.0290.
42. Miranda-Rius J, Brunet-Llobet L, Lahor-Soler E, Farre M. Salivary secretory disorders, inducing drugs, and clinical management. Int J Med Sci. 2015;12(10):811–24.
43. Kinaia BM, Chogle SM, Kinaia AM, Goodis HE. Regenerative therapy: a periodontal-endodontic perspective. Dent Clin N Am. 2012;56(3):537–47.

44. Chogle SM, Goodis HE, Kinaia BM. Pulpal and periradicular response to caries: current management and regenerative options. Dent Clin N Am. 2012;56(3):521–36.
45. Gurusamy K, Duhan J, Tewari S, Sangwan P, Gupta A, Mittal S, et al. Patient-centric outcome assessment of endodontic microsurgery using periapical radiography versus cone beam computed tomography: a randomized clinical trial. Int Endod J. 2023;56(1):3–16.
46. Chogle S, Zuaitar M, Sarkis R, Saadoun M, Mecham A, Zhao Y. The recommendation of cone-beam computed tomography and its effect on endodontic diagnosis and treatment planning. J Endodont. 2020;46(2):162–8.
47. Ahmed ZH, Almuharib AM, Abdulkarim AA, Alhassoon AH, Alanazi AF, Alhaqbani MA, et al. Artificial intelligence and its application in endodontics: a review. J Contemp Dent Pract. 2023;24(11):912–7.
48. Greiser A, Christensen J, Fuglsig J, Johannsen KM, Nixdorf DR, Burzan K, et al. Dental-dedicated MRI, a novel approach for dentomaxillofacial diagnostic imaging: technical specifications and feasibility. Dentomaxillofac Radiol. 2024;53(1):74–85.
49. Guo J, Wu Y, Chen L, Long S, Chen D, Ouyang H, et al. A perspective on the diagnosis of cracked tooth: imaging modalities evolve to AI-based analysis. Biomed Eng Online. 2022;21(1):36.
50. Jud C, Sharma Y, Gunther B, Weitz J, Pfeiffer F, Pfeiffer D. X-ray dark-field tomography reveals tooth cracks. Sci Rep. 2021;11(1):14017.
51. Hilton TJ, Funkhouser E, Ferracane JL, Gordan VV, Huff KD, Barna J, et al. Associations of types of pain with crack-level, tooth-level and patient-level characteristics in posterior teeth with visible cracks: findings from the National Dental Practice-Based Research Network. J Dent. 2018;70:67–73.
52. Hasan S, Singh K, Salati N. Cracked tooth syndrome: overview of literature. Int J Appl Basic Med Res. 2015;5(3):164–8.
53. Lee SH, Lee JJ, Chung HJ, Park JT, Kim HJ. Dental optical coherence tomography: new potential diagnostic system for cracked-tooth syndrome. Surg Radiol Anat. 2016;38(1):49–54.
54. Andreasen FM, Andreasen JO. Resorption and mineralization processes following root fracture of permanent incisors. Endod Dent Traumatol. 1988;4(5):202–14.
55. Alaugaily I, Azim AA. CBCT patterns of bone loss and clinical predictors for the diagnosis of cracked teeth and teeth with vertical root fracture. J Endodont. 2022;48(9):1100–6.
56. Gao A, Cao D, Lin Z. Diagnosis of cracked teeth using cone-beam computed tomography: literature review and clinical experience. Dentomaxillofac Radiol. 2021;50(5):20200407.
57. Mareque-Bueno MS, Nagendrababu V, Dummer PMH, Ruiz-Pinon M, Arias-Moliz T, Uroz-Torres D, et al. A retrospective clinical study to compare the ability of cone-beam computed tomographic images and periapical radiographs to reveal cracked teeth, split teeth, and teeth with vertical root fractures. J Am Dent Assoc. 2024;155(7):614–23 e2.
58. Marotti J, Heger S, Tinschert J, Tortamano P, Chuembou F, Radermacher K, et al. Recent advances of ultrasound imaging in dentistry--a review of the literature. Oral Surgery, Oral Medicine, Oral Pathology and Oral Radiology. 2013;115(6):819–32.
59. Chan KH, Tom H, Darling CL, Fried D. A method for monitoring enamel erosion using laser irradiated surfaces and optical coherence tomography. Lasers Surg Med. 2014;46(9):672–8.
60. de Oliveira BP, Camara AC, Duarte DA, Gomes ASL, Heck RJ, Antonino ACD, et al. Detection of apical root cracks using spectral domain and swept-source optical coherence tomography. J Endodont. 2017;43(7):1148–51.
61. Han SH, Sadr A, Tagami J, Park SH. Non-destructive evaluation of an internal adaptation of resin composite restoration with swept-source optical coherence tomography and micro-CT. Dent Mater. 2016;32(1):e1–7.
62. Kim JM, Kang SR, Yi WJ. Automatic detection of tooth cracks in optical coherence tomography images. J Periodontal Implant Sci. 2017;47(1):41–50.
63. Shemesh H, van Soest G, Wu MK, Wesselink PR. Diagnosis of vertical root fractures with optical coherence tomography. J Endodont. 2008;34(6):739–42.
64. Idiyatullin D, Garwood M, Gaalaas L, Nixdorf DR. Role of MRI for detecting micro cracks in teeth. Dentomaxillofac Radiol. 2016;45(7):20160150.
65. Idiyatullin D, Corum C, Moeller S, Prasad HS, Garwood M, Nixdorf DR. Dental magnetic resonance imaging: making the invisible visible. J Endodont. 2011;37(6):745–52.
66. Krell KV. Cracked teeth and vertical root fractures: a new look at a growing problem. American Association of Endodontists; 2022.
67. Dodson TB, Susarla SM. Impacted wisdom teeth. BMJ Clin Evid. 2014;2014:1302.
68. Ness G, Hechler B. Impacted teeth. In: Peterson's principles of oral and Maxillofaical surgery. 4th ed. Springer; 2022.
69. Eslami E, Barkhordar H, Abramovitch K, Kim J, Masoud MI. Cone-beam computed tomography vs conventional radiography in visualization of maxillary impacted-canine localization: a systematic review of comparative studies. Am J Orthod Dentofacial Orthop. 2017;151(2):248–58.
70. Matzen LH, Wenzel A. Efficacy of CBCT for assessment of impacted mandibular third molars: a review - based on a hierarchical model of evidence. Dentomaxillofac Radiol. 2015;44(1):20140189.
71. Nair PN. On the causes of persistent apical periodontitis: a review. Int Endod J. 2006;39(4):249–81.
72. Pogrel MA. Damage to the inferior alveolar nerve as the result of root canal therapy. J Am Dent Assoc. 2007;138(1):65–9.

73. Nitzan DW, Stabholz A, Azaz B. Concepts of accidental overfilling and overinstrumentation in the mandibular canal during root canal treatment. J Endodont. 1983;9(2):81–5.
74. Roda RGB, Johnson S. Nonsurgical retreatment: repair of perforations. Pathways of the pulp. 12th ed. Elsevier; 2021.
75. Bueno MR, Estrela C, De Figueiredo JA, Azevedo BC. Map-reading strategy to diagnose root perforations near metallic intracanal posts by using cone beam computed tomography. J Endod. 2011;37(1):85–90.
76. Shemesh H, Cristescu RC, Wesselink PR, Wu MK. The use of cone-beam computed tomography and digital periapical radiographs to diagnose root perforations. J Endodont. 2011;37(4):513–6.
77. Seltzer S, Sinai I, August D. Periodontal effects of root perforations before and during endodontic procedures. J Dent Res. 1970;49(2):332–9.
78. Fuss Z, Trope M. Root perforations: classification and treatment choices based on prognostic factors. Endod Dent Traumatol. 1996;12(6):255–64.
79. Orstavik D, Kerekes K, Eriksen HM. The periapical index: a scoring system for radiographic assessment of apical periodontitis. Endod Dent Traumatol. 1986;2(1):20–34.
80. Kirkevang LL, Orstavik D, Wenzel A, Vaeth M. Prognostic value of the full-scale Periapical Index. Int Endod J. 2015;48(11):1051–8.

Imaging of Odontogenic Pain—Heterotopic/Referred

6

Gary D. Klasser and Robert Utsman

6.1 Introduction

In the majority of dental practices, most patients present with odontogenic pain (toothache) that has its origin from pulpal tissue mainly due to carious lesions or periodontal involvement. Both these sources of pain share a common mechanism which is inflammatory in origin. However, each tissue has a distinct functionality and embryologic origin, resulting in each pain being perceived differently. Notwithstanding, these routinely acute situations are often well managed with adequate dental interventions. However, in certain instances, the symptom of toothache results from a non-odontogenic cause. This may result in misdiagnosis followed by a number of erroneous dental interventions performed by well-intentioned and caring practitioners [1, 2]. Clearly, this situation should absolutely be avoided. Furthermore, the complicated differential diagnosis in these patients can be time-consuming, and this may add to other risk factors such as anxiety and catastrophizing [3] that allow pain to become chronic.

Routinely, most cases of odontogenic pain are considered to be homotopic pain. Homotopic pain is where the site and source of pain share the same origin. More specifically, it signifies pain that originates from a dental source and is felt in the same location. However, heterotopic pain denotes a situation whereby the site where the pain is sensed or reported by the patient is not coincident with its source [4]. Traditionally, three kinds of heterotopic pain are described: central pain, projected pain, and referred pain.

In case of central pain, a lesion or event within the brain or brain stem (e.g., a cerebrovascular accident) may damage nerve tissue that somatotopically corresponds to a particular region of the body. As a consequence, pain may be experienced in, for example, the orofacial region, while the source of pain is located in the central nervous system. Projected pain occurs when a nerve is irritated or triggered at some point of its anatomical trajectory, and the pain sensation follows the anatomic course of that nerve branch. A prime example of this type of pain is the pain experienced in trigeminal neuralgia (TN) due to a neurovascular conflict at the dorsal root entry zone. The third kind of heterotopic pain, referred pain, is considered of major importance in many of the deep pain states found with orofacial pain including temporomandibular disorders (TMD) [5]. Superficial nociceptive input converges with

G. D. Klasser
Louisiana State University Health Sciences Center, School of Dentistry, Department of Diagnostic Sciences, New Orleans, LA, USA

R. Utsman (✉)
Department of Biomedical and Community Health Sciences, Division of Diagnostic Sciences & Services, James B. Edwards College of Dental Medicine, Medical University of South Carolina, Charleston, SC, USA
e-mail: utsman@musc.edu

G. A. Kaspo, G. D. Klasser (eds.), *Orofacial and Head Pain*,
https://doi.org/10.1007/978-3-032-08275-6_6

other afferent inputs from deep tissues and from cervical spinal afferents onto the second-order neurons in the trigeminal brain stem sensory nuclear complex. Concomitant release of neurochemicals results in neuroplastic changes and an increased excitability of these neurons, termed central sensitization. In addition to the underlying referred pain phenomenon, this process, if perpetuated, is considered a key factor in the genesis and continuation of chronic pain [4, 6]. The use of imaging may be an important consideration in assisting with an accurate diagnosis in these situations.

6.2 Sinonasal Origin

According to the American Academy of Otolaryngology-Head and Neck Surgery (AAO-HNS), the term “rhinosinusitis” refers to symptomatic inflammation of the nasal cavity and paranasal sinuses and is preferred over the term “sinusitis,” because inflammation of the nasal cavity nearly always accompanies inflammation of the contiguous paranasal sinuses. Rhinosinusitis (upper respiratory tract infection) may be classified as acute rhinosinusitis if symptoms last <4 weeks or as chronic rhinosinusitis if symptoms last >12 weeks [7]. From a dental perspective, it is possible that periapical infection of the maxillary teeth may lead to painful odontogenic sinusitis or potentially, in chronic form, may lead to mucosal hyperplasia of the maxillary sinuses (usually asymptomatic). Iatrogenic causes such as oroantral communication, orthognathic surgery, sinus floor elevation procedures before dental implant placement, and foreign bodies such as root fragments and endodontic filling materials may also be responsible [8]. However, the reverse is also possible whereby irritation by a sinusitis or mucosal disease of the maxillary sinuses can irritate branches of the maxillary division of the trigeminal nerve that, in addition to the maxillary teeth, also serves the maxillary sinuses and the anterior two-thirds of the nose [9, 10]. This heterotopic pain (referred pain) often presents with continuous unilateral pressure or pain of several maxillary teeth that increases while chewing, clenching, bending over, exposure to cold, physical exertion, or increased pressure in the sinuses from coughing or sneezing [11]. Often, the odontogenic pain (site of the pain) is accompanied by a (frontal) headache and otolaryngologic (ENT) symptoms like nasal congestion or discharge. In order to provide an accurate diagnosis, a thorough history and accounting for influencing factors in addition to ruling out a clear dental pathology is required. Intraoral or panoramic radiographs may be useful to exclude the dentition as being the source of the problem. The sinuses may appear cloudy, opacified, and congested on the panoramic radiograph. Importantly, advanced imaging of the area and a consultation with an otolaryngologist for further evaluation (e.g., endoscopy) and management (clearing of the sinuses, culture of nasal fluid or pus, NSAIDs or antibiotics according to the diagnosis) may be in order. Computed tomography (CT) and magnetic resonance imaging (MRI) are the primary imaging modalities used to evaluate patients with sinonasal disease. Given its detailed depiction of bony anatomy, CT can accurately demonstrate the presence of sinonasal disease, such as an increase in fluid accumulation and thickening of the sinus mucosal membranes, bony erosions, and anatomic variants, and is essential for surgical planning. Given its superior soft tissue contrast, MRI can accurately identify clinically suspected intracranial and intraorbital complications, delineate soft tissue extension of tumors, and distinguish mass from obstructed secretions [12]. This multidisciplinary approach allows for a more precise diagnosis resulting in appropriate management. The role of the dental practitioner is to be aware of the differential diagnosis and, because they are not typically trained to evaluate sinonasal structures, to arrange the proper referral [10].

6.3 Muscle Origin

The Diagnostic Criteria of Temporomandibular Disorders (DC/TMD) [13] describes myofascial pain with referral as pain of muscle origin with referral of pain beyond the boundary of the muscle being palpated. This is similarly described in the International Classification of Orofacial Pain (ICOP) [14] as chronic primary myofascial pain with referral. Classically, provocation of this pain, familiar to the patient, is most easily initiated by palpation of trigger points (defined as a hyperirritable spot in skeletal muscle that is associated with a hypersensitive palpable nodule in a taut band) [15] in the concerned muscle, while local anesthesia of these trigger points often eliminates the pain in the referred region [16]. However, the underlying concepts regarding the pathophysiology of trigger points and taut bands remain somewhat controversial. It is not uncommon for patients who experience this heterotopic pain to report odontogenic pain in the maxillary or mandibular teeth [17]. This often results in misdirected and/or unnecessary invasive procedures targeting the site of the pain rather than the source of the pain. The diagnosis of this referred pain is made by palpation of various masticatory and cervical muscles, thereby reproducing the familiar tooth pain in the patient. Local anesthesia of the involved muscle (the source of the pain) traditionally is used both in the diagnosis and management of myofascial pain, although robust evidence continues to be lacking.

Intraoral imaging may be of assistance in ruling out any pulpal or periodontal disease that may be the true source of the pain. Additionally, advanced imaging such as CT or MRI may be helpful in ruling out any occult pathologies mimicking myofascial pain.

6.4 Neuropathic Origin

Neuropathic pain is defined as "pain arising as a direct consequence of a lesion or disease affecting the somatosensory system" [18]. Nociplastic pain is defined as "pain that arises from altered nociception despite no clear evidence of actual or threatened tissue damage causing the activation of peripheral nociceptors or evidence for disease or lesion of the somatosensory system causing the pain" [19]. In other words, pain originates from abnormalities in the neural structures and not from the tissues that are innervated by those neural structures. These pains pose significant difficulty for the clinician since the structures the patient reports as painful appear clinically normal. Neuralgia is considered "pain in the distribution of a nerve or nerves" and neuropathy is "a disturbance of function or pathological change in a nerve" while neuritis relates specifically to "inflammation of a nerve or nerves" [19]. A distinction among these terms is important to ensure that conditions are accurately classified, as management strategies differ.

6.4.1 Trigeminal Neuralgia

TN is currently classified into three different types. There is a classical type which presents in either a pure paroxysmal form or concomitant with continuous facial pain usually associated with neurovascular compression typically at the trigeminal root entry/exit zone (REZ) or transition zone; a secondary type which is due to an existing underlying condition such as multiple sclerosis or a central nervous system space-occupying lesion; and an idiopathic type. It is not uncommon, more specifically, for the classical type of TN to be associated with pain referral.

TN typically exhibits unilateral attacks of short, sharp, excruciating, shock-like pain of very high intensity over the trajectory of one or multiple branches of the trigeminal nerve. The attacks may occur spontaneously but mostly are triggered by innocent stimuli like touching a trigger zone, talking, chewing, cold or wind, or even with chewing and tooth brushing. These manifestations may make a differential diagnosis, other than odontogenic pain, rather perplexing. This warrants a thorough dental examination of each patient with a tentative diagnosis of TN and, at the same time, caution from engaging in dental interventions without very convincing indication [2, 20]. Often, patients tend to blame a tooth in the involved region and urge the dentist for extraction in view of pain intensity. Unfortunately, shortly after the extraction, the pain attacks resume [21, 22].

In the circumstance of neuralgia, imaging can be very useful in discerning the source from the site of pain. Intraoral and panoramic radiographs can be utilized to rule out odontogenic sources of pain. The main purpose of neuroimaging in TN has been to identify neurovascular contact and secondary causes with the use of MRI [23].

6.4.2 Trigeminal Neuropathy

Trigeminal neuropathy can result from a biologic infection (viral, bacterial, or fungal), traumatic injury (post-traumatic trigeminal neuropathic pain, PTTNP), or unknown origin (idiopathic trigeminal neuropathic pain). In PTTNP, neuroanatomically confined somatosensory abnormalities are mandatory, and the pain is often accompanied with sensory disturbances such as hypo- or hyperesthesia [14]. This characteristic is not required for other entities that have been described more recently such as persistent idiopathic facial pain (PIFP).

The pain associated with PTTNP is mostly unilateral, confined to the dermatome of the nerve involved in the traumatic event, of moderate to severe intensity, and mostly continuous with a burning or shooting character.

PIFP (previously referred to as atypical odontalgia or atypical facial pain) involves more diverse and potentially confusing characteristics in comparison to PTTNP as it presents either with unilateral or bilateral symptoms, occurring quasi continuously, sometimes with exacerbations in attacks or without, and is mostly not confined to a particular trigeminal nerve trajectory. Due to the nature of this condition, confusion may abound regarding the source versus the site of pain. Patients may interpret the pain as originating in the dentition or surrounding structures. Imaging can be of great value to rule in or exclude odontogenic causes, thereby providing greater clarity for an accurate diagnosis.

6.5 Neurovascular Origin

Pain of neurovascular origin, otherwise known as headaches, is a group of pain disorders that are felt as cephalalgias, or pain in the head. Neurovascular pains are usually of diverse constituents that share a common anatomic region of presentation, the head, but have moderately separate pathophysiological mechanisms. Predominantly, these head pain disorders are viewed as arising from a centralized phenomenon that involves an altered sensory processing and excitability of the brain, originating in multiple brain areas and expressed predominantly in the trigeminovascular system [24]. Headache or neurovascular conditions have the potential to mimic odontogenic pain due to coactivation of adjacent trigeminal branches [25], leading to incorrect and delayed diagnoses. Imaging strategies may be an important consideration in assisting with an accurate diagnosis in differentiating these conditions, thereby avoiding unnecessary invasive dental interventions.

6.5.1 Primary Headaches

The most prevalent type of headache disorders is primary headaches, such as migraine-type headache (MTH) and tension-type headache (TTH). Migraine typically presents with mostly unilateral pulsatile attacks of moderate to severe intensity lasting 4–72 h of duration localized in the periorbital or upper cervical regions. They are aggravated by normal physical activity and commonly accompanied with nausea or vomiting, photophobia, phonophobia, or aura. TTH on the other hand is a bilateral pressing or tightening sensation of mild to moderate intensity lasting 30 min to 24 h of duration localized in the forehead, posterior head regions, and neck. They are not aggravated by normal physical activity, can be accompanied by mild nausea in chronic TTH, and are not typically accompanied with photophobia, phonophobia, or aura. The proximity of pain associated with MTH and TTH over orofacial structures such as the jaw, maxillary sinuses, and adjacent structures often leads individuals to seek evaluation by dentists, thus stressing the importance of being familiar with these concepts to avoid misdiagnosis.

After dental caries, TTH and MTH were reported as the second (20.1%) and third (14.7%)

most prevalent disorders in the world, respectively, according to the Global Burden of Disease Study 2010 [26]. The global 1-year prevalence of TTH is estimated to be 26.8%, while MTH is estimated to be 15.2% in the general population [27]. MTH is more prevalent in females, with a female-to-male ratio of 3:1 [28]. In contrast, the prevalence in TTH is more equally distributed with a female-to-male ratio of 1.2:1, possibly indicating a more pronounced influence of hormonal factors in MTH compared to TTH.

The exact cause of MTH is complex and often involves multifactorial neurovascular etiologies. MTH is thought to be initiated due to a primary neuronal dysfunction that leads to a series of changes both extra- and intracranially of the trigeminal nerve [29, 30]. The activation of the trigeminovascular system also plays a critical role in MTH, by releasing neuropeptides that cause neurogenic inflammation and pain [28, 30]. Another possible cause is imbalances in neurotransmitters, such a serotonin, that affect pain pathways and contribute to the development of MTH [30]. Genetic predisposition and environmental triggers like stress, foods, and hormonal changes also play an important role in the likelihood of experiencing MTH.

Like MTH, the pathophysiology of TTH is also unclear; however, peripheral mechanisms of pericranial tenderness, a generalized pressure pain hypersensitivity, and muscle tightness play a vital role in the development of TTH [31]. Central mechanisms expressed as central sensitivity are thought to play an important role as well. Genetic studies suggest familial aggregation of TTH and an inherited susceptibility as a role [30]. Psychological factors in many patients, particularly in patients with chronic TTH, are also critical.

Management of primary headaches involves both abortive and preventive strategies with the overall goal to reduce pain and restore function and quality of life. Management strategies should include patient education, lifestyle modifications, management of triggers, and acute or preventive pharmacology. The decision to use MRI brain scanning is a common dilemma facing clinicians, particularly as primary headache phenotypes can be triggered by secondary causes. Studies demonstrate that there is no appreciable difference in the frequency of pathological and incidental findings in common headache populations compared with the general community [32]. Imaging is therefore not routinely required where a primary headache diagnosis can be made. It is important to understand that no single treatment is effective for all patients and that proper clinical workup is fundamental in each case.

6.5.2 Trigeminal Autonomic Cephalalgias

Cluster headache (CH), paroxysmal hemicrania (PH), short-lasting unilateral neuralgiform headaches with conjunctival injection and tearing (SUNCT), short-lasting unilateral neuralgiform headaches with cranial autonomic features (SUNA), and hemicrania continua (HC) belong to a group of idiopathic headaches that involve activation of trigeminovascular nociceptive pathways along with reflex cranial autonomic activation referred to as trigeminal autonomic headaches (TACs). TACs are characterized by a lateralized symptom of prominent headache in the orbital, supraorbital, and temporal regions (but may include other sites within the trigeminal nerve distribution) and are accompanied by ipsilateral cranial autonomic features of conjunctival injection, periorbital edema, facial flushing, otic fullness, lacrimation, and rhinorrhea [14]. These disorders are distinguished by their attack duration, frequency, and response to treatment.

The localized and intense pain associated with the various trigeminal autonomic cephalalgias, particularly periorbital or maxillary pain, frequently leads to misdirected dental interventions and ultimate unnecessary loss of teeth. To avoid these unfortunate situations, brain MRI scanning should be considered in atypical features which may include abnormalities on physical examination, changes in clinical characteristics, the response to treatment, or the temporal pattern of the symptoms [33]. Additional imaging maybe considered based on specific suspicion, such as MRI of the pituitary gland and intranasal and intraorbital structures and magnetic resonance angiography (MRA) of both intracranial and cervical blood vessels.

6.6 Vascular Origin

Headaches resulting from vasodilation and contraction dysfunction of the blood vessels in the head are classified as headaches of vascular origin. According to the International Classification of Headache Disorders, third edition (ICHD-3), headaches that occur in association with the onset of new headaches, the chronicity of primary headaches, or significant exacerbation of headaches in the context of head and neck vascular diseases are classified as "headache attributed to cranial and/or cervical vascular disorders" or "cerebrovascular-related headaches" [34]. Based on etiology, vascular disorders that can mimic headaches include cerebral ischemic event (cerebral infarction), nontraumatic intracranial hemorrhage (a brain aneurysm rupture), unruptured vascular malformation (abnormal blood vessel connections), arteritis (inflammation of large arteries), carotid or vertebral artery dissection, cranial venous disorder (blood clot in brain veins), acute intracranial arterial disorder (reversible cerebral vasoconstriction syndrome), chronic intracranial vasculopathy, or pituitary apoplexy [35]. All have the potential to manifest with sudden, severe headache reaching peak intensity within seconds, sometimes described as "thunderclap" onset, a red flag for a potentially serious vascular issue that requires immediate medical attention depending on the location of the vascular issue [36].

Headache of vascular origin, for example, temporal or giant cell arteritis, can result in direful complications if not accurately diagnosed and appropriately treated. The onset of a new headache in one or both temporal regions can often be mistaken for TMD of muscle origin, hence the importance of taking an extensive headache history/exam to identify red flags or worrisome clinical features that may signify the presence of an underlying pathological condition requiring neuroimaging. Imaging studies like CT scan or MRI are crucial to identify the underlying vascular abnormality causing headaches with serious morbidity and mortality if not promptly diagnosed and treated [37].

6.7 Salivary Gland Origin

Pain of salivary gland origin is defined as pain caused by a lesion or disorder involving the salivary glands, with possible underlying causes being obstruction of the salivary duct, viral or bacterial infection, recurrent juvenile parotitis, and immunologic disorder, among others [38]. These pain conditions usually do not resemble odontogenic pain, but in cases of obstruction of the salivary duct, for example, in sialadenitis, they may cause heterotopic pain overlying the mandibular region that can be mistaken for a dental abscess. The obstruction of the salivary gland can also cause a highly intense pain caused by the attempted salivary discharge from the blocked ducts, which may be caused by salivary calculus, infection, or neoplasia [39]. On initial clinical examination, discharge and tenderness of the gland and their ducts (Stenson's duct for the parotid) may confirm that the pain is related to the salivary gland rather than odontogenic pain. Initial imaging of salivary gland disorders are done with ultrasound; however, a CT (with or without contrast) is a reliable method to detect salivary gland abnormalities when not available. Conventional sialography is another technique that requires the ability to dilate and cannulate a salivary duct orifice, which can be not only diagnostic but also therapeutic [40]. In cases of a suspected malignant salivary gland tumor, a MRI is preferred. Although no single salivary imaging modality is superior to another across most clinical scenarios, initial screening with ultrasound as the initial method of evaluation is emphasized in most cases [40].

6.8 Conclusion

Pain of sinonasal, muscle, neuropathic, neurovascular, vascular, and salivary gland origin can be sources of odontogenic pain in the orofacial region. Imaging strategies across different clinical scenarios are important to assist the clinician in discerning the source of pain, which may be quite different from the site of pain. It is important to recognize that with heterotopic pain, no single imaging is effective for all patients and that proper clinical workup is fundamental for accurate diagnosis to avoid unnecessary invasive dental interventions.

References

1. Ram S, Teruel A, Kumar SK, Clark G. Clinical characteristics and diagnosis of atypical odontalgia: implications for dentists. J Am Dent Assoc. 2009;140:223–8.
2. Von Eckardstein KL, Keil M, Rohde V. Unnecessary dental procedures as a consequence of trigeminal neuralgia. Neurosurg Rev. 2015;38:355–60.
3. Fillingim RB, Ohrbach R, Greenspan JD, Knott C, Diatchenko L, Dubner R, et al. Psychological factors associated with development of TMD: the OPPERA prospective cohort study. J Pain. 2013;14(12 Suppl):T75–90.
4. Sessle BJ. Acute and chronic craniofacial pain: brainstem mechanisms of nociceptive transmission and neuroplasticity, and their clinical correlates. Crit Rev Oral Biol Med. 2000;11:57–91.
5. Chichorro JG, Porreca F, Sessle BJ. Mechanisms of craniofacial pain. Cephalalgia. 2017;37:613–26.
6. De Laat A. Differential diagnosis of toothache to prevent erroneous and unnecessary dental treatment. J Oral Rehabil. 2020;47:775–81.
7. Rosenfeld RM, Piccirillo JF, Chandrasekhar SS, Brook I, Kumar KA, Kramper M, et al. Clinical practice guideline (update): adult sinusitis executive summary. Otolaryngol Head Neck Surg. 2015;152:598–609.
8. Sepúlveda AI, Rivas-Rodriguez F, Capizzano AA. Imaging of the Sinonasal Cavities. Dent Clin N Am. 2024;68:337–55.
9. Klasser GD, Romero Reyes M. Orofacial pain: guidelines for assessment, diagnosis, and management. 7th ed. Batavia: Quintessence Publishing Co. Inc; 2023.
10. Shueb SS, Boyer HC, Nixdorf DR. Nonodontogenic "tooth pain" of nose and sinus origin. J Am Dent Assoc. 2016;147:457–9.
11. Sharav Y, Benoliel R. Acute orofacial pain. In: Sharav Y, Benoliel R, editors. Orofacial pain and headache. 2nd ed. Chicago: Quintessence Publishing Co; 2015. p. 176–7.
12. Expert Panel on Neurological Imaging, Hagiwara M, Policeni B, Juliano AF, Agarwal M, Burns J, Dubey P, et al. ACR appropriateness criteria® Sinonasal disease: 2021 update. J Am Coll Radiol. 2022;19(5S):S175–93.
13. Schiffman E, Ohrbach R, Truelove E, Look J, Anderson G, Goulet JP, et al. Diagnostic Criteria for Temporomandibular Disorders (DC/TMD) for clinical and research applications: recommendations of the International RDC/TMD Consortium Network and Orofacial Pain Special Interest Group. J Oral Facial Pain Headache. 2014;28:6–27.
14. International Classification of orofacial pain, 1st ed. (ICOP). Cephalalgia. 2020;40:129–221.
15. Simons DG, Travell JG. Travell & Simons' myofascial pain and dysfunction: the trigger point manual. Baltimore: Williams & Wilkins; 1999.
16. Simons DG. New views of myofascial trigger points: etiology and diagnosis. Arch Phys Med Rehabil. 2008;89:157–9.
17. Wright EF. Referred craniofacial pain patterns in patients with temporomandibular disorder. J Am Dent Assoc. 2000;131:1307–15.
18. Jensen TS, Baron R, Haanpää M, Kalso E, Loeser JD, Rice ASC, et al. A new definition of neuropathic pain. Pain. 2011;152:2204–5.
19. IASP. Committee on taxonomy. International Association for the Study of Pain. IASP Publications - IASP Terminology; 2011. [cited 2024 Oct 25]. Available from: https://www.iasp-pain.org/resources/terminology/.
20. Spencer CJ, Neubert JK, Gremillion H, Zakrzewska JM, Ohrbach R. Toothache or trigeminal neuralgia: treatment dilemmas. J Pain. 2008;9:767–70.
21. Bowsher D. Trigeminal neuralgia. A symptomatic study of 126 successive patients with and without previous interventions. Pain Clinic. 2000;12:93–8.
22. Tripathi M, Sadashiva N, Gupta A, Jani P, Pulickal SJ, Deora H, et al. Please spare my teeth! Dental procedures and trigeminal neuralgia. Surg Neurol Int. 2020;11:455.
23. Watanabe M, Shrivastava RK, Balchandani P. Advanced neuroimaging of the trigeminal nerve and the whole brain in trigeminal neuralgia: a systematic review. Pain. 2024;166:282.
24. Mier RW, Dhadwal S. Primary headaches. Dent Clin N Am. 2018;62:611–28.
25. Peng KP, Benoliel R, May A. A review of current perspectives on facial presentations of primary headaches. J Pain Res. 2022;15:1613–21.
26. Vos T, Flaxman AD, Naghavi M, Lozano R, Michaud C, Ezzati M, et al. Years lived with disability (YLDs) for 1160 sequelae of 289 diseases and injuries 1990–2010: a systematic analysis for the Global Burden of Disease study 2010. Lancet. 2012;380:2163–96.
27. Institute for Health Metrics and Evaluation (IHME). GBD Results Tool [Internet], 2020 [cited 2024 Sept 10]. Available from: http://ghdx.healthdata.org/gbd-results-tool.
28. Ashina S, Mitsikostas DD, Lee MJ, Yamani N, Wang SJ, Messina R, et al. Tension-type headache. Nat Rev Dis Primers. 2021;7:24.
29. Shibata Y. Migraine pathophysiology revisited: proposal of a new molecular theory of migraine patho-

physiology and headache diagnostic criteria. Int J Mol Sci. 2022;23:13002.
30. Onan D, Younis S, Wellsgatnik WD, Farham F, Andruškevičius S, Abashidze A, et al. Debate: differences and similarities between tension-type headache and migraine. J Headache Pain. 2023;24:92.
31. Ashina S, Bendtsen L, Ashina M. Pathophysiology of tension-type headache. Curr Pain Headache Rep. 2005;9:415–22.
32. Micieli A, Kingston W. An approach to identifying headache patients that require neuroimaging. Front Public Health. 2019;7:52.
33. Wilbrink LA, Ferrari MD, Kruit MC, Haan J. Neuroimaging in trigeminal autonomic cephalgias: when, how, and of what? Curr Opin Neurol. 2009;22:247–53.
34. Headache Classification Committee of the International Headache Society (IHS). The International Classification of headache disorders, vol. 38. 3rd ed. Cephalalgia; 2018. p. 1–211.
35. Wang W, Zhu C, Martelletti P. Understanding headaches attributed to cranial and/or cervical vascular disorders: insights and challenges for neurologists. Pain Ther. 2024;13:1429–45.
36. Kapoor S. Headache attributed to cranial or cervical vascular disorders. Curr Pain Headache Rep. 2013;17(5):334.
37. Wang LL, Mahammedi A, Vagal AS. Imaging of headache attributed to vascular disorders. Neurol Clin. 2022;40:507–30.
38. Pigg M, Nixdorf DR, Law AS, Renton T, Sharav Y, Baad-Hansen L, et al. New international classification of orofacial pain: what is in it for endodontists? J Endodont. 2020;47:345–57.
39. Renton T. Tooth-related pain or not? Headache. 2020;60:235–46.
40. Benito DA, Badger C, Hoffman HT, Joshi A. Recommended imaging for salivary gland disorders. Curr Otorhinolaryngol Rep. 2020;8:311–20.

7 Overview of Imaging Modalities for Temporomandibular Disorders

Gary D. Klasser and Ghabi A. Kaspo

7.1 Introduction

Temporomandibular disorders (TMDs) are comprised of heterogeneous disorders which are commonly multifactorial in etiology, affecting the temporomandibular joint (TMJ) including the articular disc and associated attachments, the muscles involved in jaw movement, and the surrounding structures. These disorders can present with various symptoms, including pain, restricted movement, functional disturbances, and intracapsular sounds such as clicking, popping, or crunching (crepitus) sounds. TMDs are the most commonly diagnosed orofacial pains of non-dental origin, and their prevalence varies due to differences in examination methods, non-homogeneous diagnostic criteria, and study populations [1–3]. According to the World Health Organization report, TMD is the third most common stomatological disorder after dental caries and periodontal disease [4]. It has been estimated that 4.8% to 42.7% of the general population manifest some signs or symptoms of TMD [5]. Accurate diagnosis and effective management of TMDs require a comprehensive evaluation including a detailed history, thorough clinical examination, and detailed imaging to evaluate hard and soft tissues, when deemed necessary. Imaging may be of assistance in the corroboration of clinical impressions and in the confirmation of clinical diagnosis. Furthermore, imaging may be beneficial in detecting pathological changes that are not clinically detectable and provide valuable information that may influence management interventions. This chapter provides a comprehensive overview of the imaging modalities used in the assessment of TMDs, including panoramic radiography, cone beam computed tomography (CBCT), computed tomography (CT), magnetic resonance imaging (MRI), ultrasonography (US), and nuclear imaging (bone scintigraphy). Each imaging technique's principles, advantages, limitations, and clinical applications will be discussed [6–8].

7.2 Panoramic Radiography

Panoramic radiographs provide a broad image of the entire oral cavity, including the mandible, maxilla, dentition, sinuses, and surrounding bone structures in a single image. This overall two-dimensional view, a defining feature of panoramic radiography, enables a screening examination and aids dental professionals in contributing information in the diagnosis for a wide

G. D. Klasser
Louisiana State University Health Sciences Center, School of Dentistry, Department of Diagnostic Sciences, New Orleans, LA, USA

G. A. Kaspo (✉)
Henry Ford Health Systrem, Henry Ford Hospital, Department of Otolaryngology, Royal Oak, Michigan, USA

Wayne State University, Department of Psychiatry, Detroit, Michigan, USA

G. A. Kaspo, G. D. Klasser (eds.), *Orofacial and Head Pain*,
https://doi.org/10.1007/978-3-032-08275-6_7

range of dental and maxillofacial conditions [9, 10]. Panoramic images play a vital role in the early suspicion of pathologies such as cysts, tumors, infections, and bone abnormalities. By visualizing the entire dental arch and adjacent structures in one image, panoramic radiographs allow dental professionals to detect issues that might otherwise be missed with intraoral radiographs such as bitewing or periapicals, significantly enhancing patient care [10]. Additionally, these radiographs provide clear images of tooth positioning, including unerupted or impacted teeth, and are instrumental in detecting potential bone pathology [10]. This overall view is crucial for orthodontic planning, ensuring the dentitions are properly aligned with correct and adequate spacing requirements [11]. Patients with facial trauma often seek initial care in emergency departments or at oral maxillofacial surgeons' offices and may consult their general practitioners for further evaluation after discharge, especially in cases involving displaced fractures or significant injuries [12, 13].

While panoramic radiographs provide important information about the bone structure and jaw and dentition alignment, they have inherent limitations in accurately depicting vital anatomy such as the infra-alveolar nerve and the internal or external resorption of dental roots, underscoring the importance of selecting appropriate imaging techniques based on diagnostic needs. Furthermore, panoramic radiographs do not provide sufficient detail regarding the TMJ complex, including the condyles. Although they may offer an outline of the TM joints, they lack the ability to deliver a detailed and accurate view of the condyles and joint eminence, which is essential for definitive diagnosis and management planning. Due to the curved nature of the jaw and the imaging technique (transpharyngeal projection), panoramic radiographs produce distorted or overlapping images, complicating the definitive diagnostic process. Obtaining a clear panoramic radiograph requires precise patient positioning, and any movement during exposure can lead to blurred or distorted images, making diagnosis particularly challenging with young children or patients with physical or cognitive impairments. Moreover, the settings on panoramic radiograph machines are predetermined by the manufacturer, which can introduce variability in image accuracy based on the patient's head size and age, thereby affecting the quality of images of the maxillary and mandibular bones. While panoramic radiographs expose patients to less radiation than a full-mouth series of intraoral radiographs, they are not without a certain level of radiation exposure. It is essential to consider the cumulative effect of repeated radiographs, particularly for patients requiring frequent imaging, and clinicians must always follow the ALARA (As Low As Reasonably Achievable) principle to minimize radiation exposure. For comprehensive and precise TMJ evaluation, panoramic radiography has limitations in fully assessing the complex structures of the TMJs affected by conditions like degenerative joint diseases, internal derangements, and congenital anomalies. It is unable to provide a detailed and accurate view of the condyles in the fossa or effectively detect specific arthritic changes or abnormal outlines of the condyles, necessitating advanced imaging techniques like CBCT scans for a more comprehensive assessment [8, 11, 12]. Although panoramic radiography can be useful for detecting symmetrical or asymmetrical relationships of the mandible, indicating abnormal growth of the condyle or idiopathic condylar resorption [10], it offers limited diagnostic value for the TMJ complex and other orofacial pain conditions. Its contribution in assisting with the diagnosis of orofacial pain is minimal unless specific pathologies are present, leading to the conclusion that panoramic radiography should only be used as a screening image and/or considered a last resort when other imaging modalities are unavailable.

7.3 Cone Beam Computed Tomography (CBCT)

Cone beam computed tomography (CBCT) is a specialized type of CT that uses a cone-shaped X-ray (electromagnetic radiation) beam and a flat-panel detector to produce a volumetric dataset of the TMJ. It captures detailed three-dimensional images while reducing radiation exposure compared to conventional CT [14–17].

The advantages of CBCT include its ability to provide high spatial resolution, offering detailed 3D images that are especially beneficial for visualizing bony structures and dental hard tissue components. Additionally, CBCT generally involves a lower radiation dose than conventional CT, making it a safer option for repeated imaging. Another advantage is its in-office applicability, allowing clinicians to capture and evaluate images during the patient's assessment.

Similar to other modalities, CBCT has limitations. Like conventional CT, it is less effective for visualizing soft tissue structures [15]. While CBCT units are more common and less expensive than some other imaging modalities, availability and cost may still be a concern for some practices.

CBCT is commonly used for the detailed assessment of bony structures, making it useful for evaluating complex TMJ anatomy, bone morphology, and pathologies [18]. It is also frequently employed for orthodontic and surgical planning, including planning for orthodontic treatments, dental implants, and TMJ surgeries.

7.4 Computed Tomography (CT)

Computed tomography (CT) uses X-rays combined with computer processing to produce cross-sectional images of the TMJ. The CT scanner rotates around the patient, capturing multiple images from different angles, which are digitally reconstructed to create a three-dimensional image of the joint and surrounding structures [19].

One of the main advantages of CT is its ability to provide high-resolution images that are excellent for visualizing both bone structures and hard and soft tissue pathology [20]. Additionally, it offers a detailed, three-dimensional view of the TMJ and related anatomy, making it crucial for assessing complex cases. Typically, CT is not routinely used and is better reserved for more complicated situations.

Despite its advantages, CT has limitations. It involves a higher dose of ionizing radiation compared to conventional radiography and CBCT. Moreover, CT is not ideal for imaging soft tissue structures of the temporomandibular complex, such as the articular disc, which is not well defined using this modality [21, 22].

CT has several clinical applications, including the assessment of bony pathologies, where it is useful for diagnosing fractures, bone erosions, and other bony abnormalities associated with TMDs [20]. It is also valuable for pre-surgical planning, providing the detailed anatomical information necessary for evaluating TMJ disorders before surgery [20].

7.5 Magnetic Resonance Imaging (MRI)

Magnetic resonance imaging (MRI) uses strong magnetic fields and radiofrequency pulses to generate detailed images of both soft tissues and some hard tissues. It produces high-contrast images, making it especially useful for assessing the TMJ internal components, particularly the status and position of the articular disc [23].

The advantages of MRI include its ability to provide superior soft tissue imaging, making it excellent for visualizing the articular disc, ligaments, and muscles surrounding the TMJ [15]. Additionally, since MRI does not use ionizing radiation, it is particularly beneficial for patients who require multiple or sequential follow-up imaging sessions.

MRI has certain limitations. It is generally more expensive than other imaging modalities. The scan's sensitivity to movement means that any patient motion can cause artifacts, potentially compromising the image quality. The procedure is also time-consuming, requiring patients to remain still for an extended period. Furthermore, the enclosed nature of the MRI machine can lead to anxiety or claustrophobia, which may be a contraindication for some patients.

MRI has key clinical applications as it is ideal for evaluating conditions such as articular disc displacement, internal derangement, and inflammation [15, 24]. MRI is also effective in providing detailed images of the soft tissues surrounding the TMJ, aiding in the diagnosis of conditions involving inflammation such as synovitis or tendonitis [14, 25, 26].

7.6 Ultrasonography (US)

Ultrasonography (US) utilizes high-frequency sound waves to create images of the TMJ. A transducer emits sound waves that reflect off tissues and return to the transducer, producing real-time images of the TMJ and surrounding soft tissues [26].

The advantages of US include its ability to provide real-time dynamic imaging, allowing for the assessment of joint movement and function during the clinical examination. Additionally, it is non-ionizing, meaning it does not involve radiation, making it safe for repeated use.

A significant limitation associated with US is that it is less effective for imaging deeper structures, thereby limiting its ability to provide a comprehensive view of the entire TMJ [26]. The quality of the images and diagnostic accuracy are also highly dependent on the operator's experience and skill.

Clinically, US is useful for guided procedures, such as guiding joint injections or aspirations. It is also ideal for assessing superficial structures, including synovial thickening, effusion, or superficial inflammation.

7.7 Nuclear Imaging (Bone Scintigraphy)

Bone scintigraphy, commonly referred to as bone scanning, is a nuclear imaging technique that involves the injection of a radiopharmaceutical agent, typically technetium-99m-labeled diphosphonates, which has a high affinity for bone tissue. The bone absorbs radiopharmaceuticals, particularly in areas with high metabolic (osteoblastic and/or osteoclastic) activity. The emitted gamma radiation is then captured using a gamma camera, producing images that reflect the metabolic activity of the bone [27]. The sensitivity, specificity, and accuracy for detecting skeletal metastatic disease (outside of the oral region) with the use of fluorodeoxyglucose positron emission tomography (FDG PET/CT) were 97%, 98%, and 98%, respectively, and with bone scintigraphy were 83%, 98%, and 93%, respectively. The lesions that bone scintigraphy most commonly missed were located in the pelvis, spine, and sacrum. FDG PET/CT missed mostly lesions that were outside of the field of view, but in all of these cases, the patient had additional sites of skeletal metastatic disease. Bone scintigraphy falsely identified six metastatic lesions and FDG PET/CT falsely identified only three metastatic lesions [28, 29].

There are several advantages with the use of nuclear imaging due to its ability to assess metabolic changes associated with the TMJ such as osteoarthritis, systemic arthritides (a group of systemic diseases which cause inflammation) such as rheumatoid arthritis, psoriatic arthritis, and juvenile idiopathic arthritis, and other degenerative/resorptive or inflammatory diseases. Bone scintigraphy is highly sensitive to changes in bone metabolism, often detecting abnormalities before they become apparent on conventional radiographs or even MRI [30, 31]. This early detection is crucial in managing progressive conditions like osteoarthritis and systemic arthritides associated with various autoimmune disorders. Bone scintigraphy can be used for whole-body imaging, allowing for the assessment of multiple joints including the TMJ, when a systemic condition is suspected. Unlike conventional imaging modalities that primarily provide structural information, bone scintigraphy offers functional imaging, providing insights into the metabolic activity of the bone. This can be particularly beneficial in assessing the activity of disease processes within the TMJ.

Unfortunately, there are limitations to its use. While bone scintigraphy is highly sensitive, it has low specificity. Increased radiotracer uptake can be seen in numerous conditions, such as infections, tumors, or fractures, making it difficult to differentiate between pathologies based solely on nuclear imaging results. Furthermore, it does not clearly distinguish or reliably differentiate between bone deposition and/or resorption. Although the radiation dose from bone scintigraphy is relatively low, it is still a consideration, particularly in younger patients and those requiring multiple imaging studies [32]. Bone scintigraphy provides limited anatomic detail compared to imaging modalities like MRI or CT. It is often used in combination with these modalities to provide a more comprehensive evaluation of the TMJ [23, 24, 33]. Furthermore, the procedure can be more expensive than other imaging techniques, and the need for specialized equipment and radiopharmaceuticals can make it less accessible.

The use of this modality has several clinical applications. Since it is highly sensitive to changes in bone metabolism, it may be an effective tool for detecting early-stage osteoarthritis in the TMJ. This can be particularly useful in patients with joint pain and dysfunction where other imaging modalities may not show clear signs of degeneration [31]. It may be considered for the assessment of localized and systemic inflammatory conditions. An example would be its clinical utility when a suspicion of rheumatoid arthritis arises that involves the TMJ. Bone scintigraphy can help identify areas of increased metabolic activity, indicating active inflammation and bone remodeling [31]. Moreover, bone scintigraphy may be used to detect avascular necrosis of the condyle, a condition where the blood supply to the bone is compromised, leading to bone necrosis and subsequent joint dysfunction. Bone scintigraphy may also be of assistance in planning for patients undergoing surgical interventions for TMD by identifying active bone pathology. Postoperatively, it can be used to monitor the success of the treatment and the progression of bone healing.

7.8 Conclusion

Selecting an imaging modality for TMD hinges on the specific clinical question and the structures of interest. Panoramic radiography provides a fundamental assessment of bony structures, while CT and CBCT deliver detailed images of bone and joint anatomy. MRI excels in assessing soft tissue abnormalities, and ultrasonography offers real-time imaging of joint function and superficial structures. Nuclear imaging uniquely assesses bone metabolic activity. Each modality possesses its strengths and limitations, often necessitating a combination of techniques to ensure a comprehensive evaluation of TMDs. A solid understanding of these imaging modalities' capabilities and appropriate applications is vital for accurate diagnosis and effective management of TMD, thereby enhancing overall patient care.

References

1. Carlsson GE. Epidemiology and treatment need for temporomandibular disorders. J Orofac Pain. 1999;13(4):232–7.
2. Dworkin SF, Huggins KH, LeResche L, Von Korff M, Howard J, Truelove E, et al. Epidemiology of signs and symptoms in temporomandibular disorders: clinical signs in cases and controls. J Am Dent Assoc. 1990;120(3):273–81.
3. Vainionpää R, Kinnunen T, Pesonen P, Laitala ML, Anttonen V, Sipilä K. Prevalence of temporomandibular disorders (TMD) among Finnish prisoners: cross-sectional clinical study. Acta Odontol Scand. 2019;77(4):264–8.
4. Pihut M, Szuta M, Ferendiuk E, Zeńczak-Więckiewicz D. Differential diagnostics of pain in the course of trigeminal neuralgia and temporomandibular joint dysfunction. Biomed Res Int. 2014;2014:563786.
5. National Academies of Sciences, Engineering, and Medicine. Temporomandibular disorders: priorities for research and care. Washington, DC: The National Academies Press; 2020.
6. Mallya SM, Ahmad M, Cohen JR, Kaspo G, Ramesh A. Recommendations for imaging of the temporomandibular joint. Position statement from the American Academy of Oral and Maxillofacial Radiology and the American Academy of Orofacial Pain. Oral Surg Oral Med Oral Pathol Oral Radiol. 2022;134(5):639–48.
7. Kopp S. Radiographic assessment of temporomandibular disorders. J Oral Maxillofac Surg. 1990;48(6):613–20.
8. Petersson A. What you can and cannot see in TMJ imaging—an overview related to the RDC/TMD diagnostic system. J Oral Rehabil. 2010;37(10):771–8.
9. Alali Y, Mohammed WA, Aldrees AF, Alshamrani AM, Alabdullatif MA, Alhajri SA. Comparative efficacy of digital panoramic radiograph and cone beam computed tomography in locating man-

dibular foramen. Eur Rev Med Pharmacol Sci. 2024;28(8):2996–3005.
10. Cosson J. Interpreting an orthopantomogram. Aust J Gen Pract. 2020;49(9):550–5.
11. Jadaun G, Rai AB, Kharodia S, Gadhiya V. Ossifying fibroma of mandible - a case report. Indian J Dent Res. 2023;34(4):458–60.
12. De Stefano AA, Horodynski M, Bartolomucci M, Castellano M, Spota A, Galluccio G. Vertical mandibular asymmetry and hand measurements in patients in growth: cross-sectional study. Clin Ter. 2024;175(3):117–27.
13. Jacques E, Ebogo M, Eng YC, Donald N, Odile Z. Radiographic evaluation of impacted third Mandibular Molar according to the classification of Winter, Pell and Gregory in a sample of Cameroonian population. Ethiop J Health Sci. 2023;33(5):851–8.
14. Mallya SM, Ahmad M, Cohen JR, Kaspo G, Ramesh A. Recommendations for imaging of the temporomandibular joint. Position statement from the American Academy of Oral and Maxillofacial Radiology and the American Academy of Orofacial Pain. J Oral Facial Pain Headache. 2023;37(1):7–15.
15. Al-Saleh MA, Alsufyani NA, Saltaji H, Jaremko JL, Major PW. MRI and CBCT image registration of temporomandibular joint: a systematic review. J Otolaryngol Head Neck Surg. 2016;45(1):30.
16. Tsiklakis K. Cone beam computed tomographic findings in temporomandibular joint disorders. Alpha Omegan. 2010;103(2):68–78.
17. Tsai CM, Wu FY, Chai JW, Chen MH, Kao CT. The advantage of cone-beam computerized tomography over panoramic radiography and temporomandibular joint quadruple radiography in assessing temporomandibular joint osseous degenerative changes. J Dent Sci. 2020;15(2):153–62.
18. Talmaceanu D, Lenghel LM, Bolog N, Hedesiu M, Buduru S, Rotar H, et al. Imaging modalities for temporomandibular joint disorders: an update. Clujul Med. 2018;91(3):280–7.
19. Hunter DJ, Bierma-Zeinstra S. Osteoarthritis. Lancet. 2019;393(10182):1745–59.
20. Boeddinghaus R, Whyte A. Computed tomography of the temporomandibular joint. J Med Imaging Radiat Oncol. 2013;57(4):448–54.
21. Fan XD, Yang C, Wang PZ, Wang XD. The Value of CT Scanning in the Diagnosis of Temporomandibular Joint Dysfunction. Shanghai kou Qiang yi xue; Shanghai Journal of Stomatology. 1999;8(4):223–25.
22. Krennmair G, Zembic A. Computed tomography of the temporomandibular joint: a review. J Oral Maxillofac Surg. 2007;65(8):1578–84.
23. Ahmad M, Schiffman EL. Temporomandibular joint disorders and orofacial pain. Dent Clin N Am. 2016;60(1):105–24.
24. Alkhader M, Kuribayashi A, Ohbayashi N, Nakamura S, Kurabayashi T. Usefulness of cone beam computed tomography in temporomandibular joints with soft tissue pathology. Dentomaxillofac Radiol. 2010;39(6):343–8.
25. Xiong X, Ye Z, Tang H, Wei Y, Nie L, Wei X, et al. MRI of temporomandibular joint disorders: recent advances and future directions. J Magn Reson Imaging. 2021;54(4):1039–52.
26. Maranini B, Ciancio G, Mandrioli S, Galiè M, Govoni M. The role of ultrasound in temporomandibular joint disorders: an update and future perspectives. Front Med (Lausanne). 2022;9:926573.
27. Montilla-Soler JL, Makanji R. Skeletal scintigraphy. Cancer Control. 2017;24(2):137–46.
28. Chang CY, Gill CM, Joseph Simeone F, Taneja AK, Huang AJ, Torriani M, et al. Comparison of the diagnostic accuracy of 99m-Tc-MDP bone scintigraphy and 18F-FDG PET/CT for the detection of skeletal metastases. Acta Radiol. 2016;57(1):58–65.
29. Ryan JL, Aaron VD, Sims JB. PET/MRI vs PET/CT in head and neck imaging: when, why, and how? Semin Ultrasound CT MR. 2019;40(5):376–90.
30. Akdağ O, Yıldıran G, Karameşe M. Patient symptoms and magnetic resonance imaging correlation in temporomandibular joint internal derangement. Turk J Med Sci. 2018;48(6):1092–5.
31. Mupparapu M, Oak S, Chang YC, Alavi A. Quantification of TMJ rheumatoid arthritis on positron emission tomography scans using rover software. Oral Surg Oral Med Oral Pathol Oral Radiol. 2020;130(2):e65.
32. Van den Wyngaert T, Strobel K, Kampen WU, Kuwert T, van der Bruggen W, Mohan HK, et al. The EANM practice guidelines for bone scintigraphy. Eur J Nucl Med Mol Imaging. 2016;43(9):1723–38.
33. Eriksen ES, Hellem S, Skartveit L, Brun JG, Boe OE, Moen K, et al. Temporomandibular joint pain and associated magnetic resonance findings: a retrospective study with a control group. Acta Radiol Open. 2020;9(9):2058460120938738.

Cone Beam Computed Tomography for Temporomandibular Joint Disorders and Diseases

8

Ghabi A. Kaspo and Christos Angelopoulos

8.1 Introduction

Cone beam computed tomography (CBCT) has emerged as a valuable imaging tool for temporomandibular joint (TMJ) disorders, offering high-resolution, three-dimensional visualization of bony structures without superimposition [1, 2]. CBCT provides superior diagnostic accuracy compared to conventional radiography, with lower radiation exposure than multislice CT [1, 2]. It is particularly effective in detecting osseous abnormalities, including osteoarthritis, fractures, and developmental anomalies [3]. While CBCT excels in bone imaging, it has limitations in soft tissue evaluation, where MRI remains the gold standard [4]. The advantages of CBCT include cost-effectiveness, widespread availability, and improved treatment planning capabilities [5]. Despite its benefits, further research is needed to assess the impact of CBCT on patient outcomes in TMJ disorders [3].

G. A. Kaspo
Henry Ford Health Systrem, Henry Ford Hospital, Department of Otolaryngology, Royal Oak, Michigan, USA

Wayne State University, Department of Psychiatry, Detroit, Michigan, USA

C. Angelopoulos (✉)
Oral Diagnosis and Radiology, National & Kapodistrian University, Athens, Greece

8.2 Degenerative Joint Disease

Osteoarthritis is one of the most common pain-evoking and disabling diseases. Globally, it affects more than 250 million people [6]. When the TMJ is involved, degenerative joint disease (DJD), or osteoarthritis, comprises the gradual breakdown of the articular surfaces in the articulation. DJDs are the most commonly seen subtype of temporomandibular disorders (TMDs), often times leading to significant pain and dysfunction. The development of TMJ osteoarthritis (TMJOA) is characterized by progressive cartilage degradation, subchondral bone remodeling, and chronic synovial tissue inflammation. However, the precise pathogenesis and progression of TMJOA are not yet fully understood. Recent studies have increasingly focused on inflammation and subchondral bone remodeling during the early stages of TMJOA, aiming to clarify its initiation and progression mechanisms [7].

Clinical and pathological manifestations of TMJOA encompass structural and functional joint failure, including disc displacement, degeneration, subchondral bone erosions, osteophyte formation, loss of articular fibrocartilage, and synovitis. Changes in bone morphology and associated mechanical properties can alter joint mechanics, contributing to joint degeneration.

Degenerative arthritic changes in the TMJ can range from mild irregularities in the cortical

G. A. Kaspo, G. D. Klasser (eds.), *Orofacial and Head Pain*,
https://doi.org/10.1007/978-3-032-08275-6_8

surface of the condylar head to severe degenerative changes, which may include subchondral cysts and osteophytes. The occurrence of degenerative changes in the condyle alone is more common than that of degenerative changes in both the eminence and the condyle. Changes in the eminence alone are less frequently reported than the previously mentioned incidents.

Clinical signs of degenerative arthritic changes in the jaw joints include pain upon palpation of the TMJ area. The pain is aggravated by chewing, eating, and yawning. The severity of the pain can range from mild to moderate, dull, achy pain and is often associated with crepitus sounds. Most patients who visit orofacial pain clinics complain of pain and sounds. Limited mouth opening and stiffness in the jaw joints, particularly in the morning, are commonly reported. The mandibular range of motion may be limited, with jaw opening and some mild deflection to the ipsilateral side may be observed. Lateral movements will be equal bilaterally, with occasional limited movement. The patient complains of pain, which is usually reported when chewing on the contralateral side. However, the pain is less severe or may not exist when chewing on the same side.

The advent of CBCT has revolutionized the hard tissue assessment of the TMJ by providing thin sections of the anatomical areas of interest (the mandibular condyles, fossae, and eminences). Although sectional imaging was available long before the introduction of CBCT with computed tomography (CT), this was used infrequently due to inherent limitations of CT (such as slice thickness), lack of TMJ-specific image reconstructions, and increased radiation to the patient. Prior to CT and CBCT, clinicians used to rely on panoramic radiography as well as other conventional radiologic examinations for the evaluation of the TMJ. Panoramic radiographs are a form of tomographic imaging that seem to be acceptable for an initial assessment (screening) of the TMJs. Conventional TMJ imaging including variable projectional types of X-rays (postero-anterior view, reverse Towne's view, submentovertex view) and others aimed to provide visualization of the complex TMJ anatomy from different perspectives. However, the anatomic superimposition of different anatomical structures in the TMJ neighborhood was the biggest disadvantage of these diagnostic approaches.

Soon after its introduction, CBCT was established as the imaging modality of choice for the evaluation of the hard tissues of the TMJs and has become a very important tool in orofacial pain practices [1, 8–10] (Figs. 8.1, 8.2, 8.3, 8.4, 8.5, 8.6, and 8.7).

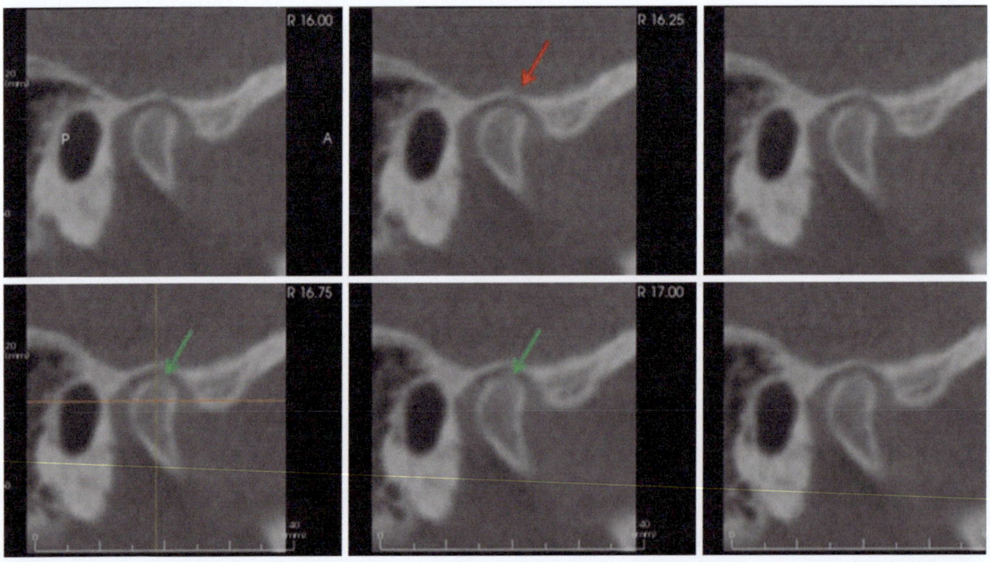

Fig. 8.1 A series of sagittal sections of the (R) TMJ showing minor condylar shape and fossa alterations by means of slight interruptions in the continuity of the cortical outlines. Small erosion in the roof of the glenoid fossa (red arrow). Small osseous projection and erosion in the condyle (green arrow)

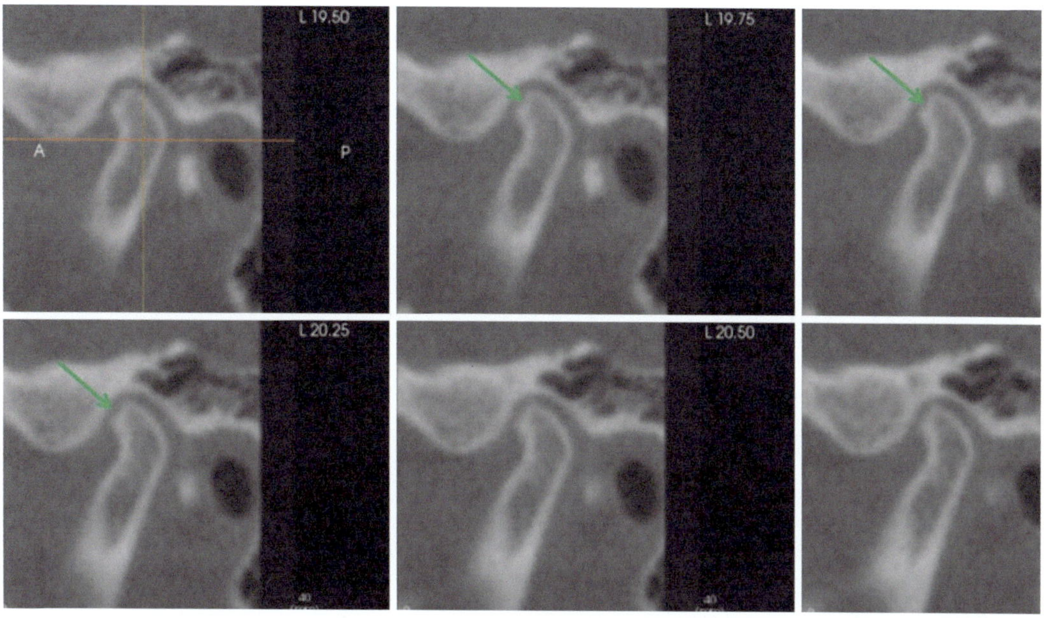

Fig. 8.2 A series of sagittal sections of the (L) TMJ showing slight irregularities in the anterior/superior aspect of the left condylar head (green arrows) in a symptomatic patient. Commonly, such minor osseous changes pose a diagnostic dilemma because of the "noise" inherently present in CBCT images. Noise may imitate the presence of osseous changes in anatomical areas that are not actually present and may lead to erroneous diagnoses, especially for the inexperienced diagnostician

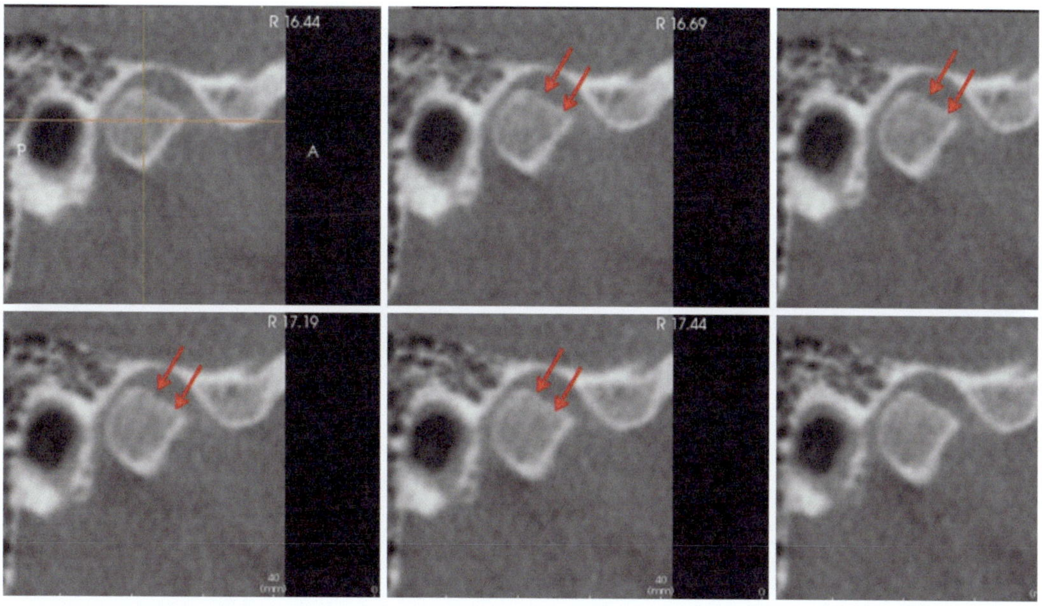

Fig. 8.3 A series of sagittal sections of the (R) TMJ showing flattening in the anterior/superior aspect of the right condylar head. Flattening of the articulating surfaces is often the first sign of osseous changes in the development of degenerative joint disease (osteoarthritis)

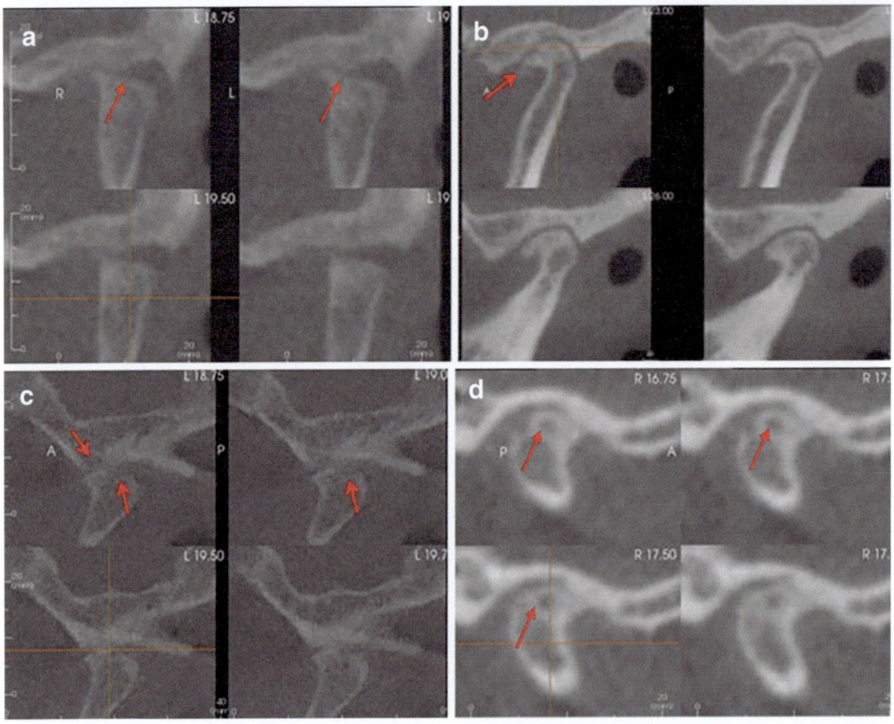

Fig. 8.4 The five most prominent manifestations (morphological changes) of degenerative joint disease (DJD) in four different case series (patients): (**a**) *Flattening* of the superior aspect of the condyle along with localized *sclerosis*. Note the coexistence of severe erosive changes and glenoid fossa shape alteration. (**b**) *Osteophyte formation* and localized *sclerosis* on the condyle along flattening and sclerosis on the anterior slope of the fossa. Also, note the small loose body (fragmented osteophyte) (arrow). (**c**) *Erosive lesions* in the superior aspect of the condyle and the articular eminence (arrows) along with flattening and sclerosis of the fossa. (**d**) *Subchondral cyst* formation along with an osteophyte and localized sclerosis in the condylar head and fossa sclerosis

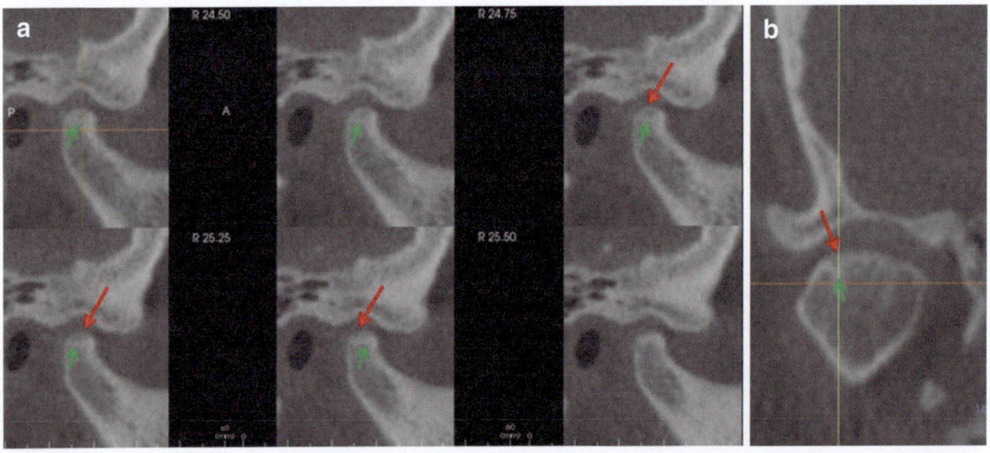

Fig. 8.5 A series of sagittal sections of the (R) TMJ (**a**) and a coronal section (**b**), showing an erosive lesion in the superior aspect of the right condyle (red arrows). This is surrounded by a thick sclerotic border (green arrows). This is often reactive sclerosis and indicates a reaction to chronic stimuli (the erosion in this case). The gravity of the various osseous findings as recognized in the diagnostic examinations (CBCT scans in this case) determines the degree of the degenerative joint disease: mild, moderate, or advanced/severe degenerative changes (mild to moderate in this case). Admittedly, this is a rather subjective classification heavily based on the diagnostician

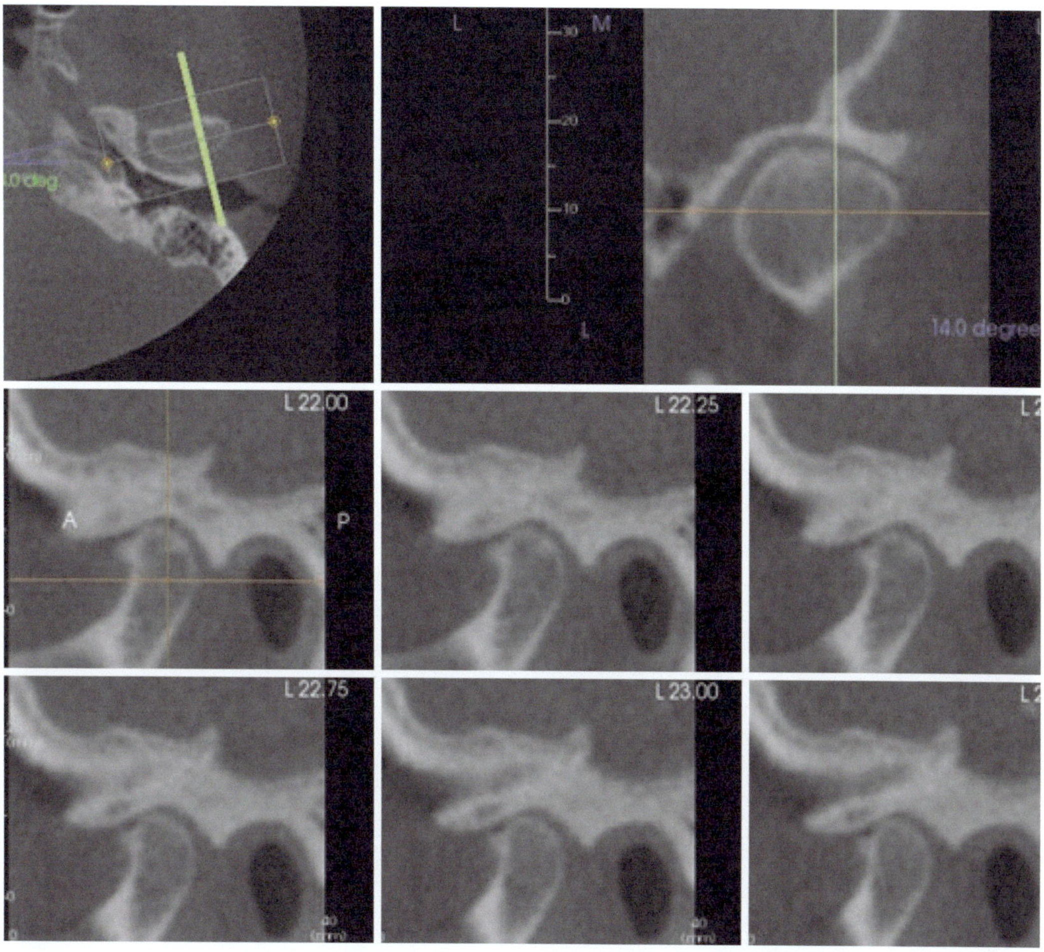

Fig. 8.6 A coronal section (above right) and a series of sagittal sections of the (L) TMJ in a symptomatic patient showing the following imaging findings: a small osteophyte in the anterior aspect of the condyle, a small erosive lesion (arrow), and marked narrowing of the left joint space. The above findings constitute mild degenerative changes in the (L) TMJ

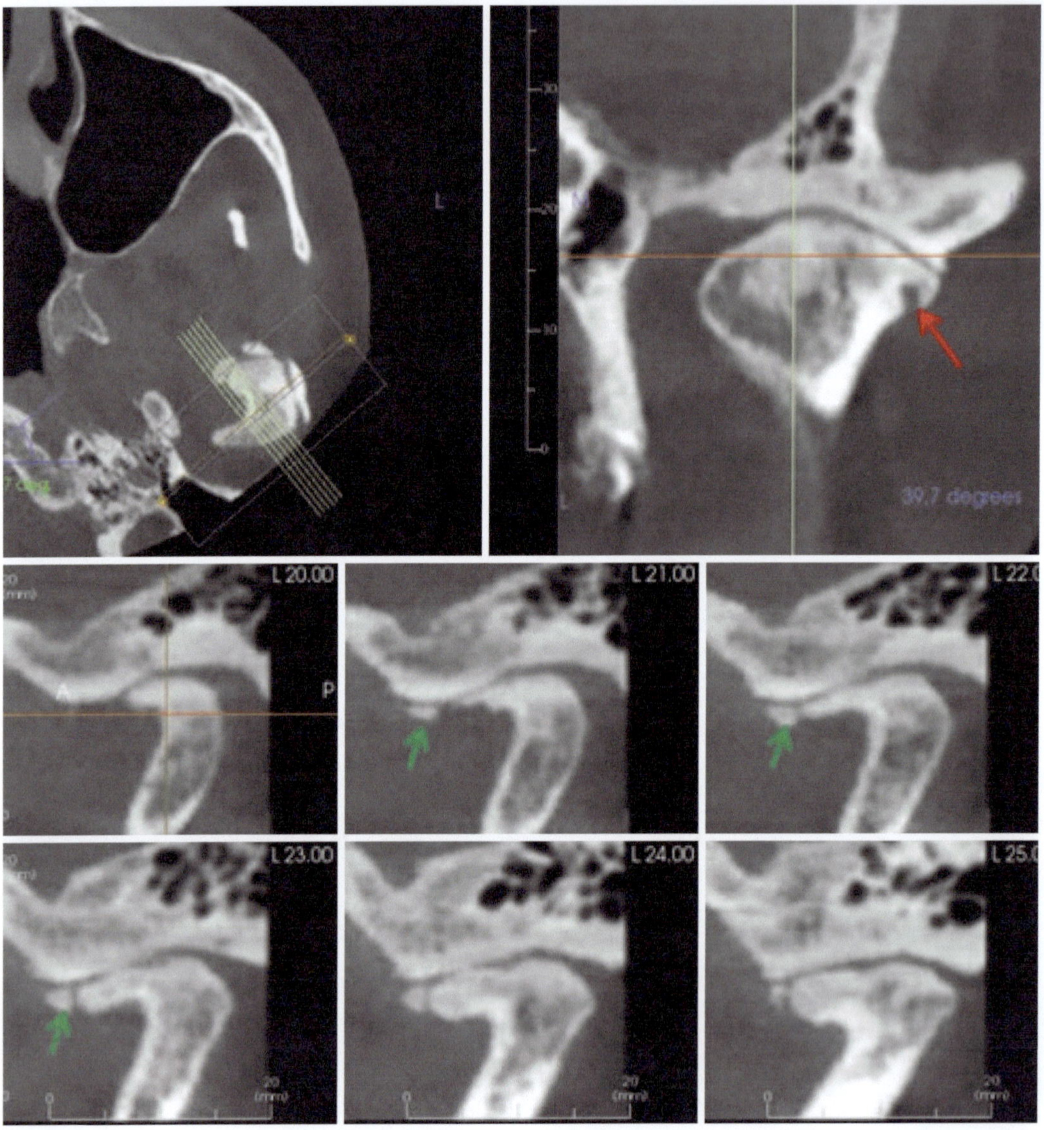

Fig. 8.7 Axial section (above left), coronal section (above right), and a series of sagittal sections of the (L) TMJ in a symptomatic patient showing the following imaging findings: a large osteophyte in the anterior aspect of the condyle, diffuse sclerosis in the condylar head, erosive lesions in its superior aspect, a subchondral cyst towards the lateral pole of the condyle (red arrow), a loose body (fractured osteophyte, green arrow) just inferior to the articular eminence, extensive flattening and sclerosis in the fossa, and lastly, total loss of the left joint space; in fact, the two articulating surfaces are in contact with one another. The above radiologic findings constitute severe degenerative changes in the (L) TMJ

8.3 Juvenile Idiopathic Arthritis

Juvenile idiopathic arthritis (JIA), formerly known as juvenile rheumatoid arthritis or juvenile chronic arthritis, represents the most prevalent pediatric rheumatological disorder. It encompasses various forms of pediatric inflammatory arthritis with unknown etiology, presenting diverse clinical and imaging manifestations. JIA is classified into oligoarticular, polyarticular (both rheumatoid factor negative and positive), psoriatic arthritis, enthesitis-related arthritis, and systemic JIA. Understanding the distinct clinical features, pathogenic mechanisms, and prognostic implications of each subtype enables a more sophisticated, imaging-based approach to diagnosis [11].

JIA is a broad term describing a clinically heterogeneous group of arthritides of unknown cause, the onset of which is prior to16 years of age, with arthritis persisting for over 6 weeks being diagnostic criteria for JIA [12, 13]. The estimated prevalence of TMJ involvement in children and adolescents with JIA varies widely, ranging from 17% to 92%, with many cases being clinically asymptomatic [14]. Pain in the temporomandibular region is relatively common, affecting about 10% of individuals over 18 years old. It predominantly affects young and middle-aged adults rather than children or the elderly and is approximately twice as prevalent in women compared to men [15]. Although few differences were observed between children with and without radiographic TMJ deformities, self-reported previous TMJ symptoms and reduced maximum unassisted opening with pain could indicate TMJ involvement. However, radiographic examinations are necessary to confirm TMJ involvement, suggesting limitations in various classification systems for targeting TMJ involvement in JIA [16].

The diagnostic criteria for TMD, which is the DC/TMD, comprise physical axis I (clinical condition) and psychosocial axis II (psychosocial distress) in its assessment. The clinical examination aligns well with consensus-based recommendations for orofacial examination in JIA, except for craniofacial deformations [17].

JIA is a diagnosis of exclusion that, when suspected, requires a complete clinical evaluation, including family to personal history and recent pathologic events, and specific attention to pain and morning stiffness. A detailed physical examination should always be performed to examine all body joints at both first evaluation and follow-up visits [33]. At the conclusion of the visit, the physician is asked to provide his/her global rating of the overall level of disease activity on a visual analog scale (VAS), ranging from 0 (no activity) to 10 (maximum activity) [33, 34]. The identification of systemic JIA may be challenging as arthritis is often not present at onset.

The radiologic examination is an essential tool for the diagnosis and management of JIA, as with TMJ disorders. The goals of TMJ imaging are to evaluate cortical integrity and trabecular architecture of the bony structures, to assess the extent of the osseous involvement, to monitor the progression of osseous changes over time, and to evaluate the response to treatment. Although conventional radiologic examinations are limited for a complete and accurate evaluation due to the anatomical complexity of the articulation and the structure superimposition observed in projectional images, they may be of some value for an initial assessment for the detection of asymmetry and gross pathology.

8.4 Rheumatoid Arthritis in Adults

Rheumatoid arthritis (RA) patients have a higher prevalence of TMD compared to healthy individuals [18–21]. TMJ involvement in RA is characterized by degenerative bone changes, including condylar resorption, joint space narrowing, and erosions [22–24]. These changes can be detected through imaging techniques such as CBCT and MRI, even in asymptomatic patients [22, 25]. Clinical symptoms of TMD in RA patients include joint pain, crepitus, and limited mandibular movement [18]. Interestingly, seronegative RA patients may have a higher prevalence of TMD pain compared to seropositive patients [21]. The duration of RA does not necessarily correlate with the severity of TMJ involvement [18, 20]. Early diagnosis and treatment are crucial to prevent structural and functional damage to the TMJ in RA patients [22] (Figs. 8.8 and 8.9).

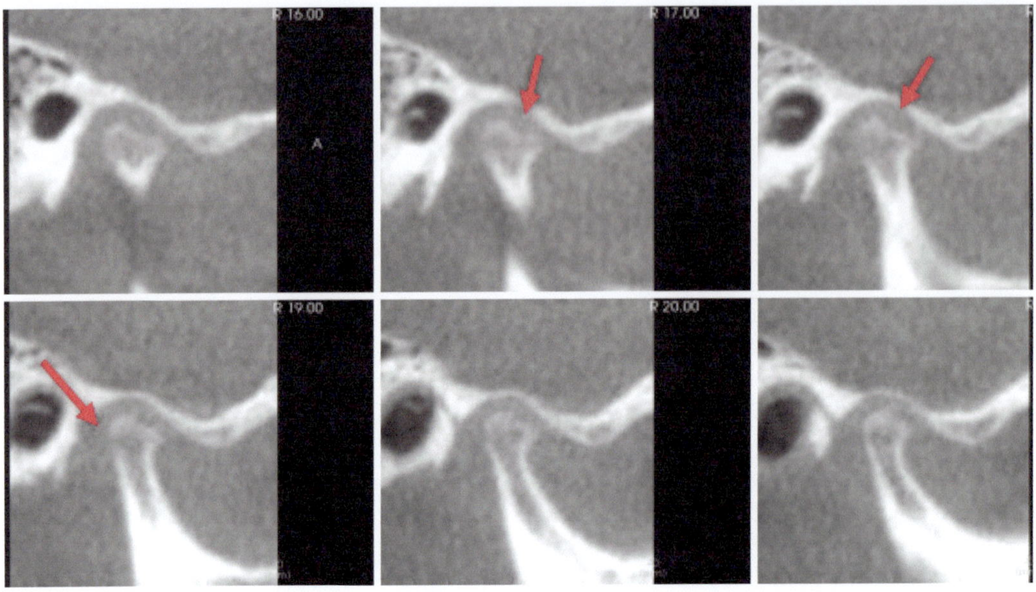

Fig. 8.8 A series of sagittal sections of the (R) TMJ towards the midcondyle (above) and towards the lateral pole (below) of 10-year-old female patient who had a confirmed diagnosis of juvenile idiopathic osteoarthritis affecting several joints. When the patient reported pain in the TMJ, a CBCT scan was ordered; the CBCT images depict early erosive changes (red arrows) in the anterior/superior aspect of the left condyle. Admittedly, in the absence of symptoms, the above findings are generally mild and could have been regarded as possible noise in the scan

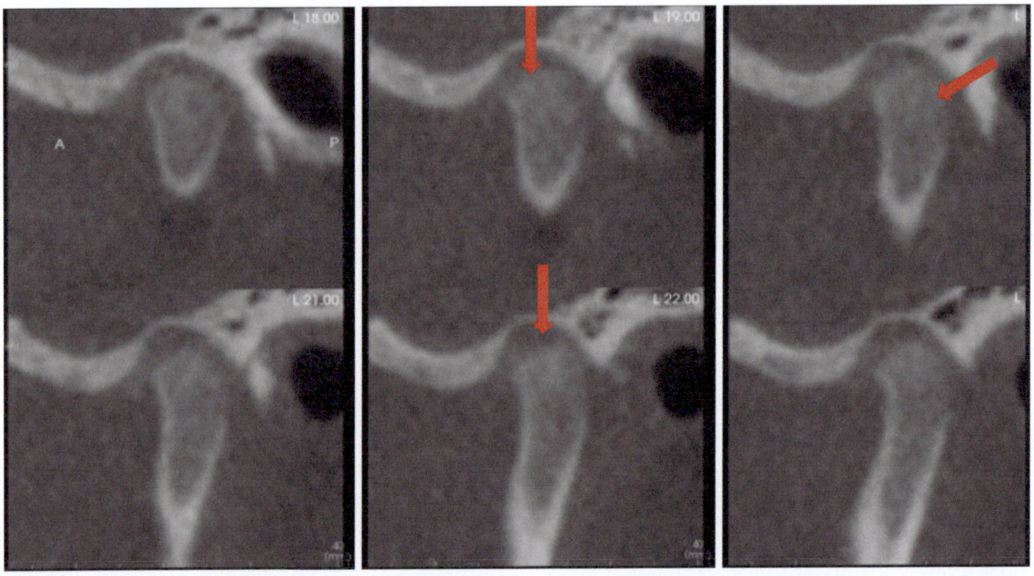

Fig. 8.9 A series of sagittal sections of the (L) TMJ of a symptomatic patient (a child) depicting erosive changes (red arrows) in the superior aspect of the left condyle causing shape alterations in the condylar head. The patient was diagnosed with JIA and the above findings regarded as involvement of the TMJs

8.5 Synovial Chondromatosis of the Temporomandibular Joint

Synovial chondromatosis (primary) is a rare, benign condition that typically affects large joints, with its occurrence in the TMJ being uncommon and more prevalent in females [16]. It is characterized by the abnormal proliferation of the synovial membrane, leading to the formation of loose cartilaginous bodies within the joint space. These nodules can vary in size and location around the condyle, both within and outside the synovial tissue. Their presence may exert pressure, potentially causing erosion of the glenoid fossa and, in severe cases, intracranial extension.

Occasionally, the degeneration of the articulating surfaces is followed by the development of multiple variable-sized loose cartilaginous or osseous bodies which are scattered within and around the articulating surfaces. This condition is known as secondary synovial chondromatosis.

In orofacial pain clinics where cone beam CT scans are utilized, the prevalence of synovial chondromatosis may be higher than previously recognized [17]. Radiographic changes indicative of synovial chondromatosis are observed in only 45% of affected patients. The increased use of CBCT scans has significantly enhanced the detection and awareness of synovial chondromatosis in the TMJ [18].

The diagnosis of synovial chondromatosis is confirmed through histopathological investigation. Grossly, hyperplastic synovium covers white multilobulated nodular projections of hyaline cartilage. Histopathological examination reveals globular masses of cartilage tissue with areas of calcification. Chondrocytes within lacunae show mild atypia, and the synovial connective tissue between the cartilages appears delicate and fibrillar. The peripheries of the globular masses exhibit cellular areas with numerous blood vessels [16] (Figs. 8.10, 8.11, and 8.12).

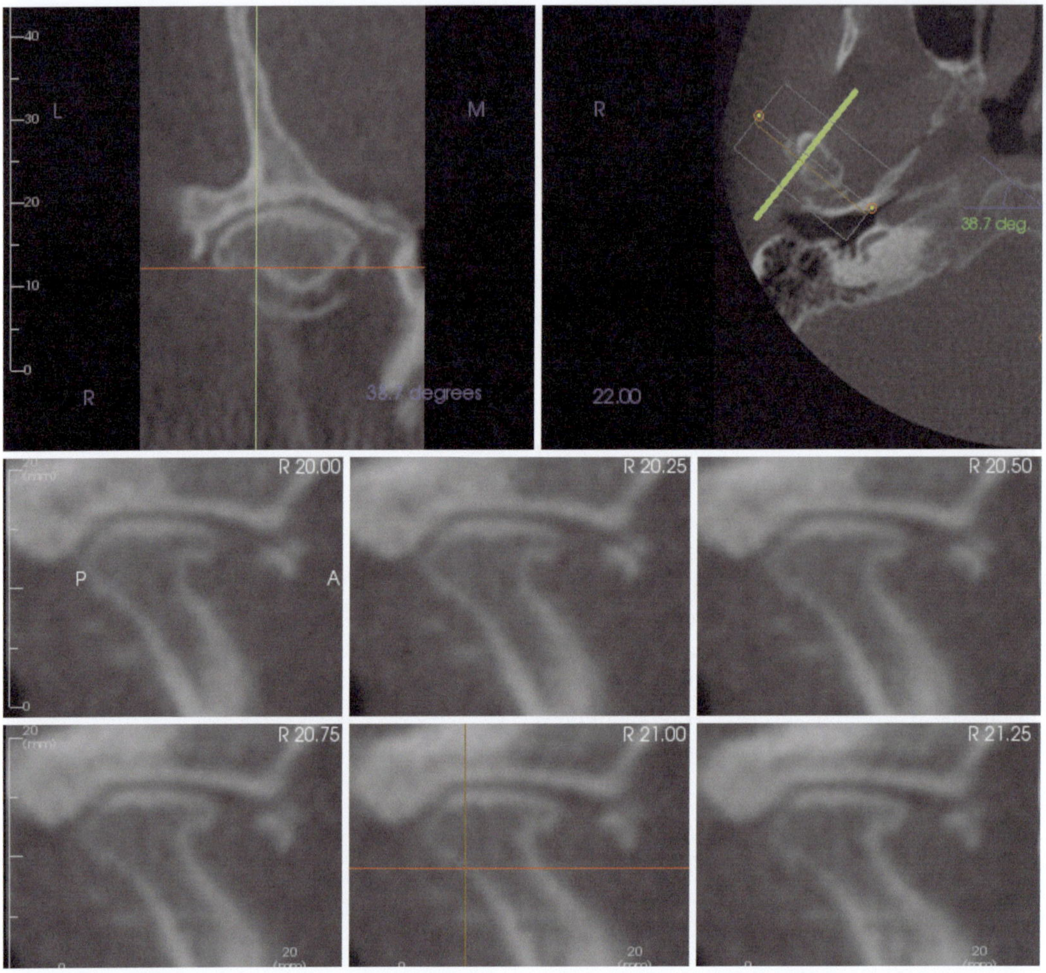

Fig. 8.10 A coronal section (above left) and a series of sagittal sections of the (R) TMJ in a symptomatic patient in which apart from the obvious radiologic findings of DJD (flattening of the condyle and the fossa, subchondral sclerosis, and narrowing of the joint space), several osseous-density loose fragments of varying size are recognized scattered around the condyle, most likely inside and outside of the joint capsule. This appearance is consistent with secondary synovial chondromatosis of the right TMJ

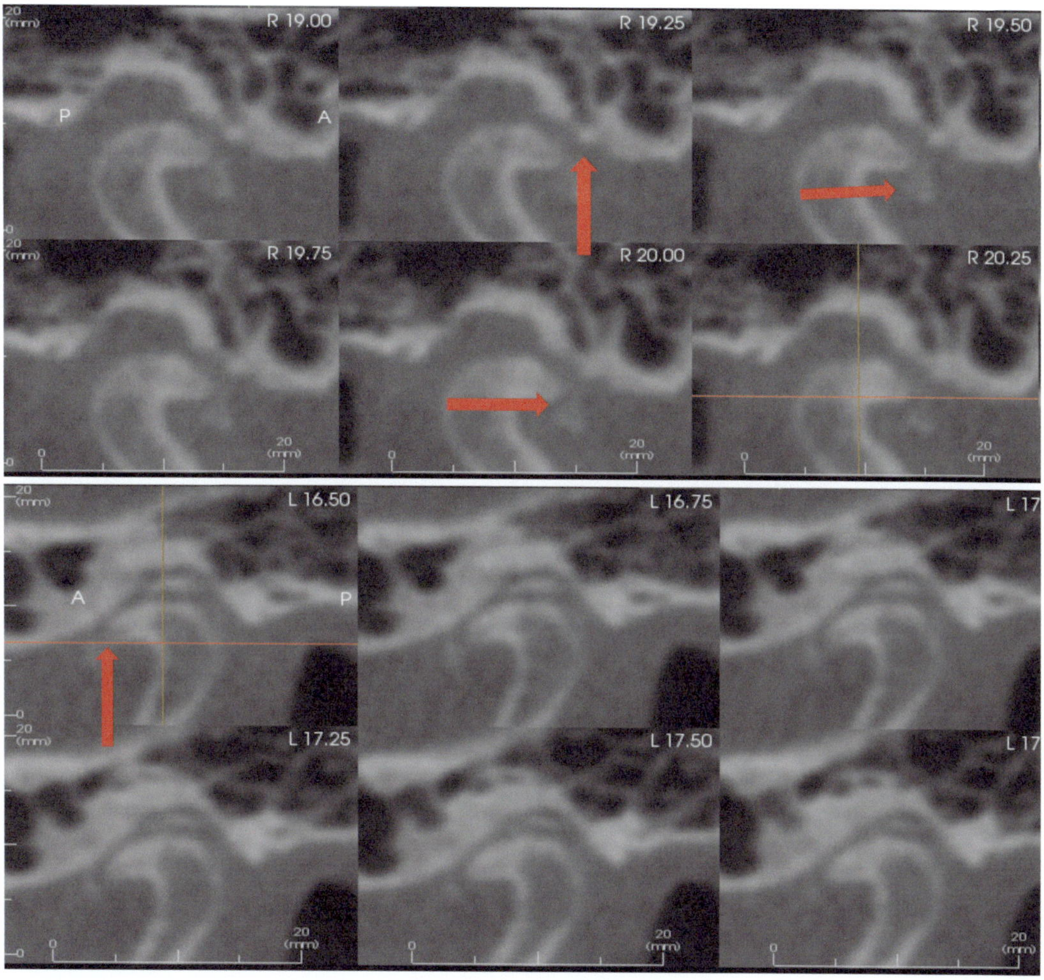

Fig. 8.11 A series of sagittal sections of the (R) TMJ (above) and the left TMJ (below) of an older symptomatic patient. The radiologic findings on both sides include multiple calcifications or loose osseous fragments of varying shapes and sizes within the joint spaces. This appearance is strongly suggestive of secondary synovial chondromatosis. Bilateral DJD is evident, with osteophyte formation bilaterally, localized sclerosis, and erosive changes in the right articular eminence (red arrows)

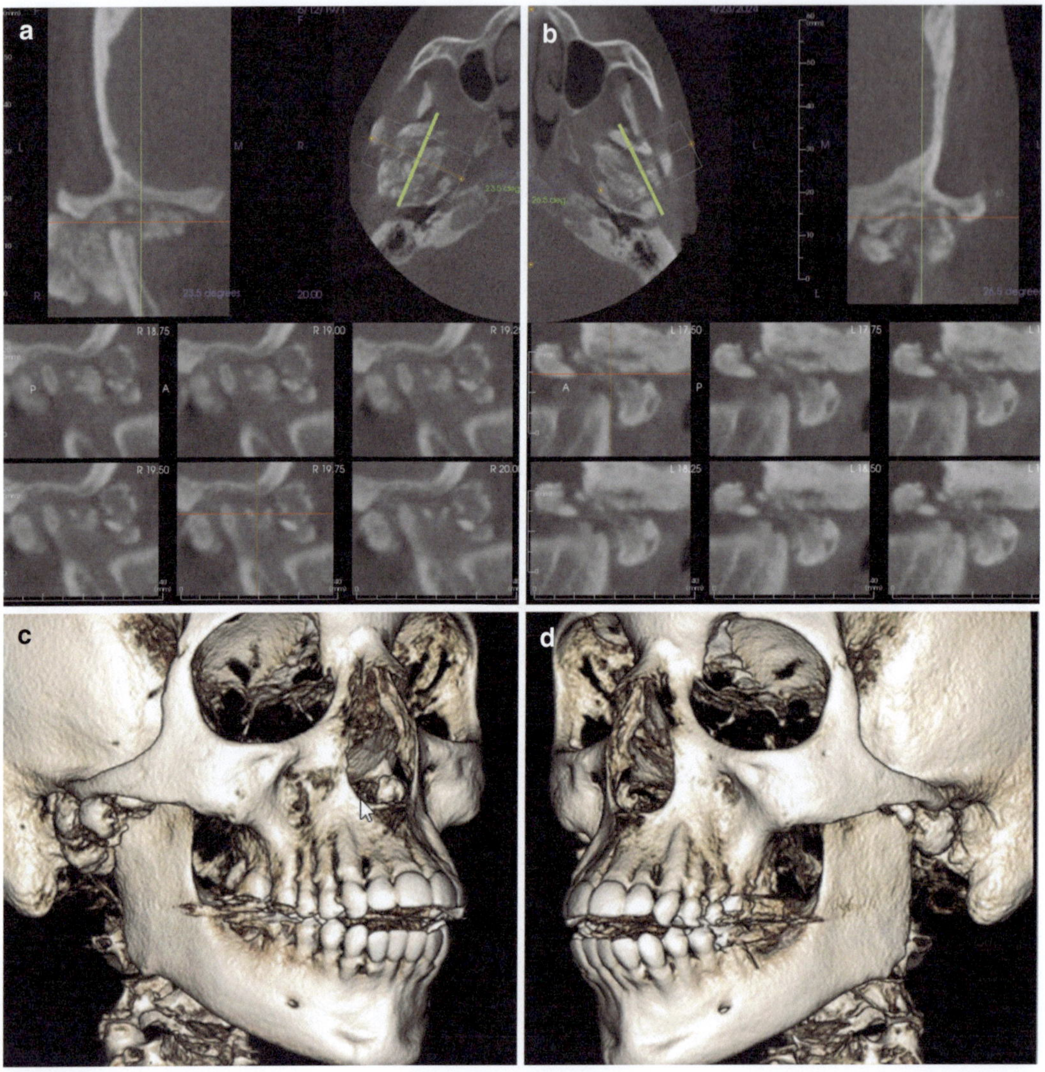

Fig. 8.12 Coronal and sagittal sections of the (R) TMJ (**a**) and similar sections of the left TMJ (**b**), along with 3D renderings of the right TMJ (**c**) and left TMJ (**d**) in a symptomatic patient. Massive, cotton-like in appearance and irregular in shape, synovial calcifications are present around the TMJs and in the peri-auricular region bilaterally. The condyles have undergone severe resorption, which has resulted in the observed anterior "open-bite." This appearance is consistent with calcium pyrophosphate dihydrate (CPPD), a metabolic condition in which calcium pyrophosphate crystals are deposited into the TM joint space

8.6 Metastatic Disease Involving the Temporomandibular Joint

Metastatic disease to the TMJ is a rather uncommon condition. High-resolution diagnostic imaging is important in order to identify infiltrative, "ill-defined" pathological entities which cause destruction of the osseous structures and do not respond to standard TMD therapeutic approaches. In such cases, periodic radiologic examinations, primarily with CBCT, are critical in order to determine possible progression (most often rapid and nonresponsive to treatment).

Two important considerations regarding TMJ metastases must be emphasized. First, their radiologic appearance can be misinterpreted as a benign entity or benign neoplastic disease (e.g., odontogenic cyst, aneurysmal cyst, simple bone cyst, hemangioma, and Langerhans cell histiocytosis). This can delay prompt diagnosis and further treatment, even though TMJ metastases usually indicate widespread disease, and treatment is often palliative. Second, they can represent the first manifestation of an undiagnosed tumor, and for this reason, a biopsy is mandatory to obtain a correct diagnosis.

The course of TMJ metastases, in general, is similar to other metastases involving the TMJ. Breast cancer as the primary tumor is most frequent, followed by lung cancer [26, 27]. Metastatic breast cancer to the condyle is rare but can masquerade as TMJ pathology. Metastatic cancer to the condyle can also masquerade as other pathologies, and it is important to be aware of the pathophysiology to ensure correct diagnosis [28]. In addition, metastatic lung cancer is rare, and the signs and symptoms associated with the presence of maxillary metastases are nonspecific. These two characteristics make the eventual diagnosis of mandibular metastases, especially condylar, difficult, leading to misdiagnosis. Therefore, a multidisciplinary approach is fundamental when faced with such conditions [27].

There are no specific clinical or radiological parameters leading to diagnosis. However, when a patient presents with TMJ-related symptoms and unusual radiological findings, especially in the context of a medical history involving malignant neoplastic disease, the possibility of metastasis should be considered. A definitive diagnosis requires biopsy and histological examination [29] (Figs. 8.13 and 8.14).

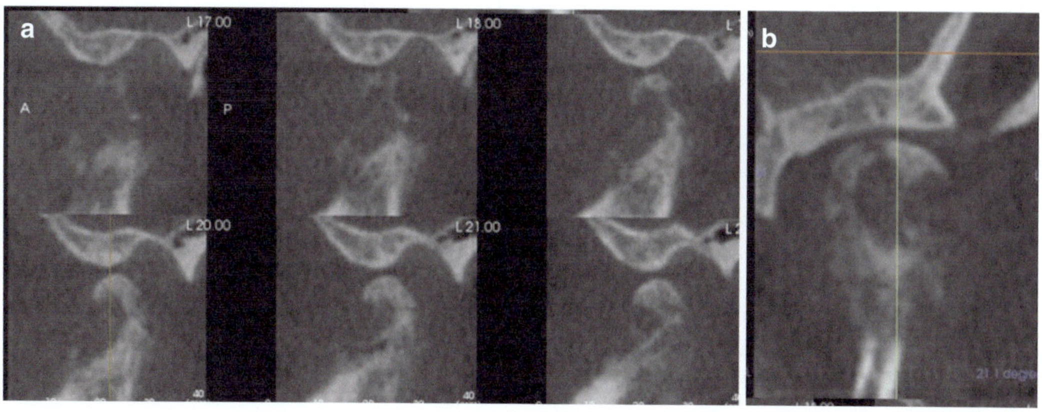

Fig. 8.13 (**a**) A series of sagittal sections (**a**) and a coronal section (**b**) of the (L) TMJ. Note the almost "explosive" or blooming appearance of the condylar head. The lack of boundary identification and the multiple "ill-defined" low-density areas indicate infiltration and extensive destruction of the osseous structures of the condylar head and neck. This deterioration of the condyloid process is strongly suspicious of an ongoing malignant entity present. The biopsy of the site confirmed a metastatic lesion from the breast, as a primary site

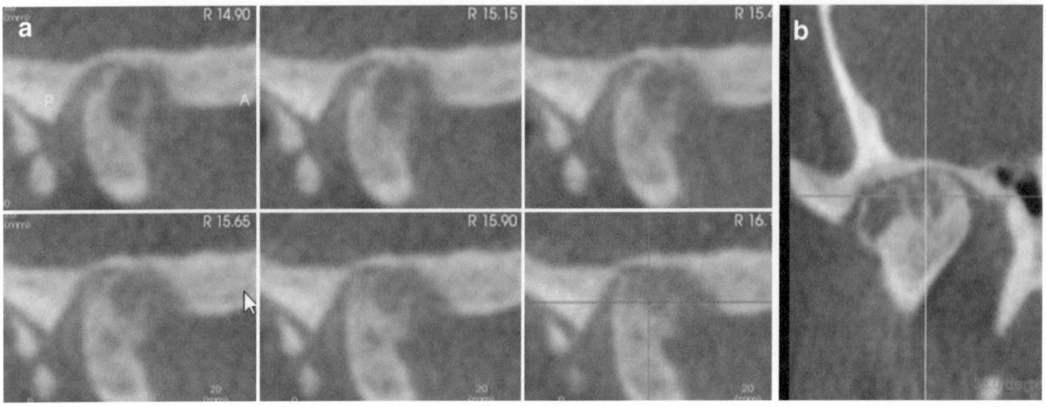

Fig. 8.14 (**a**) A series of consecutive sagittal sections (**a**) and a coronal section (**b**) of the (R) TMJ. The right condyle has suffered a rather irregular, "ill-defined" area of osteolysis (erosion) which has deteriorated its integrity and claimed the frontal half of the condylar head (at least). The overall appearance of the condyle is sclerotic as is the glenoid fossa. Furthermore, a deep erosive lesion is present in the anterior slope of the fossa. The appearance of the condyle is suspicious of an aggressive pathological entity like a malignant or a metastatic lesion

8.7 Neoplastic and Non-neoplastic Entities Affecting the Temporomandibular Joint

Tumors and pseudotumor lesions of the TMJ, though uncommon, often present symptoms similar to TMJ disorders, leading to frequent misdiagnosis and delays in treatment. Pseudotumors such as synovial chondromatosis, pigmented villonodular synovitis, eosinophilic granuloma, and osteochondroma are among the most frequently encountered [30, 31]. On average, diagnosis is delayed by 30 months, particularly in female patients, with nearly 20% of cases initially mistaken for TMJ dysfunction. Patients typically report pain, swelling, and restricted jaw movement [32]. Imaging findings vary, with benign tumors often appearing radiopaque and malignant tumors radiolucent, yet a significant percentage of cases (14.6% benign, 7.7% malignant) show no abnormalities on panoramic radiographs [31].

Imaging plays a critical role in the evaluation of TMJ tumors, aiding in diagnosis, lesion characterization, and treatment planning. Panoramic radiographs, while commonly used, may miss smaller or less calcified lesions [31]. Computed tomography (CT), particularly with contrast enhancement, is valuable for detecting bony destruction, cortical expansion, and mineralized components. Magnetic resonance imaging (MRI) is preferred for assessing soft tissue involvement, joint effusion, and marrow infiltration, though it does not always differentiate benign from malignant masses. Positron emission tomography (PET-CT) can be useful for detecting metastatic disease [33]. Histopathological evaluation remains essential for definitive diagnosis, particularly to distinguish between pseudotumors, benign tumors, and malignancies (Fig. 8.15).

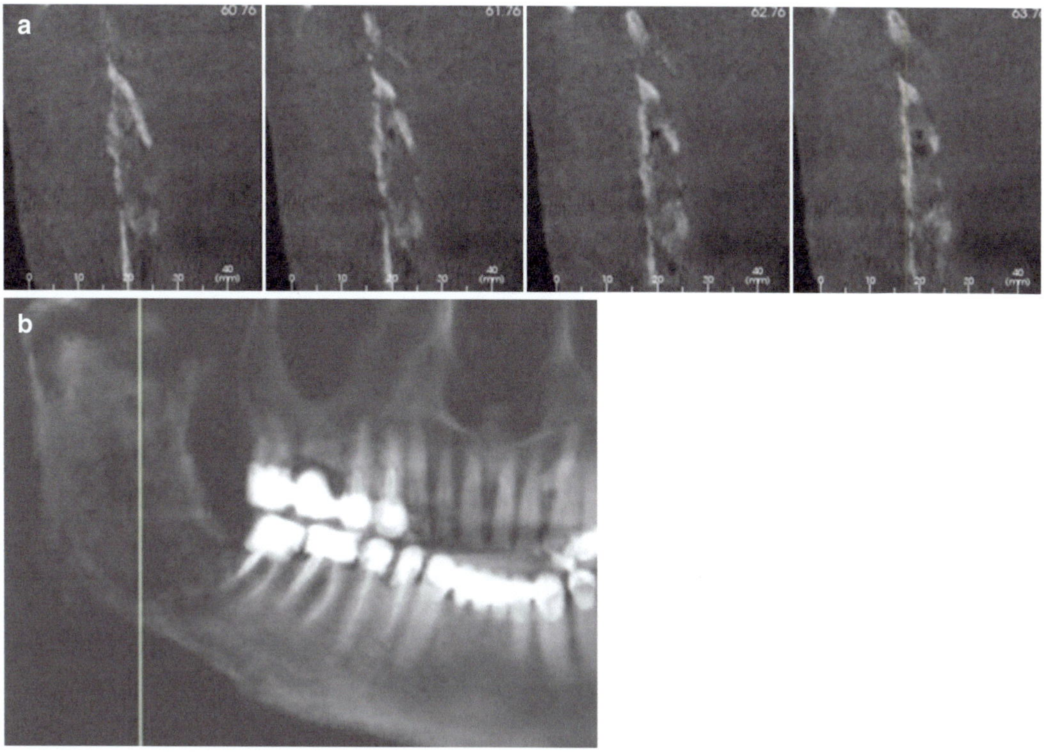

Fig. 8.15 (**a**) A series of consecutive sagittal sections (**a**) and a panoramic reconstruction (**b**) of the (R) ascending mandibular ramus. The ramus appears to be infiltrated by an osteolytic, extensive, "moth-eaten" in appearance lesion, which has deteriorated the osseous structure and compromised its cortical integrity. Moreover, it has caused pathologic fractures of the coronoid and condylar processes. These findings indicate a rather aggressive ongoing pathological entity: malignancies, osteomyelitis, radionecrosis, and MRONJ should be included in the differential diagnosis. This lesion was proven to be osteomyelitis. The similarities of the above entities to metastatic disease make them difficult to exclude from the differential diagnosis if an aggressive, infiltrating, ill-defined osteolytic lesion is presented in the TMJ region

8.8 TMJ Aneurysmal Bone Cyst

Aneurysmal bone cysts (ABCs) are rare benign lesions of bone tissue, infrequent in the craniofacial skeleton compared to other structures like long bones or the spine. They are composed of sinusoidal and vascular spaces that are blood-filled and surrounded by fibrous tissue septa. Despite their rare occurrence, ABCs have been reported in the condyle.

Aneurysmal bone cysts consist of non-neoplastic benign bony lesions which are considered pseudocysts because of the lack of an epithelial lining [34]. They are principally located in long bone metaphyses like the femur and the tibia (more than 50% of aneurysmal bone cysts) and the spine (12–30%) [35]. Although the presence of these tumors in facial bones is infrequent, they account for 2–12% of all aneurysmal bone cysts in the body [35–37]. In the case of craniofacial location, the mandible is more frequently affected than the maxilla, with a proportion from 2:1 to 11:9 [37–39]. The body and the mandibular ramus are the main locations with rare case reports in the coronoid process and the condyle [38, 40]. The age of presentation of aneurysmal bone cysts in the first two decades of life is infrequent [34, 35, 41]. There is a slight sex preponderance in females [35, 41].

Aneurysmal bone cysts often show a multilocular appearance in radiographs and should be differentiated from other multilocular entities like ameloblastoma, ossifying fibroma, and giant cell granuloma.

8.9 Conclusion

CBCT has emerged as a valuable imaging modality for TMJ disorders, offering high-resolution, three-dimensional visualization of osseous structures without superimposition of neighboring anatomical structures [1, 3]. CBCT excels in detecting early degenerative changes, including cortical bone integrity, joint space alterations, and osteophyte formation. Concordantly, it provides highly detailed evaluations of advanced degenerative changes [1, 24]. CBCT provides superior bone detail with lower radiation exposure compared to conventional CT, making it the preferred method for TMJ hard tissue assessment [8]. It is particularly useful in assessing osteoarthritis, rheumatoid arthritis, and other inflammatory conditions [2]. However, CBCT has limitations in soft tissue imaging, where MRI remains the imaging modality of choice. Despite this, CBCT's ability to provide accurate TMJ imaging has made it an essential tool for diagnosis, treatment planning, and monitoring of various TMJ pathologies [1].

References

1. Barghan S, Tetradis S, Mallya S. Application of cone beam computed tomography for assessment of the temporomandibular joints. Aust Dent J. 2012;57(Suppl 1):109–18.
2. Dhabale GS, Bhowate RR. Cone-beam computed tomography for temporomandibular joint imaging. Cureus. 2022;14(11):e31515.
3. Larheim TA, Abrahamsson AK, Kristensen M, Arvidsson LZ. Temporomandibular joint diagnostics using CBCT. Dentomaxillofac Radiol. 2015;44(1):20140235.
4. Talmaceanu D, Lenghel LM, Bolog N, Hedesiu M, Buduru S, Rotar H, et al. Imaging modalities for temporomandibular joint disorders: an update. Clujul Med. 2018;91(3):280–7.
5. Barghan S, Merrill R, Tetradis S. Cone beam computed tomography imaging in the evaluation of the temporomandibular joint. J Calif Dent Assoc. 2010;38(1):33–9.
6. Hunter DJ, Bierma-Zeinstra S. Osteoarthritis. Lancet. 2019;393(10182):1745–59.
7. Tanaka E, Detamore MS, Mercuri LG. Degenerative disorders of the temporomandibular joint: etiology, diagnosis, and treatment. J Dent Res. 2008;87(4):296–307.
8. Mallya SM, Ahmad M, Cohen JR, Kaspo G, Ramesh A. Recommendations for imaging of the temporomandibular joint. Position statement from the American Academy of Oral and Maxillofacial Radiology and the American Academy of Orofacial Pain. J Oral Facial Pain Headache. 2023;37(1):7–15.
9. Tsiklakis K. Cone beam computed tomographic findings in temporomandibular joint disorders. Alpha Omegan. 2010;103(2):68–78.
10. Tsiklakis K, Syriopoulos K, Stamatakis HC. Radiographic examination of the temporomandibular joint using cone beam computed tomography. Dentomaxillofac Radiol. 2004;33(3):196–201.
11. Tsujioka Y, Nishimura G, Sugimoto H, Nozaki T, Kono T, Jinzaki M. Imaging findings of juvenile idiopathic arthritis and autoinflammatory diseases in children. Jpn J Radiol. 2023;41(11):1186–207.
12. Giancane G, Consolaro A, Lanni S, Davì S, Schiappapietra B, Ravelli A. Juvenile idiopathic arthritis: diagnosis and treatment. Rheumatol Ther. 2016;3(2):187–207.
13. Ramanan AV, Grom AA. Does systemic-onset juvenile idiopathic arthritis belong under juvenile idiopathic arthritis? Rheumatology (Oxford). 2005;44(11):1350–3.
14. Küseler A, Pedersen TK, Gelineck J, Herlin T. A 2 year followup study of enhanced magnetic resonance imaging and clinical examination of the temporomandibular joint in children with juvenile idiopathic arthritis. J Rheumatol. 2005;32(1):162–9.
15. LeResche L. Epidemiology of temporomandibular disorders: implications for the investigation of etiologic factors. Crit Rev Oral Biol Med. 1997;8(3):291–305.
16. Collin M, Hagelberg S, Ernberg M, Hedenberg-Magnusson B, Christidis N. Temporomandibular joint involvement in children with juvenile idiopathic arthritis-symptoms, clinical signs and radiographic findings. J Oral Rehabil. 2022;49(1):37–46.
17. Schiffman E, Ohrbach R, Truelove E, Look J, Anderson G, Goulet JP, et al. Diagnostic Criteria for Temporomandibular Disorders (DC/TMD) for clinical and research applications: recommendations of the International RDC/TMD Consortium Network* and Orofacial Pain Special Interest Group†. J Oral Facial Pain Headache. 2014;28(1):6–27.
18. Witulski S, Vogl TJ, Rehart S, Ottl P. Evaluation of the TMJ by means of clinical TMD examination and MRI diagnostics in patients with rheumatoid arthritis. Biomed Res Int. 2014;2014:328560.
19. Byun SH, Min C, Choi HG, Hong SJ. Increased risk of temporomandibular joint disorder in patients with rheumatoid arthritis: a longitudinal follow-up study. J Clin Med. 2020;9(9):3005.

20. Koh ET, Yap AU, Koh CK, Chee TS, Chan SP, Boudville IC. Temporomandibular disorders in rheumatoid arthritis. J Rheumatol. 1999;26(9):1918–22.
21. Naram Khalayli DH, Jawdat Ataya, Mayssoun Kudsi, Issam Alkhouri. Temporomandibular joint in patients with rheumatoid arthritis. Int J Surg Glob Health. 2024;7:1.
22. Cordeiro PC, Guimaraes JP, de Souza VA, Dias IM, Silva JN, Devito KL, et al. Temporomandibular joint involvement in rheumatoid arthritis patients: association between clinical and tomographic data. Acta Odontol Latinoam. 2016;29(3):123–9.
23. Ardic F, Gokharman D, Atsu S, Guner S, Yilmaz M, Yorgancioglu R. The comprehensive evaluation of temporomandibular disorders seen in rheumatoid arthritis. Aust Dent J. 2006;51(1):23–8.
24. Rehan OM, Saleh HAK, Raffat HA, Abu-Taleb NS. Osseous changes in the temporomandibular joint in rheumatoid arthritis: a cone-beam computed tomography study. Imaging Sci Dent. 2018;48(1):1–9.
25. Bayar N, Kara SA, Keles I, Koç MC, Altinok D, Orkun S. Temporomandibular joint involvement in rheumatoid arthritis: a radiological and clinical study. Cranio. 2002;20(2):105–10.
26. Gupta S, Jawanda MK, Ganganna A, Basavaraju S, Kashav N, Dhawan J, et al. Jaw bone metastasis from lung cancer as sole primary source: a systematic review. J Clin Exp Dent. 2022;14(7):e573–e93.
27. Ferragina F, Sottile AR, Cristofaro MG. Unusual presentation of pulmonary adenocarcinoma metastases in the mandibular condyle: a case report. Int J Surg Case Rep. 2023;113:109058.
28. Chang VKO, Thambar S. TMJ pain as a presentation of metastatic breast cancer to the right mandibular condyle. BMJ Case Rep. 2021;14(3):e241601.
29. López-Arcas Calleja JM, Cebrián Carretero JL, González Martín J, Burgueño M. Aneurysmal bone cyst of the mandible: case presentation and review of the literature. Med Oral Patol Oral Cir Bucal. 2007;12(5):E401–3.
30. Schlund M, Roland-Billecart T, Aubert S, Nicot R. Tumors affecting the temporomandibular joint - a literature review. Bull Cancer. 2020;107(11):1186–98.
31. Poveda-Roda R, Bagán JV, Sanchis JM, Margaix M. Pseudotumors and tumors of the temporomandibular joint. A review. Med Oral Patol Oral Cir Bucal. 2013;18(3):e392–402.
32. Mostafapour SP, Futran ND. Tumors and tumorous masses presenting as temporomandibular joint syndrome. Otolaryngol Head Neck Surg. 2000;123(4):459–64.
33. Yoshitake H, Kayamori K, Nakamura R, Wake S, Harada K. Pseudotumor in the temporomandibular joint: a case report. Int J Surg Case Rep. 2015;15:5–9.
34. Kiattavorncharoen S, Joos U, Brinkschmidt C, Werkmeister R. Aneurysmal bone cyst of the mandible: a case report. Int J Oral Maxillofac Surg. 2003;32(4):419–22.
35. Perrotti V, Rubini C, Fioroni M, Piattelli A. Solid aneurysmal bone cyst of the mandible. Int J Pediatr Otorhinolaryngol. 2004;68(10):1339–44.
36. Rapidis AD, Vallianatou D, Apostolidis C, Lagogiannis G. Large lytic lesion of the ascending ramus, the condyle, and the infratemporal region. J Oral Maxillofac Surg. 2004;62(8):996–1001.
37. Bataineh AB. Aneurysmal bone cysts of the maxilla: a clinicopathologic review. J Oral Maxillofac Surg. 1997;55(11):1212–6.
38. Martins WD, Fávaro DM. Aneurysmal bone cyst of the coronoid process of the mandible: a case report. J Contemp Dent Pract. 2005;6(2):130–8.
39. Matsuura S, Tahara T, Ro T, Masumi T, Kasuya H, Yokota T. Aneurysmal bone cyst of the coronoid process of the mandible. Dentomaxillofac Radiol. 1999;28(5):324–6.
40. Motamedi MH. Destructive aneurysmal bone cyst of the mandibular condyle: report of a case and review of the literature. J Oral Maxillofac Surg. 2002;60(11):1357–61.
41. Mankin HJ, Hornicek FJ, Ortiz-Cruz E, Villafuerte J, Gebhardt MC. Aneurysmal bone cyst: a review of 150 patients. J Clin Oncol. 2005;23(27):6756–62.

MRI for Temporomandibular Joint Disorders and Diseases

9

Ghabi A. Kaspo and Mel Mupparapu

9.1 Introduction

Magnetic resonance (MR) imaging is the most reliable method for evaluating the temporomandibular joint (TMJ) in terms of both health and disease. Temporomandibular disorders (TMDs) are a heterogeneous group of neuromuscular and musculoskeletal disorders involving the joint complex and muscular and bony components. The TMJ is formed by the condyle and the mandibular (glenoid) fossa of the temporal bone. The TMJ has both hinge and gliding motions. Muscles of mastication and ligaments control the movement of this joint. The TMJ disc, also known as meniscus, is fibrocartilage that divides the joint into two compartments, a superior and an inferior joint space. The anterior translation during mouth opening occurs in the superior joint space. Rotation of the condyle happens in the inferior joint space. To evaluate the joint and the disc accurately, the MR study should have sagittal or oblique sagittal spin and gradient echo T2-weighted images or proton density (PD) images for each of the joints independently in open and closed mouth positions. The biconcave disc typically has a low signal on all sequences and is located between the temporal bone and the superior aspect of the condyle. The posterior band of the disc is located at the 12 o'clock position in the glenoid fossa. Abnormal disc morphology is generally associated with disc displacement. The displaced disc does not maintain a normal relationship with the articular surfaces throughout the opening and closing of the mouth, represented by the range of motion of the condyle. This chapter discusses the different scenarios where a disc displacement might occur and, when they do, how the MRI utilizing MR sequences in open and closed mouth positions assists the clinician in providing a definitive diagnosis of TMD related to the disc.

G. A. Kaspo
Henry Ford Health Systrem, Henry Ford Hospital, Department of Otolaryngology, Detroit, Michigan, USA

Wayne State University, Department of Psychiatry, Detroit, Michigan, USA
e-mail: drkaspo@facialpainclinic.com

M. Mupparapu (✉)
Division of Oral and Maxillofacial Radiology, University of Pennsylvania School of Dental Medicine, Philadelphia, USA
e-mail: mmd@upenn.edu

9.2 Overview of Anatomy and Imaging Evaluation for TMJ Complex

9.2.1 Anatomy of TMJ

There are several components of the joints that either contribute directly or indirectly to pain and dysfunction. The TMJ capsule is a fibrous membrane surrounding the joint and attaches to the articular eminence, the articular disc, and the

G. A. Kaspo, G. D. Klasser (eds.), *Orofacial and Head Pain*,
https://doi.org/10.1007/978-3-032-08275-6_9

neck of the condyle. The articular disc is a fibrous extension of the capsule that is located between the two articular surfaces of the condyle, thereby creating two joint spaces each with its own synovial membrane (Fig. 9.1). The disc is attached to the condyle medially and laterally by the collateral ligaments. The ligaments give passive stability to the TMJ. The temporomandibular ligament is the thickened lateral portion of the capsule consisting of two parts—an oblique outer part and a horizontal inner part (Fig. 9.2). The anterior portion of the disc attaches to the joint capsule and the superior head of the lateral pterygoid, while the posterior portion attaches to the mandibular fossa which is known as the retrodiscal tissue (RDT). Conditions that affect the integrity of these structures will lead to changes within the anatomy, leading to dysfunction. The stylomandibular ligament runs from the styloid process to the angle of the mandible. The sphenomandibular ligament runs from the spine of the sphenoid bone to the lingula of the mandible (Fig. 9.3). There are two otomandibular ligaments that arise from the malleus, namely, the discomalleolar ligament (DML) (Fig. 9.4) and the anterior malleolar ligament (AML). The AML arises from the malleus and connects with the lingula of the mandible via the sphenomandibular ligament. The DML arises from the malleus and runs to the medial retrodiscal tissue. The otomandibular ligaments are possibly related to the tinnitus associated with TMD [1]. It has been proposed that the DML and AML get elongated in TMD, affecting

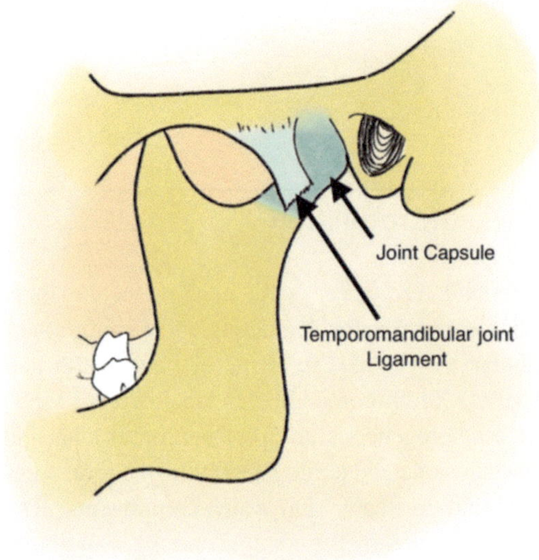

Fig. 9.2 TMJ and its ligaments—medial view. (Illustration by Nithya Vadlamudi, Royersford, Pennsylvania)

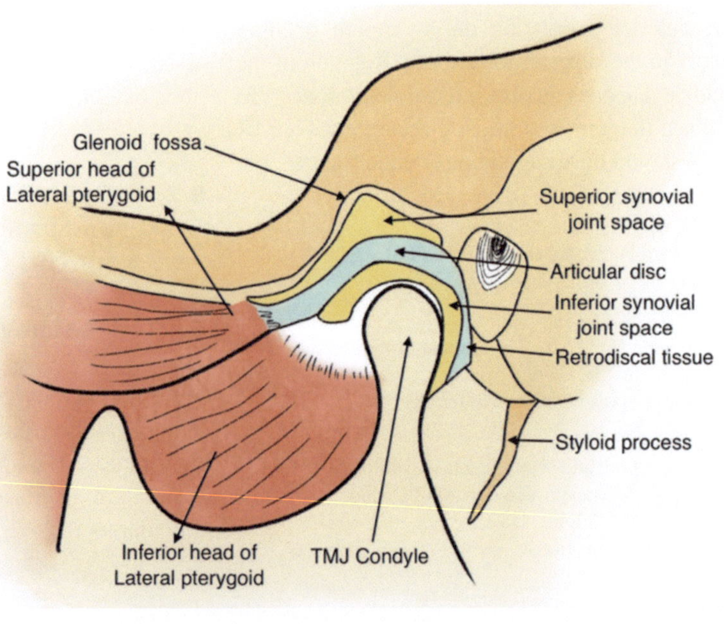

Fig. 9.1 The temporomandibular joint anatomy with labeling. (Illustration by Nithya Vadlamudi, Royersford, Pennsylvania)

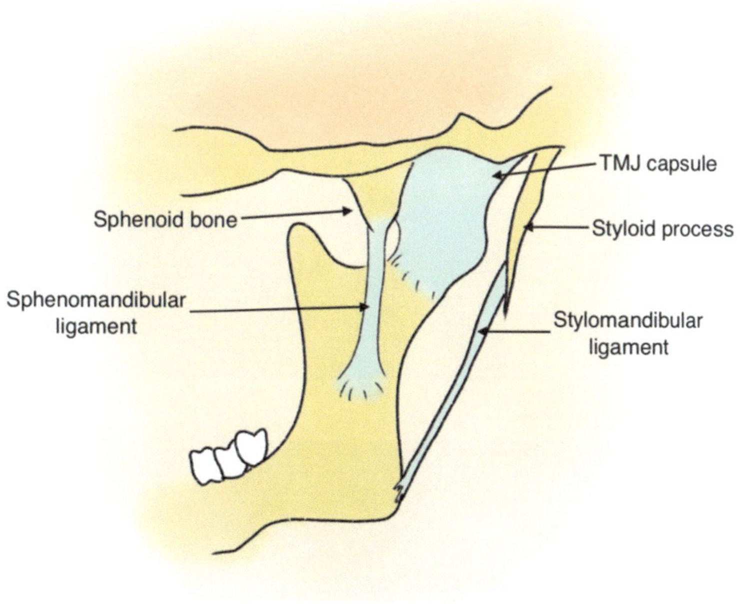

Fig. 9.3 TMJ ligament and capsule lateral view. (Illustration by Nithya Vadlamudi, Royersford, Pennsylvania)

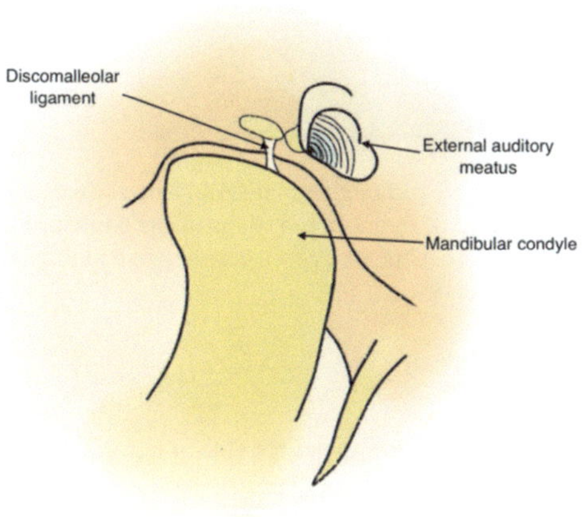

Fig. 9.4 The discomalleolar ligament and its relationship to the disc. Illustration by Nithya Vadlamudi, Royersford, Pennsylvania

the middle ear equilibrium and causing symptoms related to tinnitus, otalgia, dizziness, and hyperacusis.

9.2.2 Imaging

Although clinical examination is critical to the diagnosis of any TMD, study of the TMJ anatomy, both joint and the disc, via imaging helps the clinician to formulate a working diagnosis to plan treatment. The choice of any specific imaging test depends on the presenting complaint of the patient, the availability and affordability of the test, and clinical suspicion. The imaging data will complement the clinical data. Knowledge of each specific imaging test is essential before choosing the type of imaging [2].

Although there were several plain radiographic images that were available for evaluation of TMD, due to the unreliability of the imaging data that suffered distortions, anatomical superimposition of opposite side, and reduced sharpness of the area of interest, techniques like trans-cranial, trans-pharyngeal and trans-orbital TMJ views became largely outdated. Panoramic radiography survived the test of time as the tomographic cuts gave a better view of the joints bilaterally without any superimpositions, along with reduced dose to the patient. Digital panoramic radiography replaced film-based panoramic radiography (Fig. 9.5). The positioning of the patient within the machine's focal trough is the key to obtaining accurate panoramic radiographs. If the object falls outside of the focal trough, the objects get distorted and even ghosted. Since anatomical variations may be misdiagnosed as pathology, a good knowledge of the panoramic radiographic

Fig. 9.5 A digital panoramic radiograph showing partially edentulous mandible and maxilla. Condyles are bilaterally seated within the fossa demonstrating changes consistent with mild to moderate DJD within the fossa and condyles

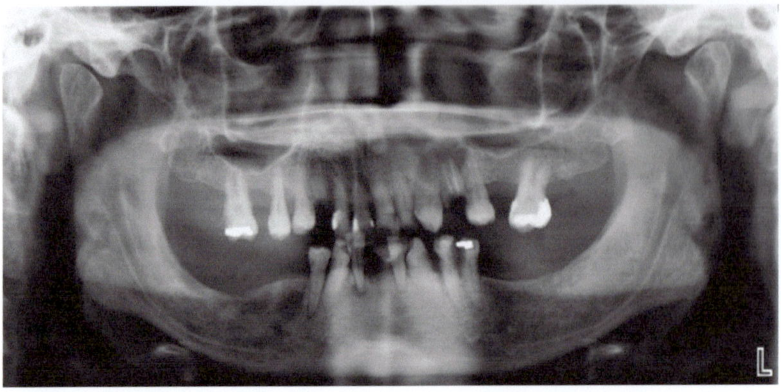

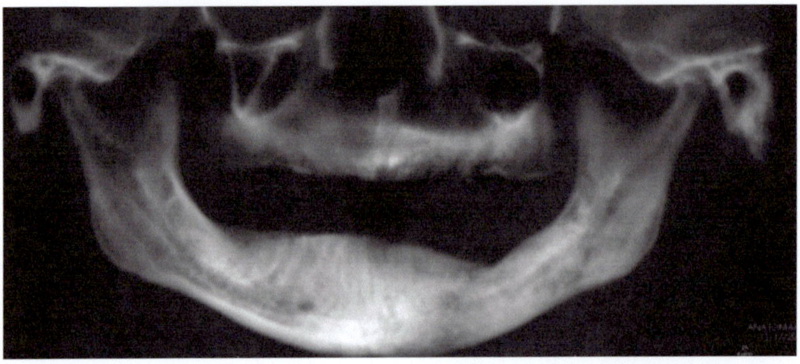

Fig. 9.6 CBCT-panoramic reconstruction showing edentulous maxilla and mandible along with bilateral condyles in view. The TMJ spaces appear uneven, but the assessment is difficult as the patient is edentulous. The condyles appear to be seated within the fossa bilaterally and appear well corticated, although generative changes like sclerosis, flattening of the posterior slope of the eminence, and mild anterior beaking suggest a degenerative joint disease radiographically

anatomy becomes necessary before the interpretation [3].

Cone beam computed tomography (CBCT), a CT technique introduced to dentistry at the beginning of the millennium, has the advantage of not duplicating the structures, the ability to view the condyles and fossa in three dimensions (Figs. 9.6 and 9.7) at a reduced dose compared with multidetector computed tomography (MDCT). The disadvantage of using panoramic, CBCT, or CT imaging is their inability to accurately evaluate the fibrocartilaginous disc. MRI can detect the disc and its precise location within the joint space. The MR study uses various pulse sequences and protocols to demonstrate the bony and soft tissue components of the TMJ [3–5].

The evaluation of the TMJ and its components via MRI starts with the study of anatomy of the joint via pulse sequences. The fibrocartilage disc is biconcave in shape and is attached to the TMJ capsule except posteriorly. The anterior and posterior bands are essentially transverse thickenings of the disc. Between the two bands, there is the intermediate zone. There are several attachments to the TMJ. Anteriorly, the capsule is attached to and blends with the superior belly of lateral pterygoid muscle. Medially and laterally, the capsule forms the boundary. Posteriorly, the capsule blends with the retrodiscal tissue. The disc has low signal intensity in T1-weighted (W) images and can be easily identified within the joint space which has a brighter signal compared to the disc [3].

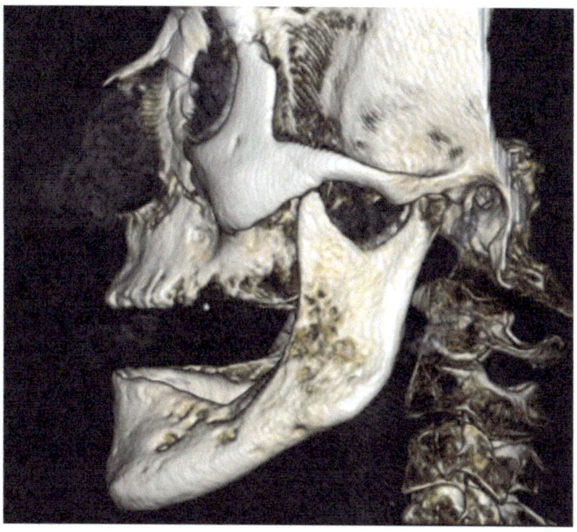

Fig. 9.7 CBCT 3D reconstruction showing edentulous maxilla and mandible. The left condyle is noted within the fossa

The anterior band and the intermediate zone have low signal intensity in T2W and proton density (PD) sequences. The posterior band and the retrodiscal tissue are intermediate to hyperintense in T2W and PD sequences. Any inflammatory exudate or fluid collection appears hyperintense in T2W sequences and is seen well compared to surrounding tissues that are hypointense in this sequence. The fluid collection within the joint spaces is seen much better if the sequence is fat suppressed essentially eliminating any other bright signal in the area. The anterior band is noted well in both open and closed sagittal or oblique sagittal views, while the posterior band and retrodiscal zone are noted well in the closed mouth views. While the normal disc is biconcave, it gets altered due to pathology and may appear thickened, irregular, thin, or perforated [3].

9.2.3 Internal Derangements

The TMJ is a ginglymoarthrodial joint that allows a hinge-like movement combined with an arthrodial gliding motion. The hinge-like movement represents the first half of the mouth opening, whereas the sliding movement represents the second half and the protrusion and lateral movements. TMDs encompass various conditions involving the TMJ and related structures. Typical TMD symptoms include pain, limited mouth opening, and joint sounds [6].

TMD is most common in young and middle-aged women (20–50 years old), with a female-to-male ratio ranging from 3:1 to 9:1. Women also seek treatment three times more frequently than men [7].

The most common emerging symptom is pain, typically felt in the preauricular area or in the muscles used for chewing. Patients often experience restricted jaw movement and TMJ noises, which may be described as "popping," "clicking," "grating," or "crepitus." They also commonly report earache, headache, jaw pain, and facial discomfort. Additionally, related issues may be related to nonpainful enlargement of the masticatory muscles and unusual wear on the teeth due to oral parafunctions like grinding and clenching.

The condyle articulates with the mandibular fossa of the temporal and tympanic bones at the base of the skull. Unlike most joints in the body, which are lined with hyaline cartilage, the condyle and fossa are covered with fibrous connective tissue. This tissue type generally withstands damage better over time and has superior repair properties [8].

An articular disc made of dense fibrous connective tissue is situated between the condyle and fossa with the posterior band located at the 12 o'clock position (Figs. 9.8 and 9.9). The disc is biconcave in shape, with its thinnest part at the center. Its posterior border is thicker than the anterior border, and the medial border is thicker than the lateral border. These thicker borders help keep the disc properly positioned on the rounded condylar head [8].

The articular disc is further stabilized by additional soft tissues that surround it. Posteriorly, the retrodiscal tissue consists of three main components while securing the disc. The superior section contains elastic fibers in the superior retrodiscal lamina, which connects the disc to the tympanic plate. The inferior section, made of collagenous fibers in the inferior retrodiscal lamina, attaches the disc to the mandibular condyle. The

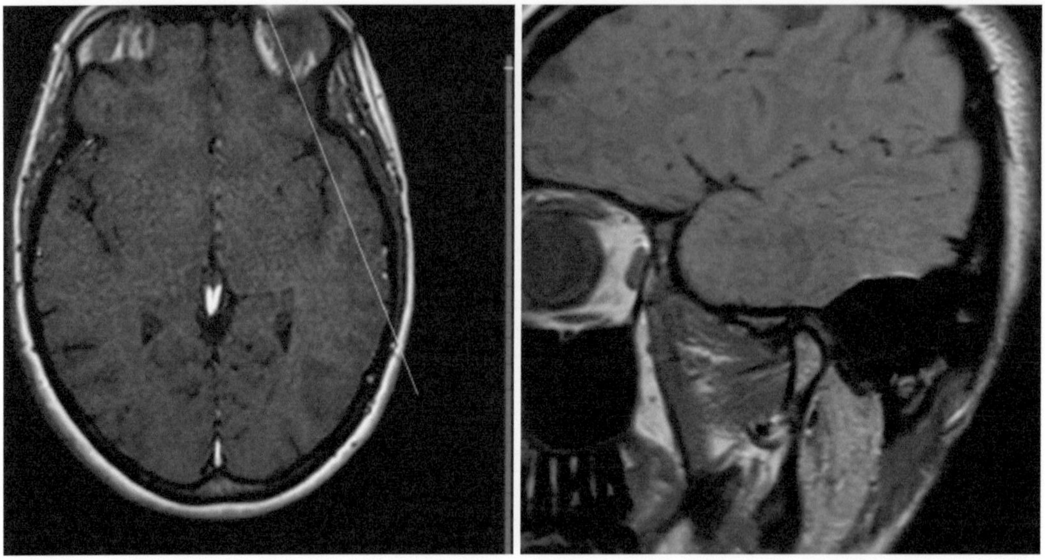

Fig. 9.8 Left TMJ closed mouth, sagittal MR proton density: TMJ MR showing the posterior band of the disc at 12 o'clock position interposed between the fossa and the head of the condyle. The axial MR image depicts the orientation of the slice reconstructed sagittally

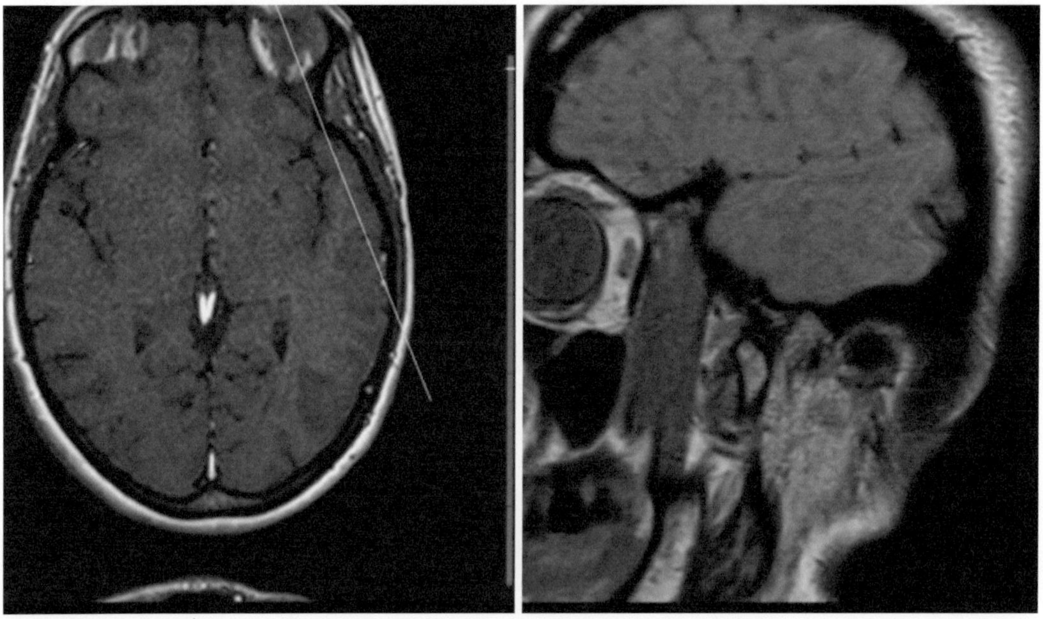

Fig. 9.9 Left TMJ open mouth, sagittal MR proton density. Note the anterior translation of the condyle. The disc is stuck superiorly in the open mouth position (stuck disc). Stuck disc is an immobile disc in relation to the glenoid fossa and articular eminence and is thought to be related to adhesions. The axial MR image depicts the orientation of the slice reconstructed sagittally

venous plexus, located between these two laminae, fills with blood during mandibular protrusion [10]. Anteriorly, the articular disc is composed of three main attachments: the superior section connects to the temporal bone via collagenous fibers, the inferior section attaches to the condyle also via collagenous fibers, and the lateral pterygoid muscle is situated between these two attachments [10]. Collateral or discal ligaments connect the medial and lateral sides of the articular disc to the condyle. Other ligaments associated with the TMJ are not discussed here, as they are not directly involved in internal derangements [10].

The etiology of TMJ internal derangements is multifactorial, involving traumatic injury, anatomical variations, and parafunctional habits such as bruxism. These factors contribute to disc position, morphology, or integrity alterations, resulting in symptoms such as clicking, popping, or locking sensations during jaw movement [10].

In 1978, Wilkes developed criteria for internal derangement of the TMJ using clinical symptoms and surgical and radiological findings. These criteria were later combined with MRI findings of the TMJ internal derangement [11].

Previous studies have shown an association between joint pain, dysfunctional symptoms, and disc displacement. Additionally, the results of these studies demonstrated that disc deformity and bone degenerative changes in the complex tissues of the TMJ are also associated with TMJ disc displacement [12–14].

According to Wilkes's criteria, internal derangement is considered a progressive disease. Wilkes described the radiological stages, starting from symptom-free normal joints with slight forward displacement to progressive cases with bone degenerative changes and severe clinical symptoms [15]. There are other investigators who believe that disc derangement can be present without any progression and persists for years without any significant radiographic changes within the joint [16].

Internal derangements of the TMJ can present in various ways. Partial derangement causes slight abnormal movement of the disc during mouth opening, while complete disc displacement can happen with or without reduction [17].

With reduction, the disc goes back to its place with a clicking sound when the mouth is opened, while without reduction, the disc remains displaced in front, leading to clicking or locking, especially when the mouth is opened wide. Another variation involves a delayed click after the jaw has opened, often associated with excessive movement and partial dislocation of the condyle, resulting in a delayed clicking sound towards the end of the mouth opening. Internal derangement without reduction means the disc is wholly displaced anteriorly, leading to elongation of ligaments and increased pain when the mouth is opened due to the mandible pushing against the displaced disc [15–17]. It is very uncommon for the disc to get displaced posteriorly, behind the condyle; in these cases, patients will hear clicking on closing only (Figs. 9.9, 9.10 and 9.11).

In summary, internal derangement of the TMJ presents a complex clinical scenario with various causes and symptoms. The best approach involves accurate diagnosis, personalized treatment, and patient-centered care to improve outcomes and the overall well-being of affected individuals.

The disc can be displaced or dislocated in any direction, but anteromedial or anterolateral are the two most common directions for its displacement. The anterior disc displacement is the most common seen in up to a third of the joints [12, 18]. The disc is interposed between the condyle and the eminence but is no longer moving with anterior movement of the condyle.

Posterior disc displacement is noted when the disc is (posterior attachment) towards the retrodiscal tissue area and, when fully displaced, causes pain upon closure or even an open lock. Stuck disc (when the disc fails to displace in open or closed mouth position and becomes sort of fixed to the temporal bone due to adhesion) is also a common finding in the MRI of the TMJ.

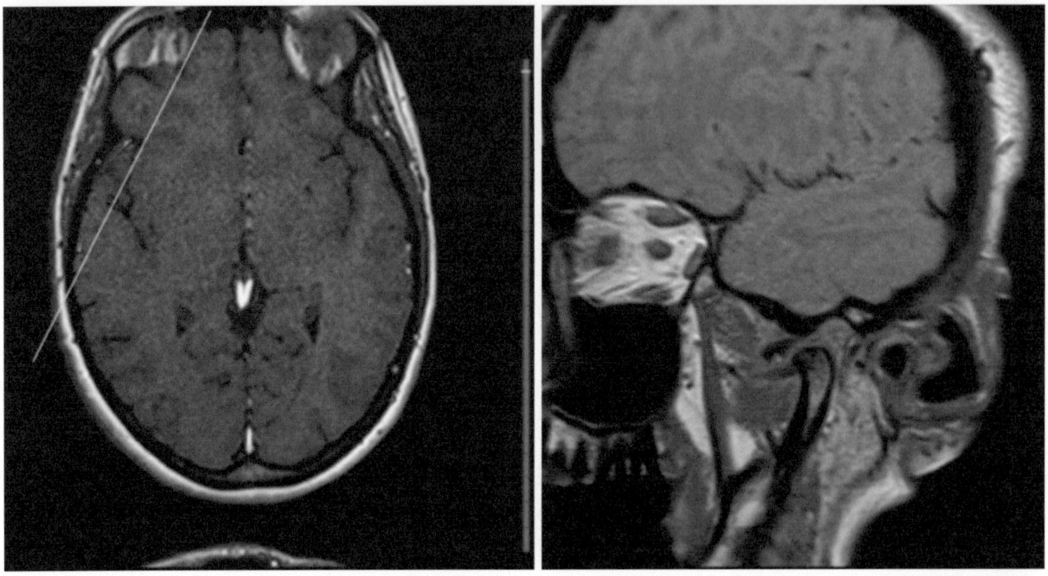

Fig. 9.10 Right TMJ open mouth, sagittal MR proton density. Anterior disc displacement noted in the right condyle. (The disc no longer maintains its anatomical integrity). The axial MR image depicts the orientation of the slice reconstructed sagittally

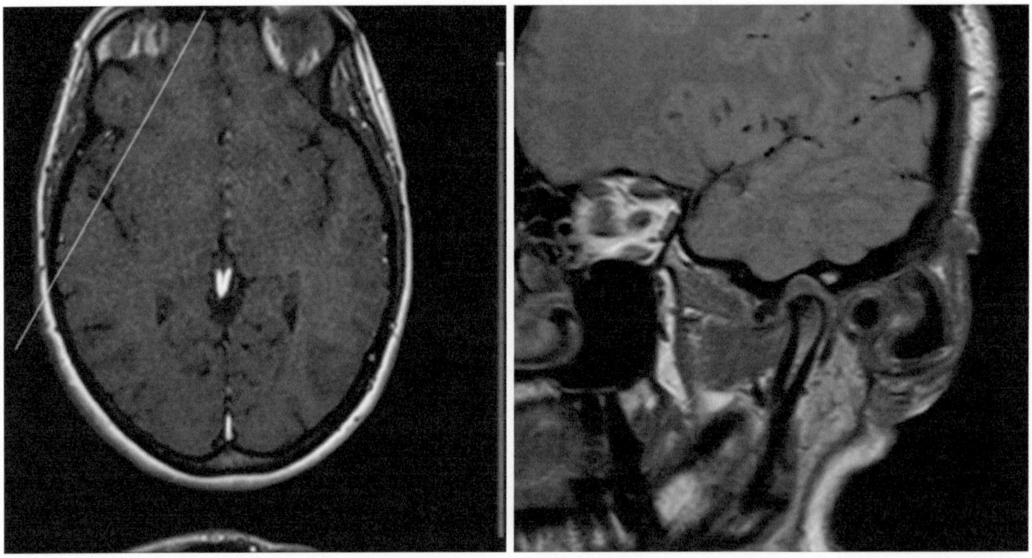

Fig. 9.11 Right TMJ closed mouth, sagittal MR proton density. Anterior disc displacement non-reduction upon closure. The axial MR image depicts the orientation of the slice reconstructed sagittally

Wilkes's [15] Clinical Stages of Internal Derangement

Stage	Clinical features	Pathologic features
I	Clicking during opening; No pain or reduced motion	Normal morphology
II	Increased clicking, occasional locking; Pain, tenderness, headaches	Anteriorly displaced disc
III	Multiple episodes of pain; Major mechanical symptoms	Displaced disc with deformity; No osseous changes
IV	Chronic symptoms, reduced motion	Increased disc deformity; bone changes with osteophytes
V	Decreased motion, reduced function	Gross degenerative changes

Schellhas's [13] Classification of Disc Displacement Combined with MR Features

Stage	MR features
I	Anterior disc displacement, reduces with opening
II	Disc displacement and deformity, reduces with opening
	+/− signal changes in disc, +/− joint effusion
III	Disc displacement and deformity, no reduction with opening
	+/− Joint effusion
IV	Severe disc deformity and displacement, no reduction with opening
	Joint effusion, Osseous changes
V	Severe disc deformity, no reduction with opening
	Disc perforation, progressive osseous deformity

9.2.4 Joint Effusion

Effusion in the TMJ refers to the abnormal fluid accumulation within the joint space. This condition can arise from various underlying causes and typically presents with distinctive clinical signs, necessitating specific diagnostic procedures for accurate evaluation and management.

TMJ effusion can occur due to several factors, including inflammatory processes, trauma, degenerative joint diseases, and systemic conditions. Inflammatory causes may involve arthritis (e.g., rheumatoid arthritis, psoriatic arthritis) or synovitis, where inflammation increases synovial fluid production. Traumatic injuries, such as direct blows to the jaw or prolonged dental procedures, can also induce joint effusion by disrupting the joint capsule or causing bleeding into the joint space. Degenerative joint diseases like osteoarthritis may contribute to chronic inflammation and fluid accumulation within the TMJ. Additionally, systemic conditions such as autoimmune disorders (e.g., systemic lupus erythematosus) or infections (e.g., septic arthritis) can potentially lead to TMJ effusion through systemic inflammatory responses affecting joint health [9, 11, 19].

The clinical presentation of TMJ effusion varies depending on the underlying cause and the severity of fluid accumulation. Common signs and symptoms include the following:

Pain: Patients may experience localized pain around the TMJ area, exacerbated by jaw movement or palpation of the joint.

Swelling: Visible or palpable swelling around the TMJ, indicating fluid accumulation within the joint capsule (Figs. 9.12 and 9.13).

Clicking or Crepitus: Some patients may report clicking sounds or crepitus during jaw move-

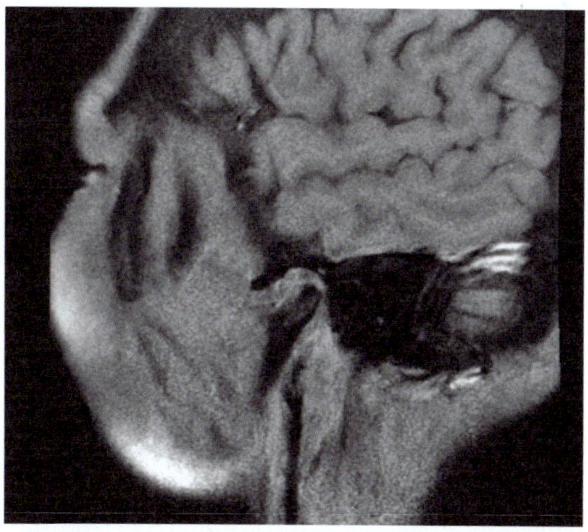

Fig. 9.12 Sagittal T1W FS MR image showing enlarged TMJ space anterior to the head of the condyle and erosion of the posterior slope of the articular eminence and glenoid fossa. Note the destruction of the head of the condyle especially anteriorly and superiorly. Fat signal is suppressed in this MR image

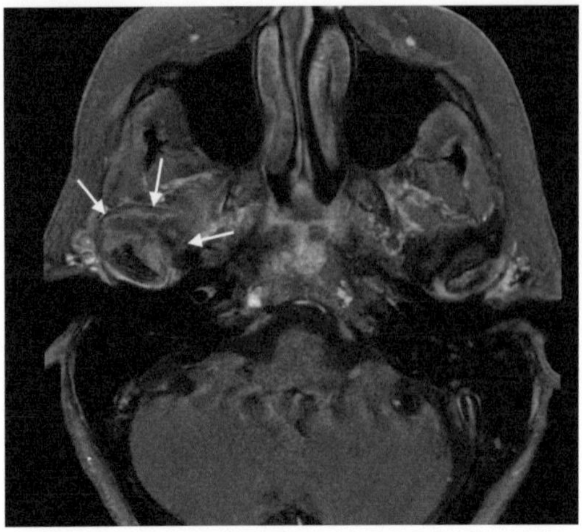

Fig. 9.13 Axial T1W MR image showing enlarged right TMJ space antero-posteriorly and increased signal within the joint space indicative of fluid or vascular aggregation (arrows) when compared with the left side. Fat signal is suppressed in this MR image

ment, indicating mechanical disturbances within the joint due to fluid buildup.

Systemic Symptoms: In cases of systemic involvement or infection, patients may present with fever, malaise, or signs of systemic inflammation.

Accurate diagnosis of TMJ effusion involves a combination of clinical evaluation, imaging studies, and, occasionally, laboratory tests to determine the underlying cause. Diagnostic procedures commonly employed include the following:

Clinical Examination: A thorough examination of the TMJ by a healthcare professional to assess for signs of swelling, tenderness, range of motion, and joint sounds and ipsilateral separation of posterior teeth (e.g., clicking, crepitus).

Limited Jaw Movement: Effusion can restrict normal jaw movement, causing stiffness or difficulty opening and closing the mouth [8, 19].

Radiographic imaging, such as panoramic radiographs and CBCT, is unreliable for this issue. The best diagnostic modality is MRI with contrast to enhance the fluid in the synovial tissue. MRI provides detailed visualization of TMJ anatomy, disc position, and the presence of effusion. MRI is beneficial for assessing soft tissue changes and detecting fluid accumulation within the joint space [9, 20–23].

A change in occlusion is noted in cases where either of the bands becomes hypertrophic with or without effusion [24].

In summary, TMJ effusion is a clinical condition characterized by abnormal fluid accumulation within the TMJ stemming from various inflammatory, traumatic, degenerative, or systemic causes. Accurate diagnosis through clinical evaluation, imaging studies, and sometimes arthrocentesis is crucial for appropriate management. Early identification assists in early intervention and alleviates symptoms and improves outcomes for patients affected by TMJ effusion.

9.3 Non-inflammatory Conditions Affecting TMJ

9.3.1 Degenerative Joint Disease (DJD)

MRI plays a crucial role in understanding DJD completely including the disc location, characterization, and the stage of DJD [25].

9.4 Inflammatory Conditions Affecting TMJ

MR findings associated with the inflamed joints unfortunately appear similar. Although adequate to diagnose the inflammation within the joint, the MR findings will not be able to distinguish the different types of inflammatory conditions. They all share a similar spectrum of imaging findings. Common findings are effusion, joint space narrowing, disc destruction or displacement, bone marrow edema, and cortical erosions [26].

The inflammatory synovial pannus destroys the articular disc and bilaminar zone, resulting in abnormal disc position, commonly superior. There can even be complete destruction of the disc in some cases. Proton density fat-saturated images may show varying degrees of condylar erosion depending on the chronicity of the arthritis, joint effusion, enhancing synovitis, absence of normal appearing disc, and areas of pannus formation. Pannus formation and synovitis are distinguished from TMJ effusion via contrast administration. Soft tissue swelling and edema as noted on STIR are more pronounced in the retrodiscal tissue.

9.4.1 Rheumatoid Arthritis

Pain and limitation of opening are common features. Based on MR features, Lin and co-workers classified RA into different grades. Grade 0 represents normal condyle and joint. Grade 1 represents mild RA involvement with morphological change or irregularity in the condyle, osseous changes or destruction, and minimal joint space narrowing. Grade 2 represents moderate RA changes like significant condylar erosion or destruction and joint space narrowing. Grade 3 is a severe form of RA and may show complete destruction of the condyle and joint space narrowing or loss [27–29].

9.4.2 Juvenile Idiopathic Arthritis

This is the most commonly diagnosed rheumatologic condition in children. TMJ is a very susceptible synovial joint compared to other synovial joints due to the fact that the growth plate of the condylar head is located in close proximity to the area of synovial inflammation [28, 29]. Early diagnosis of the synovitis and treatment can prevent joint damage or deformity and functional limitations to the growing condyle. It is interesting to note that despite the high prevalence of radiographic evidence of TMD in patients with JIA, most children have little or no evidence of TMJ symptoms at the time of examination [29]. MRI with gadolinium-based contrast material is the most sensitive tool for detecting TMJ arthritis in patients with JIA. Common MRI features in JIA are condylar head erosion, flattening of articular surface, synovial enhancement, joint effusion, deformed or dislocated disc in both open and closed mouth positions, bone marrow edema, glenoid fossa sclerosis, sclerosis of condylar head, and presence of osteophytes. There are several juvenile inflammatory subtypes.

Subtype 1: Extended oligoarticular
Subtype 2: Polyarticular Rh factor negative
Subtype 3: Psoriatic
Subtype 4: Systemic
Subtype 5: Polyarticular Rh factor positive
Subtype 6: Persistent oligoarticular
Subtype 7: Enthesitis-related arthritis (ERA)
Subtype 8: Unclassified JIA

References

1. Kuttila S, Kuttila M, Le Bell Y, et al. Recurrent tinnitus and associated ear symptoms in adults. Int J Audiol. 2005;44(3):164–70.
2. Kim IH, Singer SR, Hong DJ, et al. Fundamentals of radiographic interpretation for the dentist. Dent Clin N Am. 2021;65(3):409–25.
3. Singer SR, Mupparapu M. Temporomandibular joint imaging. Dent Clin North Am. 2023;67(2):227–41.
4. Mupparapu M, Nadeau C. Oral and maxillofacial imaging. Dent Clin North Am. 2016;60(1):1–37.
5. de Boer EW, Dijkstra PU, Stegenga B, et al. Value of cone-beam computed tomography in the process of diagnosis and management of disorders of the temporomandibular joint. Br J Oral Maxillofac Surg. 2014;52:241–6.
6. Dym H, Israel H. Diagnosis and treatment of temporomandibular disorders. Dent Clin North Am. 2012;56(1):149–61.
7. Vervaeke K, Verhelst PJ, Orhan K, et al. Correlation of MRI and arthroscopic findings with clinical outcome in temporomandibular joint disorders: a retrospective cohort study. Head Face Med. 2022;18(1):2.
8. Okeson J. Management of Temporomandibular Disorders and Occlusion. Philadelphia: Elsevier Health Sciences; 2019.
9. Ahmad M, Schiffman EL. Temporomandibular joint disorders and orofacial pain. Dent Clin N Am. 2016;60(1):105–24.
10. Laskin DM, Green CS, Hylander W. TMDs an evidence-based approach to diagnosis and treatment. 1st ed. Singapore: Quintessence Books; 2006.
11. Schiffman E, Ohrbach R, Truelove E, et al. Diagnostic criteria for temporomandibular disorders (DC/TMD) for clinical and research applications: recommendations of the international RDC/TMD consortium network and orofacial pain special interest group. J Oral Facial Pain Headache. 2014;28(1):6–27.
12. Katzberg RW, Westesson PL, Tallents RH, et al. Anatomic disorders of the temporomandibular joint disc in asymptomatic subjects. J Oral Maxillofac Surg. 1996;54(2):147–53; discussion 53–5.

13. Schellhas KP. Internal derangement of the temporomandibular joint: radiologic staging with clinical, surgical, and pathologic correlation. Magn Reson Imaging. 1989;7(5):495–515.
14. Taşkaya-Yilmaz N, Oğütcen-Toller M. Magnetic resonance imaging evaluation of temporomandibular joint disc deformities in relation to type of disc displacement. J Oral Maxillofac Surg. 2001;59(8):860–5; discussion 5–6.
15. Wilkes CH. Internal derangements of the temporomandibular joint. Pathological variations. Arch Otolaryngol Head Neck Surg. 1989;115(4):469–77.
16. de Leeuw R. Internal derangements of the temporomandibular joint. Oral Maxillofac Surg Clin North Am. 2008;20(2):159–68.
17. Chang CL, Wang DH, Yang MC, et al. Functional disorders of the temporomandibular joints: internal derangement of the temporomandibular joint. Kaohsiung J Med Sci. 2018;34(4):223–30.
18. Ribeiro R, Tallents R, Katzberg R, et al. The prevalence of disc displacement in symptomatic and asymptomatic volunteers aged 6 to 25 years. J Orofac Pain. 1997;11(1):37–47.
19. Klasser GD, Reyes MR. Orofacial pain: guidelines for assessment, diagnosis, and management, AAOP the American Academy of orofacial pain. 7th ed. Quintessence Publishing; 2023. p. 1–368.
20. Mallya SM, Ahmad M, Cohen JR, et al. Recommendations for imaging of the temporomandibular joint. Position statement from the American Academy of Oral and maxillofacial radiology and the American Academy of orofacial pain. J Oral Facial Pain Headache. 2023;37(1):7–15.
21. Xiong X, Ye Z, Tang H, et al. MRI of temporomandibular joint disorders: recent advances and future directions. J Magn Reson Imaging. 2020;54(4):1039–52.
22. Roth C, Ward RJ, Tsai S, et al. MR imaging of the TMJ: a pictorial essay. Appl Radiol. 2005;34:9–16.
23. Okeson JP, de Leeuw R. Differential diagnosis of temporomandibular disorders and other orofacial pain disorders. Dent Clin N Am. 2011;55(1):105–20.
24. Mupparapu M, Parisi E, DeRossi SS. Temporomandibular joint disc disfigurement and abnormal thickening of the posterior band. Gen Dent. 2003;51(3):256–8.
25. Resnick CM, Vakilian PM, Breen M, et al. Quantifying temporomandibular joint synovitis in children with juvenile idiopathic arthritis. Arthritis Care Res (Hoboken). 2016;68(12):1795–802.
26. Tomas X, Pomes J, Berenguer J, et al. MR imaging of temporomandibular joint dysfunction: a pictorial review. Radiographics. 2006;26:765–81.
27. Lin YC, Hsu ML, Yang JS, et al. Temporomandibular joint disorders in patients with rheumatoid arthritis. J Chin Med Assoc. 2007;70(12):527–34.
28. Hauer RL, Semidey MI. Diagnosis and treatment of temporomandibular disorders. Am Fam Physician. 2015;91(6):378–86.
29. Cayón-Somacarrera S, Gutiérrez-Rodríguez R, Muñoz-Guerra MF, Rodríguez-Campo FJ, Escorial-Hernández V, Ocón-Alonso EM. Unlocking the temporomandibular joint: CT, MRI, and arthroscopic correlation. Radiographics. 2024;44(10):e240025.

Otolaryngologic Causes of Orofacial Pain

10

Sandeep Uppal and Chew Lip Ng

10.1 Introduction

Orofacial pain is a complex and multifaceted condition affecting the head, face, and neck regions, often causing diagnostic and therapeutic challenges for healthcare professionals [1]. It may arise from a variety of sources, including sinonasal, dental, musculoskeletal, neurovascular, and psychogenic origins. Radiological imaging plays a crucial role in the evaluation of orofacial pain, providing valuable insights into the underlying causes, assisting in diagnosis, and guiding therapeutic interventions [2, 3]. This chapter delves into the radiological approach to orofacial pain, emphasizing the importance of targeted imaging modalities, key pathologies, and diagnostic protocols used to investigate and manage these conditions [4].

S. Uppal
The ENT Clinic, Singapore, Singapore

C. L. Ng (✉)
Department of Otolaryngology-Head and Neck Surgery, Ng Teng Fong General Hospital, National University Health System, Singapore, Singapore
e-mail: chew_lip_ng@nuhs.edu.sg

10.2 Otolaryngologic Causes of Orofacial Pain

Otolaryngologic causes can be classified into various categories based on its site and etiology. These include sinonasal disease which arises from sinus infections, neoplasms, or aberrant nasal anatomy; otologic diseases involving the external ear, middle ear, mastoid, and the inner ear, which are common sites of pain due to conditions ranging from infections to neoplasms; temporomandibular disorders (TMD) involving the musculoskeletal and articular structures of the jaw and salivary glands such as the parotid, submandibular, sublingual, and minor salivary glands, which can be afflicted by conditions such as sialolithiasis, infections, or neoplasms that cause pain.

Clinicians must be aware of the wide differential diagnosis for otolaryngologic causes of orofacial pain and select imaging strategies accordingly.

10.2.1 Imaging Modalities

Several imaging modalities are available for evaluating orofacial pain, each with its own strengths, limitations, and clinical indications. The choice of imaging depends on the suspected cause and anatomical region involved [3, 5].

G. A. Kaspo, G. D. Klasser (eds.), *Orofacial and Head Pain*,
https://doi.org/10.1007/978-3-032-08275-6_10

10.2.1.1 Conventional Radiography

Conventional radiography consists of sinus radiographs which allows for evaluation of the presence of sinus infections. Panoramic radiography (orthopantomogram, OPG) is commonly used as an initial screening tool, providing a broad overview of the teeth, maxillary sinuses, mandible, and temporomandibular joints (TMJ) [6]. This radiograph is useful in identifying dental pathologies (e.g., caries, abscesses, cysts, fractures) and joint abnormalities (e.g., degenerative changes) [7]. Periapical radiography offers detailed views of individual teeth and surrounding alveolar bone, aiding in the diagnosis of localized dental issues such as periapical abscesses, cysts, and fractures [8].

10.2.1.2 Cone Beam Computed Tomography

Cone Beam Computed Tomography (CBCT) is widely used for dental and maxillofacial imaging, offering high-resolution, 3D imaging with relatively low radiation exposure. It is particularly useful in evaluating the following: dentoalveolar pathology such as assessing impacted teeth, root fractures, cysts, and bone lesions; TMJ as it provides detailed imaging of joint spaces, disc position, condylar morphology, and bony changes; maxillofacial trauma including the detection of fractures of the maxilla, mandible, and other facial bones, which may not be visible on conventional radiographs [6].

10.2.1.3 Computed Tomography

There are various types of computed tomography (CT) which aid in assisting in diagnosis. These include high-resolution CT which is often employed when higher-resolution (1-mm cuts or better) imaging of the bony structures of the face and skull is required, particularly in complex trauma (Figs. 10.1, 10.2 and 10.3), tumor evaluation, and inflammatory conditions [9]. It offers excellent bony detail, allowing assessment of fractures, osteomyelitis, and tumors. CT angiography (CTA) is applicable for the evaluation of vascular causes of orofacial pain, such as vascular malformations, aneurysms, and dissections [10].

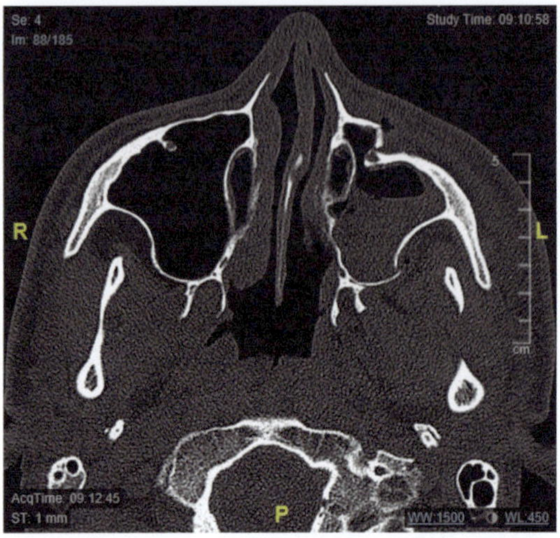

Fig. 10.1 CT facial bones (axial view) showing left-sided zygomaticomaxillary complex (ZMC) displaced fractures. There is posteromedial displacement of the ZMC fragment and blood within the maxillary sinus

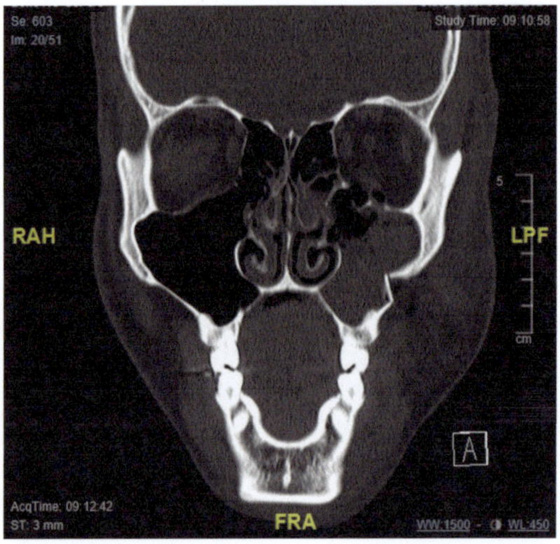

Fig. 10.2 CT facial bones (coronal view) displaying left-sided zygomaticomaxillary complex (ZMC) displaced fractures. There is posteromedial displacement of the ZMC fragment and blood within the maxillary sinus

10.2.1.4 Magnetic Resonance Imaging

Magnetic resonance imaging (MRI) is invaluable for evaluating soft tissues and neural structures, making it the modality of choice for conditions involving the temporomandibular joint, muscles of mastication, and neurogenic pain syndromes. MRI is valuable when the clinician needs to visualize the articular disc, joint effusion, synovitis,

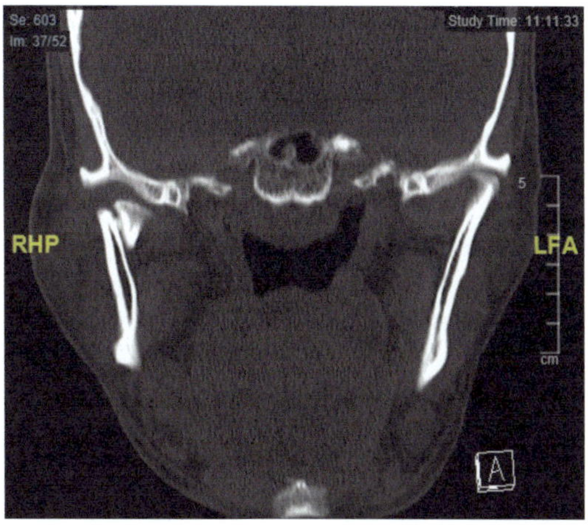

Fig. 10.3 CT facial bones showing right mandibular condyle displaced fracture

and retrodiscal tissues, identifying disc displacement and degenerative changes [11, 12]. In conditions such as trigeminal neuralgia, MRI can assess the trigeminal nerve, brainstem, and surrounding vessels. High-resolution, T2-weighted imaging is often used to detect neurovascular compression or demyelinating lesions [13]. It can be of assistance for assessing soft tissue pathology such as tumors, cysts, and inflammatory processes, as the salivary glands, muscles, and other soft tissues of the head and neck can be effectively visualized [14]. It plays a role in distinguishing between fungal and bacterial sinusitis [15].

10.2.1.5 Ultrasound

Ultrasound (US) is a noninvasive, low-cost imaging modality with increasing applications in the assessment of superficial structures such as salivary glands, muscles, and lymph nodes [16, 17]. It is particularly useful in the evaluation of salivary gland disorders in identifying stones, ductal dilatation, cysts, and tumors [18]. Furthermore, it can be applicable for muscle and soft tissue lesions in visualizing inflammatory changes, muscle tears, and superficial masses and for guided injections and aspiration procedures [16].

10.2.1.6 Bone Scintigraphy

Bone scintigraphy is used to detect osteoblastic activity in cases of osteomyelitis, bone metastasis, and temporomandibular joint pathology [19]. Positron emission tomography (PET) either PET-CT or PET-MRI may be utilized in complex cases of orofacial pain associated with malignancy, detecting metabolic activity of tumors and metastatic disease [20, 21].

10.3 Sinonasal Diseases

Sinusitis, or inflammation of the sinus cavities, is a common condition that can lead to significant pain and discomfort. It occurs when the mucous membranes lining the sinuses become inflamed, often due to infection (viral, bacterial, or fungal), allergies, or irritants. Sinusitis can be classified as acute, subacute, chronic, or recurrent, depending on its duration and frequency of episodes. Understanding the drainage pathways and identifying the causes of obstruction are important as obstruction of drainage leads to stasis within the affected sinuses, superimposed infection, and sinusitis [22]. Restoration of drainage and ventilation of the sinuses are the central tenets of functional endoscopic sinus surgery [22].

The human skull houses several pairs of paranasal sinuses, which include the maxillary, frontal, ethmoid, and sphenoid sinuses. The maxillary sinus is the largest of the sinuses. Infections can present as cheek tenderness or upper molar sensitivity; often the most commonly affected sinuses, the maxillary sinus can also be affected by odontogenic infections via upper molar roots [23, 24]. The maxillary sinuses drain through the maxillary sinus ostium, which opens into the middle meatus of the nasal cavity, just above the uncinate process. The maxillary sinus ostium is situated high on the medial wall of the sinus, rendering drainage more difficult than if it were situated lower. Ciliary movement propels mucus against gravity to drain through the ostium. Impaired ciliary movement leads to mucus stasis. The frontal sinus is located in the forehead, above the eyes. Infection can lead to frontal headaches and pressure. The frontal recess (or frontonasal duct) runs posteriorly and inferiorly from the frontal sinus, merging with the maxillary sinus drainage at the hiatus semilunaris, located in the middle meatus. There are cells around the frontal recess that may narrow it [24]. These cells may be removed in surgery for frontal sinusitis to widen the recess. These cells can be anatomically classified into anteriorly based cells (agger nasi and cells that lie superior to the agger nasi), posteriorly based cells (supra-bulla and frontal bulla cells, which are cells located superior to the ethmoidal bulla), medially based cells (inter-sinus septal cell which develops within the septum between the frontal sinuses), and laterally based cells (supra-orbital ethmoid cell). The ethmoid sinus is positioned between the orbits laterally, inferior to and attached to the skull base, and between the frontal and sphenoid sinuses. There are multiple small air cells that can get infected and contribute to pain, pressure, and headaches. The air cells can be divided into anterior and posterior ethmoid cells by the posterior turn of the middle turbinate (basal lamella). Anterior ethmoid cells are smaller and more numerous than posterior ethmoid cells. Anterior ethmoid cells drain into the middle meatus in the region of the ethmoidal bulla. Posterior ethmoid cells drain into the superior meatus. The sphenoid sinus is the most posterior of the sinuses. Infection can cause deep, central headache and referred pain in the head and neck [25]. The sphenoid sinus drains through the sphenoethmoidal recess, which is situated posteriorly in the nasal cavity in the region of the superior turbinate [26]. Sensory innervation of these sinuses is primarily from branches of the trigeminal nerve (CN V).

Sinusitis-induced pain arises from several mechanisms: inflammation, increased mucus production, nerve stimulation, and referred pain. Inflammation and swelling of the sinus lining lead to obstruction of sinus ostia and outflow tracts, which lead to an accumulation of mucus and superimposed infection. This increases pressure within the sinuses, resulting in localized pain. Mucosal swelling and blockage of sinus drainage pathways can cause fluid accumulation, further increasing pressure [27, 28]. Since the sinuses are innervated by sensory nerves, including branches of the trigeminal nerve, inflammation can activate these nociceptors, leading to pain sensation. Pain from the sinuses can radiate to surrounding areas, such as the teeth, jaw, and even the ears, due to the shared nerve pathways [29].

Patients with sinusitis may experience a range of symptoms, including facial pain and pressure often localized to the affected sinuses and often exacerbated by bending forward or lying down; headaches commonly associated with the frontal or maxillary sinus result from pressure changes and inflammation [30]. Deep central headaches may occur in sphenoid sinusitis. Nasal congestion due to obstruction of airflow through the nasal passages may lead to difficulty breathing. Rhinorrhea, which implies increased nasal discharge, may be purulent due to an underlying bacterial infection. Loss of smell (hyposmia or anosmia) can occur due to mucosal swelling, and cacosmia (sensation of foul smell) may be present. Fever and fatigue due to systemic symptoms may accompany acute sinusitis [31].

10.3.1 Diagnosis of Sinusitis

Diagnosis of sinusitis involves clinical and radiographic assessment. It requires a thorough history including the symptoms listed above, their duration, and any prior episodes of sinusitis. Often, sinusitis is preceded by a bout of upper respiratory tract infection (URTI) which causes the sinus drainage pathways to be occluded from mucosal edema. Acute sinusitis is considered to be less than 6 weeks, while chronic sinusitis lasts more than 6 weeks. A nasal examination to assess for signs of inflammation, tenderness over the sinuses, epistaxis, and nasal discharge should ensue [32]. Nasoendoscopy is helpful in determining the presence of sinusitis. Nasoendoscope findings include presence of edema, nasal polyps, mucopus, and blood within the middle and superior meati, nasal cavity, or nasopharynx [33].

10.3.2 Imaging Studies

Most acute sinusitis can be effectively managed without imaging. When symptoms are persistent or complicated, imaging may be necessary [34]. CT is a common modality for assessing sinus disease. CT scan of the paranasal sinuses can provide detailed images of the sinuses, revealing mucosal thickening, fluid levels, and anatomical variations. Imaging sequences that are compatible with image-guidance systems used intraoperatively are helpful for cases that will require sinus surgery. Findings from CT may include mucosal thickening, sinus opacification, nasal polyposis, bone changes, and osteomeatal complex/unit obstruction. Thinning or thickening of the mucosa lining the sinuses is a hallmark sign. Mild mucosal thickening may indicate acute sinusitis, while more pronounced thickening may be seen in chronic cases. Opacification of one or more sinuses suggests fluid accumulation due to infection. This can appear as complete opacification or partial opacification with air-fluid levels [35, 36]. Nasal polyposis involves globular soft tissues occupying spaces within the sinuses, in the meati, and in the nasal cavity, leading to obstruction of sinus drainage pathways. Additionally, erosion of surrounding bony structures may indicate complications, especially in invasive fungal sinusitis or spread of infection to adjacent structures. This is critical for diagnosing conditions such as orbital cellulitis or intracranial abscesses. Furthermore, it should be noted that the osteomeatal complex is a key drainage pathway for the frontal, maxillary, and anterior ethmoid sinuses [37]. Obstruction in this area can contribute to sinusitis and is often a target for surgical intervention. Other considerations are anatomic anomalies and dental causes [38]. Anatomic anomalies such as a deviated nasal septum, large concha bullosa, and prominent frontal sinus cells may lead to obstruction of sinus drainage pathways. These anomalies can be detected on CT and corrected surgically to relieve the obstruction. Odontogenic infections from decayed upper premolars and molars can spread via their roots into the maxillary sinus. Typically, periapical lucencies can be seen on CT.

10.4 Otologic Conditions

Otologic conditions encompass a range of conditions that can lead to significant pain, impacting quality of life and overall well-being. These conditions primarily affect the outer, middle, or inner ear and can arise from various etiologies. These may include vascular issues and biologic components involving bacterial, viral, and fungal pathogens. Additionally, some etiologies are idiopathic in nature. Understanding the mechanisms by which these various conditions cause pain is essential for accurate diagnosis and effective management [39, 40].

10.4.1 Tinnitus

Tinnitus is described as a perception of sound in the absence of an external source of sound. Tinnitus is characterized by various auditory sensations, including ringing, buzzing, hissing, or clicking sounds. It can be classified into subjective and objective tinnitus [41]. Subjective tinnitus is the most common form, perceived only by the affected individual. It is often related to auditory system damage or dysfunction. Objective tinnitus is uncommon and can be heard by both the patient and the examiner, typically due to vascular issues or muscular clicking [42]. Tinnitus affects a significant portion of the population, with varying degrees of severity. It can lead to psychological distress, anxiety, depression, and difficulties with concentration, sleep, and social interactions. Tinnitus has been reported as having an association with chronic pain, but the mechanisms linking the two perceptions are not clear. Tinnitus has also been compared as an analogy to pain to help understand the pathophysiology and psychological impact of pain, as both are unpleasant, perceived only by the patient and cannot be objectively measured.

Individuals with tinnitus may report concurrent pain, particularly in some head and neck areas. Cervical and TMJ pain may be associated with tinnitus in TMJ disorders, where joint dysfunction leads to muscle tension and pain in the jaw, neck, and head [43]. Headaches such as tension-type headaches and migraines have been reported more frequently in tinnitus patients, suggesting a possible link between the two conditions. Otalgia and ear discomfort can accompany tinnitus.

A comprehensive assessment of tinnitus patients may include an evaluation of pain symptoms. Validated questionnaires such as the Tinnitus Handicap Inventory are commonly used to assess the severity of tinnitus. Clinicians should consider the potential for overlapping conditions, particularly in patients presenting with both tinnitus and orofacial pain. Imaging of the brain and internal acoustic meatus may be considered, particularly in unilateral cases that are associated with facial palsy or vestibular weakness [44].

10.4.2 Otologic Infections

Otologic infections include otitis externa, otitis media, mastoiditis, malignant otitis externa, and labyrinthitis. The pain associated with otologic infections can be attributed to several factors: inflammation, pressure, nerve irritation, muscle spasms, and biologic entities (bacterial, viral, and fungal pathogens). Inflammatory mediators such as prostaglandins and cytokines increase sensitivity in the nociceptive pathways, leading to heightened pain perception [45]. In middle ear infections, fluid accumulation creates pressure against the eardrum, resulting in significant discomfort. Infections can irritate the trigeminal (CN V) and glossopharyngeal (CN IX) nerves, contributing to referred pain patterns [45]. In some cases, the muscles around the ear may spasm in response to infection, further exacerbating pain.

10.4.2.1 Otitis Externa (Swimmer's Ear)

Otitis externa is an infection of the external auditory canal (EAC), often caused by water exposure, trauma from ear picking, or dermatitis. Common pathogens include *Pseudomonas aeruginosa* and *Staphylococcus aureus* [46]. The infection leads to inflammation and swelling of the canal, which can cause significant pain. Symptoms include itch, pain, discharge (purulent and foul-smelling), sensation of blocked ear, and hearing loss in some cases [47]. Imaging may show soft tissue density within the EAC [48].

10.4.2.2 Otitis Media

Otitis media is an infection of the middle ear, commonly occurring in children. It can be acute or chronic, with acute otitis media often resulting from a viral upper respiratory infection that leads to Eustachian tube dysfunction and subsequent bacterial infection (e.g., *Streptococcus pneumoniae*, *Haemophilus influenzae*). Symptoms include sensation of blocked ear, hearing loss, otalgia in some cases, and fluid discharge if the tympanic membrane perforates. In children, acute otitis media may present with fever, ear-tugging, and irritability [49].

10.4.2.3 Mastoiditis

Mastoiditis is a serious complication of untreated or inadequately treated otitis media. The infection spreads to the mastoid bone, leading to inflammation and bone destruction (Fig. 10.4). Common pathogens include those associated with otitis media. Symptoms include severe otalgia, often deep and throbbing, retroauricular swelling and erythema, fever, and ear discharge. Intracranial involvement may occur and present with symptoms of meningitis and encephalitis [50–52].

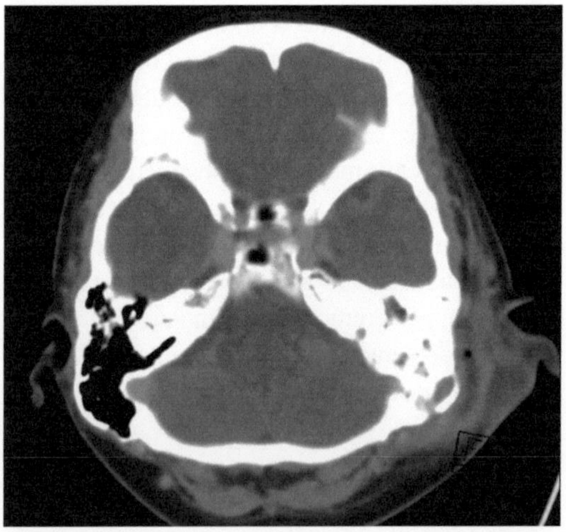

Fig. 10.4 Axial view of CT temporal bone demonstrating left acute mastoiditis with abscess formation. Note the opacification of mastoid air cells, cortical bone breaches, and post-auricular soft tissue swelling

10.4.2.4 Malignant Otitis Externa

Malignant otitis externa (MOE), or necrotizing external otitis, is a skull base osteomyelitis that begins as an infection in the EAC or middle ear and progresses due to failure of local defense mechanisms, allowing for invasion into deeper tissues including the temporal bone and skull base and involving adjacent cranial nerves (commonly VII and less commonly V, VI, IX, and X nerves) which portends a poorer prognosis [53]. Though not malignant in the neoplastic sense, the condition was named for its aggressive behavior that can be life-threatening. MOE can present with severe otalgia and craniofacial pain that mimics or overlaps with other causes of orofacial discomfort, necessitating its inclusion in a differential diagnosis. MOE most commonly affects elderly individuals, particularly those with poorly controlled diabetes mellitus or other forms of immunosuppression. The condition is uncommon in immunocompetent individuals. The most frequently implicated pathogen is *Pseudomonas aeruginosa*, although other organisms such as *Staphylococcus aureus*, *Aspergillus* species, and polymicrobial flora may also be involved.

The most typical presentation is a severe, deep-seated otalgia, often disproportionate to findings on physical exam. Pain may radiate to the TMJ, mastoid, or temporal region. Otorrhea is common, with granulation tissue seen in the EAC. Hearing loss is conductive in early stages and may progress to mixed or sensorineural if deeper structures are affected [54]. Trismus or jaw pain can occur due to spread to adjacent masticatory muscles. Cranial nerve palsies can present with the facial nerve (VII) being the most commonly involved. This often leads to facial weakness or paralysis. Constitutional symptoms of fever, fatigue, and weight loss may present in more advanced cases [55].

Early recognition is critical to reduce morbidity and prevent progression. Diagnosis is based on clinical suspicion, imaging, and microbiological testing. Imaging involving CT, MRI, and nuclear scans (e.g., gallium-67 or technetium-99) may be of assistance in assessing disease activity and treatment response [56, 57].

10.4.2.5 Labyrinthitis

Labyrinthitis is an infection of the inner ear, usually secondary to otitis media or meningitis. It can be viral (e.g., after a viral upper respiratory infection) or bacterial. The infection affects the vestibular and cochlear systems, leading to balance and hearing issues. Vertigo lasting hours to days, sudden sensorineural hearing loss (SSNHL) and/or tinnitus, nausea, and vomiting are typical symptoms. Pain is not a prominent symptom [58].

10.5 Ear Tumors

There are two main types of tumors: benign and malignant (Figs. 10.5, 10.6 and 10.7). Benign tumors include vestibular or facial schwannomas, paragangliomas/glomus tympanicum, and adenomas. Vestibular or facial schwannomas usually do not present with pain. Common presentations include asymmetric hearing loss, facial weakness, and vestibular weakness. Paragangliomas/glomus tympanicum are neuroendocrine tumors arising from Jacobson's nerve at the cochlear promontory. They are the commonest benign middle ear tumors, are hypervascular, and can cause pulsatile tinnitus. Adenomas arise from glandular tissue and can occur in the outer ear or

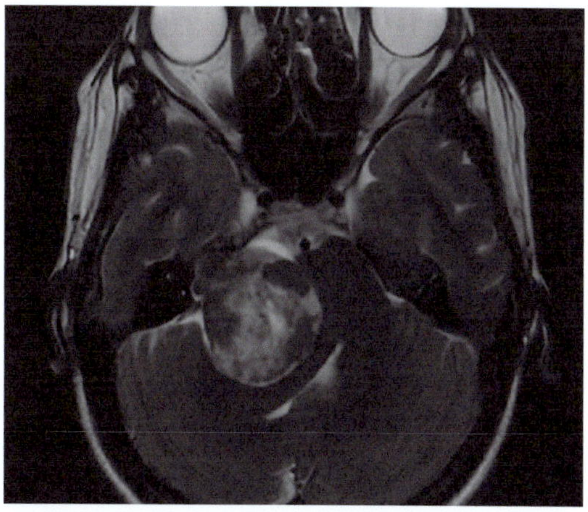

Fig. 10.5 MRI axial T2 view of the internal auditory meatus (IAM) demonstrating a large right vestibular schwannoma with mass effect on the cerebellum and brain stem, leading to midline shift and ventricular dilatation

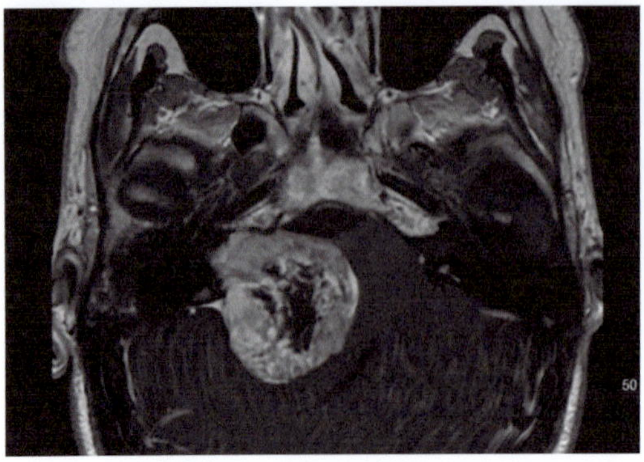

Fig. 10.6 MRI with contrast T1 axial view of the internal auditory meatus (IAM) demonstrating a large right vestibular schwannoma with mass effect on the cerebellum and brain stem, leading to midline shift and ventricular dilatation

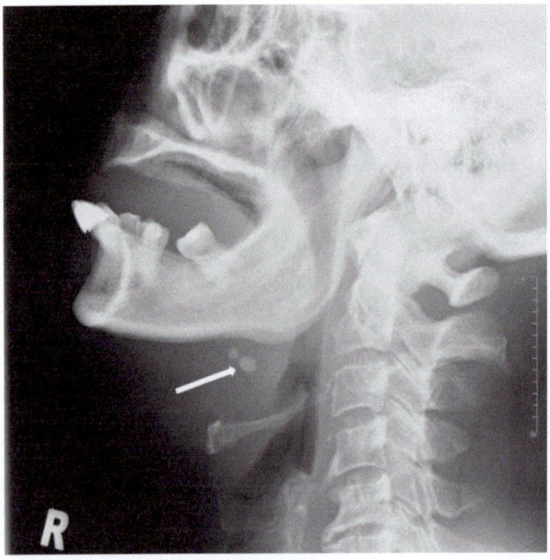

Fig. 10.7 Right submandibular sialolithiasis demonstrated on lateral plane film radiograph

the middle ear. Malignant tumors include squamous cell carcinoma, adenoid cystic carcinoma, and adenocarcinoma. Squamous cell carcinoma is a form of skin cancer that can occur in the outer ear and can be associated with pain, especially as it invades surrounding tissues. Adenoid cystic carcinoma is a rare cancer that can originate in the salivary glands around the ear, leading to painful swelling and potentially affecting hearing. Adenocarcinoma arises from glandular tissues within the middle ear which is lined by mucosa [59].

Pain associated with ear tumors can arise from several mechanisms. This can result from the effects directly related to the tumor, such as pressure on surrounding tissues, including nerves and blood vessels, and invasion of nearby tissues. The pain may be due to an inflammatory response as tumors may directly affect cranial nerves, particularly the trigeminal or facial nerves, leading to neuropathic pain. This type of pain can be sharp, shooting, or burning and may not respond well to typical pain medications. Moreover, ear pain can sometimes be referred from other areas, such as the jaw, teeth, or throat. This can complicate the diagnosis and management of ear tumors [29, 45].

Overall, the pain may be acute or chronic, and either localized or radiating. The intensity can vary from mild discomfort to severe, debilitating pain. Hearing loss often accompanies pain, particularly with tumors affecting the middle or inner ear. Pulsatile tinnitus can occur in vascular neoplasms like paragangliomas. Non-pulsatile tinnitus may occur in tumors that occlude the middle ear or external auditory canal, or in inner ear tumors such as vestibular schwanommas. In cases of infection, there may be an associated discharge from the ear, which may be purulent or bloody.

Accurate diagnosis of ear tumors involves a combination of medical history, physical examination, and imaging studies. CT and MRI scans provide detailed views of the ear structures, helping to identify the location and extent of tumors [60, 61].

10.6 Salivary Gland Diseases

Salivary glands are divided into major and minor glands, each playing a distinct role in saliva production. The major salivary glands are the parotid, submandibular, and sublingual glands. The parotid gland is located anterior to the ear, extending from the zygomatic arch to the angle of the mandible. Drainage of the gland is via Stensen's duct which opens into the vestibule of the oral cavity opposite the second maxillary molar. It primarily produces a serous secretion. The submandibular gland is located beneath the floor of the mouth, medial to the body of the mandible. Drainage is via Wharton's duct, which is tortuous and opens at either side of the lingual frenulum. It produces both serous and mucinous secretions, with a predominance of mucinous. The submandibular gland is prone to sialolithiasis as its secretions are mucinous and flow against gravity in a tortuous duct. The sublingual gland is located beneath the floor of the mouth along the inner surface of the mandible, anterior to the submandibular gland. It drains through multiple small ducts that open into the floor of the mouth [62, 63]. They produce mucinous, viscous secretions. The minor salivary glands are distributed throughout the oral cavity, including the labial, buccal, palatine, and glossopharyngeal glands. They primarily secrete mucinous saliva. The glands receive parasympathetic fibers from the glossopharyngeal nerve (CN IX) for the parotid gland and the facial nerve (CN VII) for the submandibular and sublingual glands. There are also sympathetic fibers that originate from the superior cervical ganglion and help regulate glandular blood flow and saliva secretion [64].

10.6.1 Sialolithiasis

Sialolithiasis occurs when substances in saliva consisting primarily of calcium, phosphate, and carbonate crystallize and form stones. The exact etiology of stone formation is multifactorial and can include dehydration as reduced fluid intake can lead to concentrated saliva, promoting stone formation; reduced salivary flow; altered saliva composition as changes in the electrolyte balance or protein content of saliva may contribute to crystallization; and ductal obstruction as blockages due to mucus, bacteria, or previous stone formation can lead to stagnant saliva, fostering stone development [65, 66].

The most commonly affected gland is the submandibular gland, which accounts for approximately 80% of sialolithiasis cases [67]. This prevalence is attributed to the nature of the saliva it produces and the anatomical configuration of its duct, which is longer and has a more acute angle compared to the parotid gland. The clinical manifestations of sialolithiasis can vary based on the location and size of the stone, as well as the duration of the obstruction. Patients often experience unilateral pain and recurrent swelling in the affected gland, especially during meals when salivary secretion increases. Recurrent infections are common. Blocked saliva can lead to sialadenitis, characterized by inflammation, pus, and systemic symptoms such as fever. If there is an associated infection, patients may report a foul taste in the mouth and halitosis. Abscess formation is not uncommon, particularly in immunocompromised patients such as diabetics.

Imaging may be helpful with the objectives being to establish a diagnosis and determine the number, size, and location of calculi. Location and size are of particular importance as they determine the modality for treatment. Ultrasound may be considered a first-line imaging modality that can effectively identify stones and assess gland size and structure. CT scans provide detailed images of the salivary glands and can help detect stones that are not visible on ultrasound or sialography. MRI is occasionally used, especially in cases where soft tissue involvement is suspected. Sialography involves injecting contrast material into the salivary ducts to visualize the extent of obstruction and stone location. It is less commonly done now due to the widespread availability of CT scans and ultrasound [68–70] (Figs. 10.7, 10.8 and 10.9).

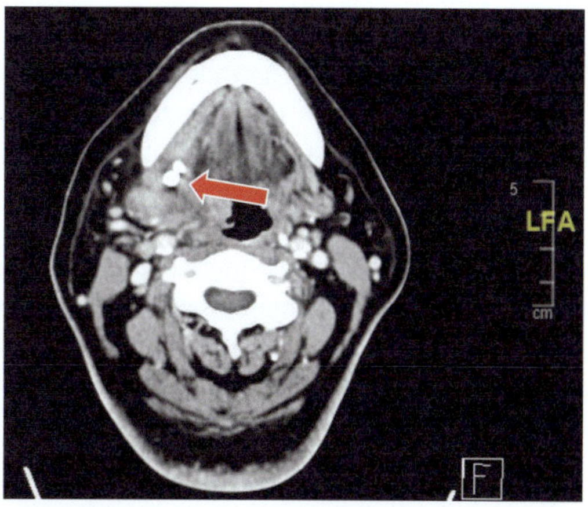

Fig. 10.8 CT axial view of a right submandibular sialolithiasis

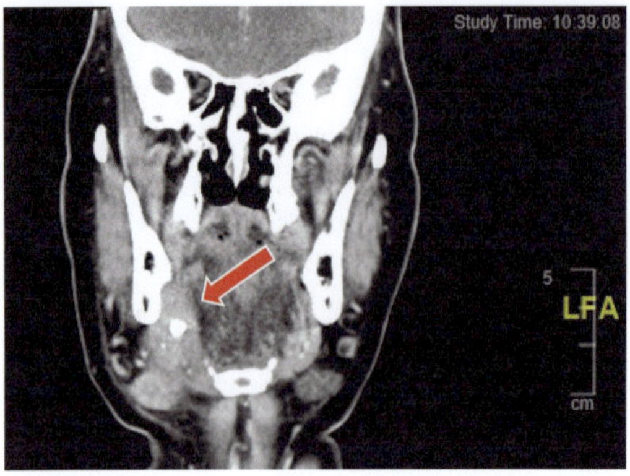

Fig. 10.9 CT coronal view of a right submandibular sialolithiasis

10.7 Sialadenitis

Sialadenitis can result from various factors. These factors may be related to infectious causes (bacterial, viral, fungal) or non-infectious (ductal obstruction, autoimmune disorders, radiation therapy) [63, 71].

Bacterial infections are most commonly caused by *Staphylococcus aureus* or *Streptococcus* species, often following duct obstruction. Viral infections such as the virus associated with parotitis (mumps) is a classic cause, particularly in unvaccinated populations. Fungal infections are rare but can occur, especially in immunocompromised patients [72].

Duct obstruction may involve stones (sialolithiasis) or strictures that can lead to stagnant saliva and subsequent inflammation. Autoimmune disorders such as Sjögren's syndrome may result in chronic inflammation and enlargement of the glands. Radiation therapy for treatment of head and neck cancers can lead to chronic sialadenitis.

Patients with sialadenitis may present with a variety of symptoms, including swelling and pain worse during meals when salivary flow is stimulated. Purulent discharge indicates an infective process. Systemic signs of infection, such as fever and malaise, may be present. Dry mouth may occur in autoimmune conditions [73].

When evaluating a patient with suspected sialadenitis, a differential diagnosis should consider the following conditions: sialolithiasis, tumors (benign or malignant), autoimmune disorders, and viral infections (especially when there is bilateral parotid gland involvement).

10.7.1 Imaging Modalities

The choice of imaging modality depends on the clinical scenario, but several options are commonly used in the evaluation of sialadenitis [74]. Ultrasound is commonly the first-line imaging modality for suspected sialadenitis due to its accessibility, cost-effectiveness, and effectiveness in soft tissue evaluation. Typical findings include enlargement of the gland, with the affected gland appearing hypoechoic due to edema. The main duct may be dilated, particularly in the presence of stones or strictures. Abscess formation may occur and appear as anechoic or hypoechoic areas within the gland. Sialography can be useful for assessing ductal anatomy and obstructions. It involves cannulating the duct through its natural opening and contrast administration into the ductal system for mapping of the ductal system. Findings may include stenosis or filling defects, indicating the presence of stones or strictures. Ductal dilation may be observed proximal to an obstruction. CT scans are a common imaging modality for salivary gland diseases, especially when a detailed evaluation of surrounding structures is needed. Findings include gland enlargement with possible stranding of surrounding fat. Abscess and phlegmon collections can be detected as low attenuation areas. Calculi may be visible within the duct or gland [75]. Neoplasms will be detected as well, and its appearance will give an indication of its nature. MRI is helpful in evaluating soft tissue structures and distinguishing between infectious and neoplastic processes. MRI can also visualize ductal anatomy and complications like abscess formation. Edema appears hyperintense, while stones appear hypointense in T2-weighted images [76].

10.8 Benign and Malignant Neoplasms of the Salivary Glands

Salivary gland neoplasms encompass a diverse group of tumors that can arise from the major and minor salivary glands. While most of these tumors are benign, some can be malignant, with significant implications for patient management. Pain, although not a universal symptom, can be a critical factor influencing the presentation, diagnosis, and treatment of these neoplasms [77].

10.8.1 Benign Salivary Gland Neoplasms

Benign salivary gland tumors typically have a favorable prognosis and are often asymptomatic or present with mild discomfort. The most common types include pleomorphic adenoma, also known as "mixed benign tumor." This is the most common benign salivary gland tumor often arising in the parotid and submandibular glands. Warthin's tumor, also known as papillary cystadenoma lymphomatosum, is a benign tumor in the parotid gland often seen in older males and characterized by a cystic appearance. Pleomorphic adenomas have malignant potential, while Warthin's tumors do not.

Pleomorphic adenoma often presents as a painless, slow-growing mass which feels firm and knobbly. Pain can occur if the tumor compresses surrounding structures or undergoes rapid enlargement. Warthin's tumor typically presents as a painless doughy or cystic swelling, often bilateral and in the lower pole of the parotid gland. Pain may arise if there is secondary infection [78].

10.8.1.1 Radiological Features of Pleomorphic Adenoma

Ultrasound findings for pleomorphic adenoma display well-circumscribed, hypoechoic lesions with heterogeneous internal echogenicity [79]. CT imaging appears as a well-defined, homogeneous mass that may be nodular. Borders are generally smooth and well-circumscribed, although they may be irregular in some cases. On noncontrast CT, pleomorphic adenomas typically appear as hypodense due to their predominantly cystic or mixed composition. They may exhibit some degree of enhancement with contrast. Calcifications may be present, often appearing as punctate, scattered foci within the mass [10, 80]. There is usually no significant invasion into surrounding tissues. However, displacement of adjacent structures may be noted. MRI features on T1-weighted images typically appear isointense to slightly hypointense compared to muscle. On T2-weighted images, they may be hyperintense due to their cystic components [81].

A defined capsule is often visible, reflecting the tumor's benign nature. Pleomorphic adenomas generally show homogeneous enhancement but may also be heterogenous. They may exhibit both cystic and solid areas, with the cystic component appearing hyperintense on T2-weighted images and the solid component being iso- to hypointense. Similar to CT findings, there is typically no invasion into surrounding tissues. The mass may displace adjacent structures rather than infiltrate them [81].

10.8.1.2 Radiological Features of Warthin's Tumor

Warthin's tumor is typically located in the parotid gland, often in the tail region, and on CT scans, it appears as a well-defined, lobulated mass with smooth margins. The tumor may be somewhat heterogeneous due to varying cystic and solid components. The CT features demonstrate generally low attenuation (hypodense) due to its cystic nature. It may exhibit areas of higher attenuation related to solid components or surrounding lymphoid tissue. Cystic areas are often noted, which can range from small cysts to larger fluid-filled spaces. After the administration of contrast material, the solid components may show mild to moderate enhancement, while cystic areas usually do not enhance. The tumor is typically well-circumscribed with no significant infiltration into surrounding tissues, although mild displacement of adjacent structures may occur [82] (Fig. 10.10). On T1-weighted MR images, Warthin's tumors are usually isointense

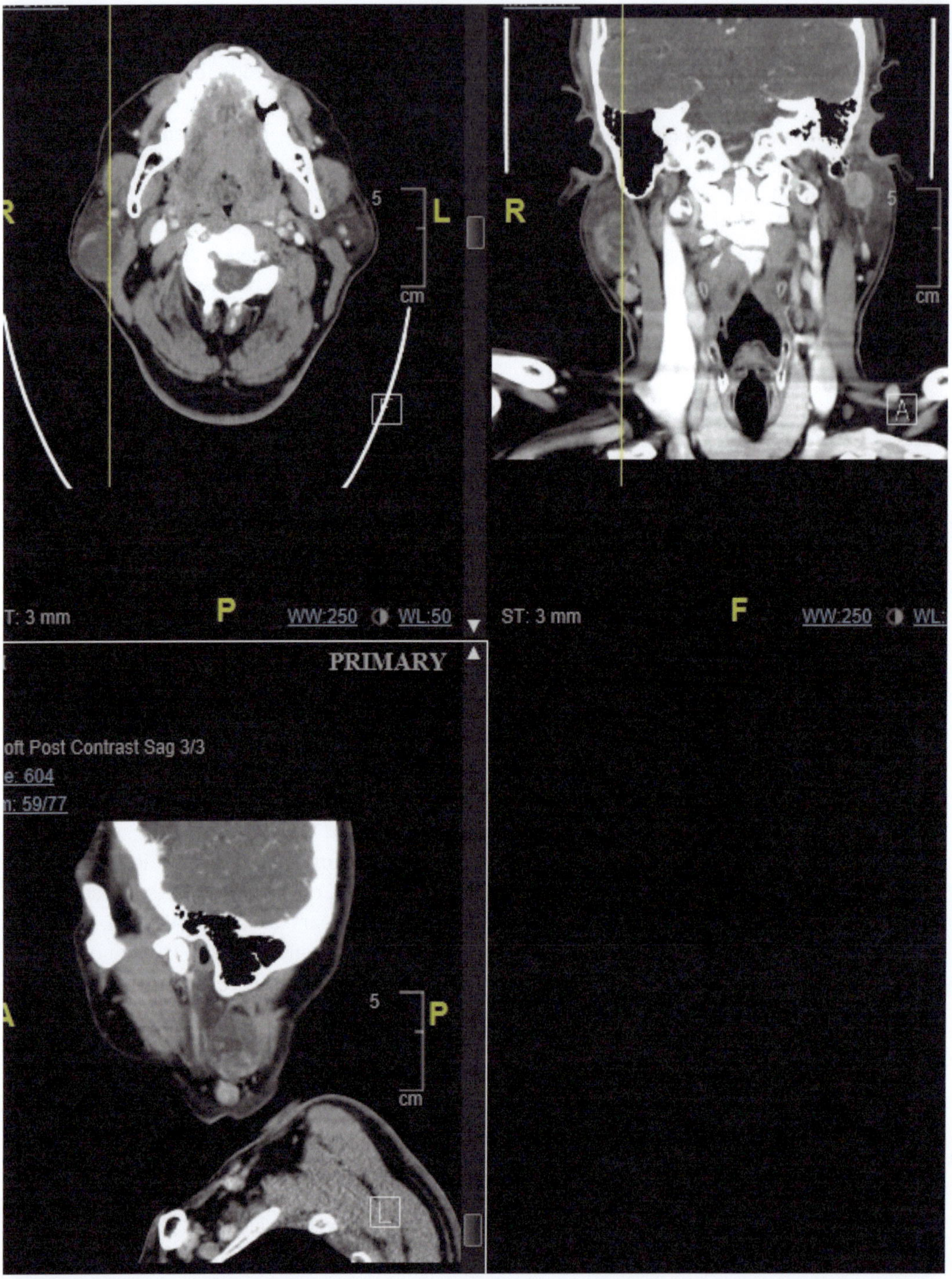

Fig. 10.10 CT salivary glands demonstrating a right Warthin's tumor. Note the well-circumscribed lesion with prominent cystic components. The location is commonly in the inferior half of the parotid gland

to slightly hypointense compared to muscle. On T2-weighted images, they typically appear hyperintense due to the presence of cystic components [83]. The tumor is often predominantly cystic with thin, smooth walls and may contain internal solid components. Solid areas may show varying signal intensity, often iso- to hypointense on T2-weighted images. Following contrast administration, the solid components of the tumor exhibit homogeneous enhancement. Cystic regions remain non-enhancing. Well-defined margins help differentiate it from malignant processes, with no evidence of infiltration into adjacent tissues [84].

10.8.2 Malignant Salivary Gland Neoplasms

Malignant salivary gland tumors are less common than benign tumors but can be more aggressive and symptomatic. Common malignant neoplasms include mucoepidermoid carcinoma, the most common malignant salivary gland tumor; adenoid cystic carcinoma, known for its slow growth but high propensity for perineural invasion and recurrence; and acinic cell carcinoma, which typically presents in the parotid gland. These enlarging irregular masses are often associated with facial weakness (due to facial nerve involvement) and pain. The presence of lymphadenopathy may suggest malignancy [85, 86].

10.8.2.1 Radiological Features

Ultrasound often displays these malignant tumors as irregular, infiltrative masses with heterogeneous echogenicity [87]. CT scans typically show ill-defined margins, infiltrative growth patterns, and may involve adjacent structures. Lymph node metastasis may also be visible. MRI generally shows heterogeneous signal intensity with possible enhancement after contrast administration. Perineural spread may be indicated by encasement of nerve, especially for adenoid cystic carcinoma. Again, lymph node metastasis may also be visible [88].

References

1. Sarlani E, Balciunas BA, Grace EG. Orofacial Pain–Part II: assessment and management of vascular, neurovascular, idiopathic, secondary, and psychogenic causes. AACN Clin Issues. 2005;16(3):347–58.
2. Whyte A, Matias M. Imaging of orofacial pain. J Oral Pathol Med. 2020;49(6):490–8.
3. Liang H. Imaging in orofacial pain. Dent Clin N Am. 2018;62(4):533–51.
4. Hunter A, Kalathingal S. Diagnostic imaging for temporomandibular disorders and orofacial pain. Dent Clin N Am. 2013;57(3):405–18.
5. Schellhas KP. Medical imaging in the evaluation of facial pain. Semin Neurol. 1988;8(4):265–71.
6. Suomalainen A, Pakbaznejad Esmaeili E, Robinson S. Dentomaxillofacial imaging with panoramic views and cone beam CT. Insights Imaging. 2015;6(1):1–16.
7. Sawas M, Alqasoumi O, Alesawi L, Alaqeeli M, Naser A, Aldowian M, Alkhamjani A, Rawah S, Alanazi F, Alshahrani R, Alahmadi SM. Anatomical features and pathologies in Orthopantomogram. J Healthc Sci. 2022; https://doi.org/10.52533/JOHS.2022.21009.
8. Vera Widyastuti AA, Epsilawati L. Sensitivity of panoramic radiographs in diagnosing maxillary sinusitis: a scoping review. Jurnal Radiologi Dentomaksilofasial Indonesia. 2021; https://doi.org/10.32793/jrdi.v5i3.703.
9. Sung EK, Nadgir RN, Sakai O. Computed tomographic imaging in head and neck trauma: what the radiologist needs to know. Semin Roentgenol. 2012;47(4):320–9.
10. Brant-Zawadzki MN, Minagi H, Federle MP, Rowe LD. High resolution CT with image reformation in maxillofacial pathology. AJR Am J Roentgenol. 1982;138(3):477–83.
11. Orhan K, Aksoy S. Magnetic resonance imaging of TMJ. In: Imaging of the temporomandibular joint; 2018.
12. Larheim TA. Role of magnetic resonance imaging in the clinical diagnosis of the temporomandibular joint. Cells Tissues Organs. 2005;180(1):6–21.
13. Seeburg DP, Northcutt B, Aygun N, Blitz AM. The role of imaging for trigeminal neuralgia: a segmental approach to high-resolution MRI. Neurosurg Clin N Am. 2016;27(3):315–26.
14. Rodriguez JD, Selleck AM, Abdel Razek AAK, Huang BY. Update on MR imaging of soft tissue tumors of head and neck. Magn Reson Imaging Clin N Am. 2022;30(1):151–98.
15. Groppo ER, El-Sayed IH, Aiken AH, Glastonbury CM. Computed tomography and magnetic resonance imaging characteristics of acute invasive fungal sinusitis. Arch Otolaryngol Head Neck Surg. 2011;137(10):1005–10.
16. Kotecha S, Bhatia P, Rout PG. Diagnostic ultrasound in the head and neck region. Dent Update. 2008;35(8):529–30, 33-4.

17. Evirgen Ş, Kamburoğlu K. Review on the applications of ultrasonography in dentomaxillofacial region. World J Radiol. 2016;8(1):50–8.
18. Lee YY, Wong KT, King AD, Ahuja AT. Imaging of salivary gland tumours. Eur J Radiol. 2008;66(3):419–36.
19. Ferreira RI, de Almeida SM, Bóscolo FN, Santos AO, Camargo EE. Bone scintigraphy as an adjunct for the diagnosis of oral diseases. J Dent Educ. 2002;66(12):1381–7.
20. Wassef HR, Colletti PM. Nuclear medicine imaging in the Dentomaxillofacial region. Dent Clin N Am. 2018;62(3):491–509.
21. van Kroonenburgh AMJL, Bothof RJP, Tilburg MV, Tongeren JV, Postma A. Advanced imaging techniques in Skull Base osteomyelitis due to malignant otitis externa. Curr Radiol Rep. 2018; https://doi.org/10.1007/s40134-018-0263-y.
22. Chan Y, Kuhn FA. An update on the classifications, diagnosis, and treatment of rhinosinusitis. Curr Opin Otolaryngol Head Neck Surg. 2009;17(3):204–8.
23. Lafci Fahrioglu S, Van Kampen N, Andaloro C. Anatomy, head and neck, sinus function and development. In: StatPearls. Treasure Island (FL): StatPearls Publishing. Copyright © 2025, StatPearls Publishing LLC; 2025.
24. Riad H. Anatomy of frontal recess and opening. Online J Otolaryngol Rhinol. 2020;
25. Zinreich S, Kuhn F, London N, Kennedy D, Solaiyappan M, Hosemann W. 3D CT stereoscopic imaging: an improved anatomical understanding of the anterior ethmoid sinus and frontal sinus drainage pathway. Rhinology Online. 2020; https://doi.org/10.4193/rhin20.061.
26. Millar DA, Orlandi RR. The sphenoid sinus natural ostium is consistently medial to the superior turbinate. Am J Rhinol. 2006;20(2):180–1.
27. Evans KL. Diagnosis and management of sinusitis. BMJ. 1994;309(6966):1415–22.
28. Rohr AS, Spector SL. Paranasal sinus anatomy and pathophysiology. Clin Rev Allergy. 1984;2(4):387–95.
29. Benoliel R, Biron A, Quek SY, Nahlieli O, Eliav E. Trigeminal neurosensory changes following acute and chronic paranasal sinusitis. Quintessence Int. 2006;37(6):437–43.
30. Khalaf QJ. Evaluating symptoms of chronic rhino sinusitis and most common sinuses affected. Diyala J Med. 2023; https://doi.org/10.26505/djm.v25i1.1032.
31. Jones NS. Sinus headaches: avoiding over- and misdiagnosis. Expert Rev Neurother. 2009;9(4):439–44.
32. Lim G, Lee J. Diagnosis and treatment of acute and chronic sinusitis. J Med Life Sci. 2011;
33. Osguthorpe JD. Adult rhinosinusitis: diagnosis and management. Am Fam Physician. 2001;63(1):69–76.
34. Joshi VM, Sansi R. Imaging in Sinonasal Inflammatory Disease. Neuroimaging Clin N Am. 2015;25(4):549–68.
35. Okuyemi KS, Tsue TT. Radiologic imaging in the management of sinusitis. Am Fam Physician. 2002;66(10):1882–6.
36. Bolger WE, Butzin CA, Parsons DS. Paranasal sinus bony anatomic variations and mucosal abnormalities: CT analysis for endoscopic sinus surgery. Laryngoscope. 1991;101(1 Pt 1):56–64.
37. Aramani A, Karadi RN, Kumar S. A study of anatomical variations of Osteomeatal complex in chronic Rhinosinusitis patients-CT findings. J Clin Diagn Res. 2014;8(10):Kc01-4.
38. Patel NA, Ferguson BJ. Odontogenic sinusitis: an ancient but under-appreciated cause of maxillary sinusitis. Curr Opin Otolaryngol Head Neck Surg. 2012;20(1):24–8.
39. Ong YK, Chee G. Infections of the external ear. Ann Acad Med Singap. 2005;34(4):330–4.
40. Hans S, Brasnu D. Pain as a symptom in otolaryngology conditions. Ann Otolaryngol Chir Cervicofac. 2007;124(Suppl 1):S11–5.
41. Vajsakovic D, Maslin M, Searchfield GD. Principles and methods for psychoacoustic evaluation of tinnitus. Curr Top Behav Neurosci. 2021;51:419–59.
42. Crummer RW, Hassan GA. Diagnostic approach to tinnitus. Am Fam Physician. 2004;69(1):120–6.
43. Moller AR. Similarities between severe tinnitus and chronic pain. J Am Acad Audiol. 2000;11(3):115–24.
44. De Meulemeester K, Meeus M, Dhooge I, Taevernier A, Van Elslander M, Cagnie B, et al. Comparing tinnitus, pain, psychosocial and cognitive factors between patients with tinnitus and pain: A systematic review. J Psychosom Res. 2023;168:111201.
45. Norris CD, Koontz NA. Secondary otalgia: referred pain pathways and pathologies. AJNR Am J Neuroradiol. 2020;41(12):2188–98.
46. Stone KE. Otitis externa. Pediatr Rev. 2007;28(2):77–8. discussion 8.
47. Jackson EA, Geer K. Acute otitis externa: rapid evidence review. Am Fam Physician. 2023;107(2):145–51.
48. Rosenfeld RM, Schwartz SR, Cannon CR, Roland PS, Simon GR, Kumar KA, et al. Clinical practice guideline: acute otitis externa. Otolaryngol Head Neck Surg. 2014;150(1 Suppl):S1–s24.
49. Schilder AG, Chonmaitree T, Cripps AW, Rosenfeld RM, Casselbrant ML, Haggard MP, et al. Otitis media. Nat Rev Dis Primers. 2016;2(1):16063.
50. Mustafa A, Debry C, Wiorowski M, Martin E, Gentine A. Treatment of acute mastoiditis: report of 31 cases over a ten year period. Rev Laryngol Otol Rhinol (Bord). 2004;125(3):165–9.
51. Wilson E, Jenner L, Paul SP. Mastoiditis: on the rise again? Br J Nurs. 2017;26(10):542.
52. Bridwell RE, Koyfman A, Long B. High risk and low prevalence diseases: acute mastoiditis. Am J Emerg Med. 2024;79:63–9.
53. Hickham M, Amedee RG. Malignant otitis externa. J La State Med Soc. 1996;148(12):511–3.
54. Marina S, Goutham MK, Rajeshwary A, Vadisha B, Devika T. A retrospective review of 14 cases of malignant otitis externa. J Otol. 2019;14(2):63–6.

55. Reñé R, Mas A, Villabona C, Ricart MC, Bassa A, Tolosa F. Otitis externa maligna and cranial neuropathy. Neurologia. 1990;5(7):222.
56. Sudhoff H, Rajagopal S, Mani N, Moumoulidis I, Axon PR, Moffat D. Usefulness of CT scans in malignant external otitis: effective tool for the diagnosis, but of limited value in predicting outcome. Eur Arch Otorrinolaringol. 2008;265(1):53–6.
57. Rubin J, Curtin HD, Yu VL, Kamerer DB. Malignant external otitis: utility of CT in diagnosis and follow-up. Radiology. 1990;174(2):391–4.
58. Nurhadi F. Otitis media complications: Labyrinthitis. KESANS Int J oHealth Sci. 2022;1:467.
59. Dehner LP, Chen KT. Primary tumors of the external and middle ear. Benign and malignant glandular neoplasms. Arch Otolaryngol. 1980;106(1):13–9.
60. Dubernard X, Kleiber JC, Brenet E, Louges MA, Veleine Y, Labrousse M, et al. The tumors of the ear. Presse Med. 2017;46(11):1079–88.
61. Veillon F, Moulin G, Roedlich M, Blonde E, Tongio J. Imaging of tumors and pseudotumors of the ear. J Radiol. 1999;
62. Robinson M, Pemberton M, Sloan P. Salivary gland diseases, Soames' & Southam's Oral Pathology, Fifth Edition. https://doi.org/10.1093/oso/9780199697786.003.0009.
63. Ogle OE. Salivary gland diseases. Dent Clin N Am. 2020;64(1):87–104.
64. Proctor GB, Carpenter GH. Salivary secretion: mechanism and neural regulation. Monogr Oral Sci. 2014;24:14–29.
65. Su YX, Zhang K, Ke ZF, Zheng GS, Chu M, Liao GQ. Increased calcium and decreased magnesium and citrate concentrations of submandibular/sublingual saliva in sialolithiasis. Arch Oral Biol. 2010;55(1):15–20.
66. Bakshi SS. A hard calculus: submandibular Sialolithiasis. Am J Med. 2017;130(2):161–2.
67. Stelmach R, Pawłowski M, Klimek L, Janas A. Biochemical structure, symptoms, location and treatment of sialoliths. J Dent Sci. 2016;11(3):299–303.
68. Zenk J, Constantinidis J, Kydles S, Hornung J, Iro H. Clinical and diagnostic findings of sialolithiasis. HNO. 1999;47(11):963–9.
69. Rzymska-Grala I, Stopa Z, Grala B, Gołębiowski M, Wanyura H, Zuchowska A, et al. Salivary gland calculi – contemporary methods of imaging. Pol J Radiol. 2010;75(3):25–37.
70. Manomani B, Jesudas PC, Kumar SK, Ilanila M, Priscilla PJS. Imaging modalities in Sialolithiasis. Glob J Res Anal. 2022; https://doi.org/10.36106/gjra/7407015.
71. Lenka S, Subudhi SK, Padihary S. Sialadenitis: a review of the literature. Indian J Forensic Med Toxicol. 2020;
72. Michael J, Kim AM, Gerold DJ. Salivary gland disorders: rapid evidence review. Am Fam Physician. 2024;109(6):550–9.
73. Francis CL, Larsen CG. Pediatric sialadenitis. Otolaryngol Clin N Am. 2014;47(5):763–78.
74. Zenk J, Iro H, Klintworth N, Lell M. Diagnostic imaging in sialadenitis. Oral Maxillofac Surg Clin North Am. 2009;21(3):275–92.
75. Yousem DM, Kraut MA, Chalian AA. Major salivary gland imaging. Radiology. 2000;216(1):19–29.
76. Abdel Razek AAK, Mukherji S. Imaging of sialadenitis. Neuroradiol J. 2017;30(3):205–15.
77. Bradley PJ. Frequency and histopathology by site, major pathologies, symptoms and signs of salivary gland neoplasms. Adv Otorhinolaryngol. 2016;78:9–16.
78. Borner U, Stow NW, Landis BN. Pleomorphic adenoma of the parotid gland. Am J Med. 2016;129(1):e1–2.
79. Yuan WH, Hsu HC, Chou YH, Hsueh HC, Tseng TK, Tiu CM. Gray-scale and color Doppler ultrasonographic features of pleomorphic adenoma and Warthin's tumor in major salivary glands. Clin Imaging. 2009;33(5):348–53.
80. Bogaert J, Hermans R, Baert AL. Pleomorphic adenoma of the parotid gland. J Belg Radiol. 1993;76(5):307–10.
81. Palacios E, Valvassori G. Parotid mass: pleomorphic adenoma (mixed tumor). Ear Nose Throat J. 1999;78(10):746–7.
82. Woo SH, Choi DS, Kim JP, Park JJ, Joo YH, Chung PS, et al. Two-phase computed tomography study of warthin tumor of parotid gland: differentiation from other parotid gland tumors and its pathologic explanation. J Comput Assist Tomogr. 2013;37(4):518–24.
83. Ikeda M, Motoori K, Hanazawa T, Nagai Y, Yamamoto S, Ueda T, et al. Warthin tumor of the parotid gland: diagnostic value of MR imaging with histopathologic correlation. AJNR Am J Neuroradiol. 2004;25(7):1256–62.
84. Minami M, Tanioka H, Oyama K, Itai Y, Eguchi M, Yoshikawa K, et al. Warthin tumor of the parotid gland: MR-pathologic correlation. AJNR Am J Neuroradiol. 1993;14(1):209–14.
85. Rodriguez CP, Parvathaneni U, Méndez E, Martins RG. Salivary gland malignancies. Hematol Oncol Clin North Am. 2015;29(6):1145–57.
86. Young A, Okuyemi OT. Malignant salivary gland tumors. In: StatPearls. Treasure Island (FL): StatPearls Publishing. Copyright © 2025, StatPearls Publishing LLC.; 2025.
87. Cantisani V, David E, Sidhu PS, Sacconi B, Greco A, Pandolfi F, et al. Parotid gland lesions: multiparametric ultrasound and MRI features. Ultraschall Med. 2016;37(5):454–71.
88. Wang Y, Guo X, Yu K, Shen X, Liu J, Zhao T, et al. Adenoid cystic carcinoma of head and neck: summary and review of imaging findings. Heliyon. 2023;9(11):e21901.

11 Imaging for Osseous Pathology of the Maxillofacial Skeleton: Osteomyelitis, Jaw Tumors, Osteoradionecrosis, and Medicine-Related Osteonecrosis of the Jaw

Cameron J. Szelesi, Benjamin T. Barbetta, and Jerold E. Armstrong

11.1 Introduction

When evaluating patients with orofacial pain and temporomandibular joint disorder (TMJD), it is critically important that the practitioner expands their clinical focus to include diseases of the maxillofacial skeleton and systemic conditions which either present with or are directly or indirectly related to jaw pain and pathology. Bone infections, tumors, osteoradionecrosis (ORN), and medicine-related osteonecrosis of the jaw (MRONJ) are often discovered through systematic detailed patient interviews. Limiting the focus of a history and physical examination to the head and neck region can be problematic as it may result in an incomplete picture of the patient's health and well-being. Pairing a comprehensive history and physical exam with well-selected imaging provides the astute practitioner the information essential to form a complete clinical picture for an individual patient. This chapter provides a broad overview of the imaging for diseases including osteomyelitis, jaw tumors, ORN, and MRONJ.

C. J. Szelesi (✉)
Henry Ford Health – Henry Ford Hospital, Detroit, MI, USA
e-mail: cszeles1@hfhs.org; BBarbet1@hfhs.org

B. T. Barbetta · J. E. Armstrong
Henry Ford Health – Henry Ford Hospital, Detroit, MI, USA

Michigan State University, East Lansing, MI, USA
e-mail: joejarmstr8@hfhs.org

11.2 Anatomy and Physiology

Comprehensive understanding of the anatomy and physiology of the maxillofacial skeleton is a prerequisite to understand its interrelationship with the myriad of medications and diseases that affect this region. The maxillofacial skeleton provides a foundational role in facilitating human life and sensation. The skeleton of the head and neck supports the body's respiratory system and allows for the exchange of gases. The skull provides a conduit via the ear canal where air and bone interface to transform sound waves into electrical signals which we perceive as hearing. It encloses the orbits and transmits cranial nerves responsible for vision, smell, taste, and touch. The face, skull, and cervical vertebra protect the brain and spinal cord which is the epicenter of conscious thought, movement, and sensation. Additionally, the ginglymoarthrodial temporomandibular joint provides a complicated articulation with the temporal bone. In conjunction with the oral cavity, teeth, tongue, trachea, vocal

G. A. Kaspo, G. D. Klasser (eds.), *Orofacial and Head Pain*,
https://doi.org/10.1007/978-3-032-08275-6_11

cords, and salivary glands, it facilitates mastication of food and speech. The additional complex interrelationship of glands, nerves, blood vessels, tendons, muscle, fat, and other tissues makes the head and neck the most complex portion of the human anatomy. The intricacy of this system is a benefit, as comprehension of these systems aids in the diagnosis and treatment of diseases in this region when abnormalities arise. Paired with sophisticated imaging, accurate and detailed diagnosis can be performed.

11.3 Bone

Macroscopically, bone appears as an invariable organ. Composed of a thick and regular outer cortex overlying a softer meshwork of medullary bone, imaging studies focus on identifying disruptions of this pattern. However, at the microscopic level, bone is continuously being modified, repaired, and replaced. Bone is a porous substance composed of cylindrically arranged osteons. Further magnification will reveal multiple concentric osteocytes containing lamellae which surround a central Haversian canal. This shelters the lacunocanilicular network of bone cells critical for bone physiology [1]. Homeostasis of bone metabolism relies on a continuous and powerful process of resorbing old or damaged bone by osteoclasts and laying down of a new osteoid matrix produced by osteoblasts, with immature osteoid subsequently becoming fully mineralized bone. Remodeling of bone is a tightly regulated process involving numerous multifunctional growth factors (BMP family, PDGF), regulators (calcium), the osteoprotegerin (OPG) and NF-κB (RANK)/NF-κB ligand (RANKL) system, and calciotropic hormones (parathyroid hormone, sex steroids, etc.). The OPG/RANK/RANKL pathway is the dominating regulatory pathway involved in osteoclast differentiation, a pathway that begins with macrophage colony-stimulating factor (M-CSF) [2]. Osteoblasts are a checkpoint in the process of osteoclast differentiation as they control the membrane presentation of RANKL where an osteoclast's RANK membrane receptor will bind and promote bone resorption. OPG also maintains a critical role as a decoy that binds RANKL in the place of RANK inhibiting osteoclastic activation. The ratio of OPG:RANKL is often used to determine whether bone is undergoing maturation or resorption. Additionally, estrogen plays a key function in the pathway as it increases the OPG:RANKL ratio, favoring a state of bone formation. Postmenopausal loss of estrogens can lead to osteoporotic changes. The use of antiresorptive drugs including bisphosphonates and RANKL inhibitors (denosumab) have been important tools in the fight against osteoporotic fractures and have found additional benefit in the adjunctive treatment of patients with bone cancer, multiple myeloma, Paget's disease, and others [3, 4]. Antiresorptive medication choices have also expanded with focus on the OPG/RANK/RANKL system with the development of targeted monoclonal antibody pharmacologic therapy [5]. These relationships have the unfortunate side effect of predisposing patients to the development of MRONJ via disruption of the osteoblastic and osteoclastic activity in normal bone physiology. The role of parathyroid hormone (PTH) in bone metabolism is critical and is associated with the rate at which PTH is expressed in vivo. A continuous rate of PTH secretion, as seen in primary hyperparathyroidism, leads to a decrease in OPG:RANKL ratio, thus promoting osteoclastic differentiation [6]. This is in contrast to pulsatile PTH secretion which promotes bone anabolism [6]. Bone morphogenic proteins (BMPs) are a family of growth factors that are involved in regulation of bone metabolism. The highest studied BMPs, notably −2, −4, −5, −6, −7 and −9, have not only been shown to cause bone-inducing ability but bone resorption as well, thus impacting overall bone homeostasis [7]. BMPs are part of a much bigger family of the TGFβ superfamily [7]. This dual effect seen in BMP signaling is involved in the pathological disorders causing inflammatory infiltration impacting bones and joints. Disruptions of the process of bone metabolism and homeostasis lead to pathological processes which require intervention to reduce morbidity and mortality in patients with head and neck pathology.

11.4 Imaging Choices

Cysts, tumors, bony lesions, infections, and bone necrosis of the maxilla and mandible often have the opportunity to be detected utilizing panoramic radiography [8]. It is an image advantageous in detecting pathology, surgical planning, and follow-up. Its advantages include the minimal cost and widespread availability, minimal radiation dose, the ability to view a single image providing information for a large portion of the maxillofacial skeleton [9], the ability to focus an image in a "focal trough," minimal impact of metallic artifact on the film which is common with dental restorative materials, and relative ease in obtaining. It is estimated that over 320 million dental imaging procedures were completed in the United States in 2016, which comprises nearly 46% of all diagnostic imaging and nuclear medicine procedures nationwide, a portion of which include panoramic films [10]. Additionally, panoramic radiographs deliver between 19 and 75 μSv of ionizing radiation, compared to adult cone beam computed tomography (CBCT) with a large field of view which delivers between 68 and 1073 μSv and conventional CT delivering 860–1500 μSv [10]. With these factors in mind, panoramic radiography is a clear best choice as a first-line radiograph in multiple clinical presentations. In fact, due to the ubiquity of panoramic radiography as an imaging modality, there have been a number of projects related to real-time object-detecting deep convolutional neural networks evaluating panoramic images. This work represents multiple attempts at creating artificial intelligence (AI) programs aimed at identifying abnormalities on the study, using pattern recognition to alert providers of the possibility of abnormal findings [11]. This type of AI may become more reliable and integrated in the future. Panoramic radiography does have some disadvantages. It is impractical to obtain panoramic radiographs on critically ill patients, as the exam is non-portable and requires proper patient positioning to achieve a diagnostic quality image. Patients must be able to stand or be positioned in a wheelchair for the study. Also, overlying structures and projection of these structures onto the final image, along with distortion by the imaging modality, make accurate estimation of the size and position of items of interest difficult to precisely and reliably acquire. Panoramic radiographs also do not provide reliable interpretation of soft tissue structures [11]. In fact, CBCT also has very poor differentiation of facial soft tissue, making panoramic radiographs and CBCT both poor choices when evaluation of soft tissue is required [12]. Alternatively, contrast-enhanced CT [12], MRI, [13], and nuclear medicine studies, i.e., positron emissions tomography (PET) CT [14], provide far better utility for soft tissue imaging and should be considered when that is required. While ultrasound is used extensively as an adjunct for treatment of patients with head and neck abnormalities, the diagnostic use of ultrasound for head and neck pathology including cysts, tumors, bony lesions, infections, and bone necrosis of the maxilla and mandible has limited utility. Notable exceptions to this include identification of extracranial vascular anomalies of the head and neck region [15], evaluation of lymph nodes [16, 17], and imaging of the thyroid [18, 19], parathyroid [20, 21], and salivary glands, particularly the parotid gland [22, 23]. Whenever possible, the practitioner should refer to the American College of Radiology (ACR) Appropriateness Criteria to help select imaging for a particular indication. The ACR provides criteria for both diagnostic and interventional therapy.

11.5 Osteomyelitis

Osteomyelitis simply stated means bone infection. The World Health Organization (WHO) describes osteomyelitis as an infection that occurs in both children and adults which can originate from various sources. Osteomyelitis can have many forms including hematogenous acute osteomyelitis which is predominately found in children or subacute or chronic infection that develops secondary to an open injury of bone, more common in adults [24]. Subacute hematogenous, chronic recurrent, unifocal, and multifocal osteomyelitis forms exist with some relationship to autoimmune diseases including granulomatosis with polyangiitis (formerly Wegner's granulomatosis), psoriasis, and inflammatory bowel disease [24]. When imaging patients with presumed osteomyelitis, findings such as lytic changes, sclerosis, periosteal bone formation are key [25]. Subperiosteal bone reaction/formation is an important finding. Classically referred to as "Garrè's osteomyelitis," periostitis adjacent to infected bone results in the formation of parallel layers of vital bone which are arranged parallel to the surface of the affected bone [26]. While this can occur in pathologic conditions other than osteomyelitis, it is a response to inflammation of the bones' overlying periosteum and is not a normal architectural feature.

It can be difficult to appreciate periosteal bone formation on panoramic imaging, particularly when it presents lateral to the jaw or in the same plane to the panoramic image. However, lytic changes and sclerosis can be easily identified and compared immediately to the uninvolved side.

Figure 11.1 is a panoramic radiograph obtained on a 58-year-old female who presented to the oral and maxillofacial clinic with an 8-month history of right-sided jaw pain and limited opening. Eight months prior, the right mandibular second molar tooth was removed, and despite this treatment, the patient continued to be symptomatic. The patient has been experiencing progressively worsening mouth opening for 2 months. Figure 11.2 represents a sclerotic-appearing bone present in the right mandibular angle and ascending ramus, near the horizontally impacted right mandibular wisdom tooth. There are subtle lytic changes in the right ascending ramus. The extraction socket of the right mandibular second molar demonstrates bony fill. CT scans were obtained immediately following the panoramic radiograph (Figs. 11.3, 11.4 and 11.5).

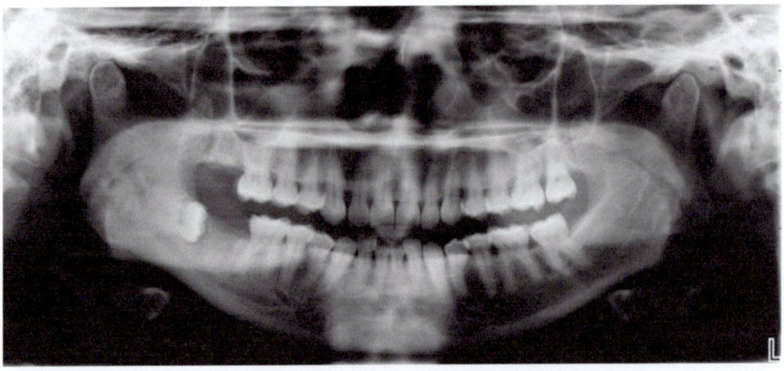

Fig. 11.1 Initial panoramic radiograph obtained on a 58-year-old female who presented to the oral and maxillofacial clinic with an 8-month history of right-sided jaw pain and limited opening

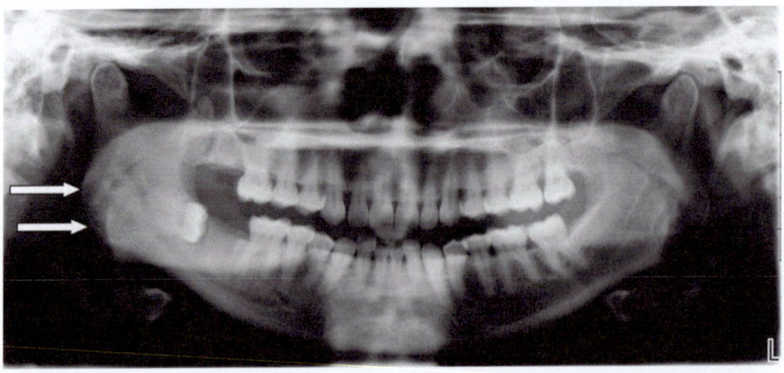

Fig. 11.2 Panoramic radiograph of sclerotic-appearing bone present in the right mandibular angle and ascending ramus, near the horizontally impacted right mandibular third molar. There are subtle lytic changes in the right ascending ramus. The extraction socket of the right mandibular second molar demonstrates bony fill

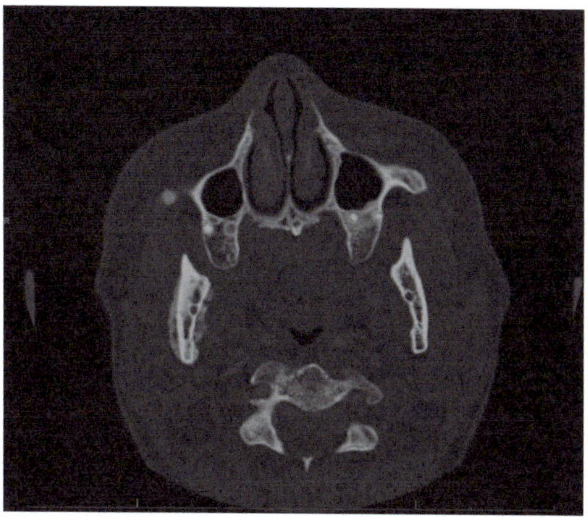

Fig. 11.3 CT scan obtained immediately following the panoramic radiograph

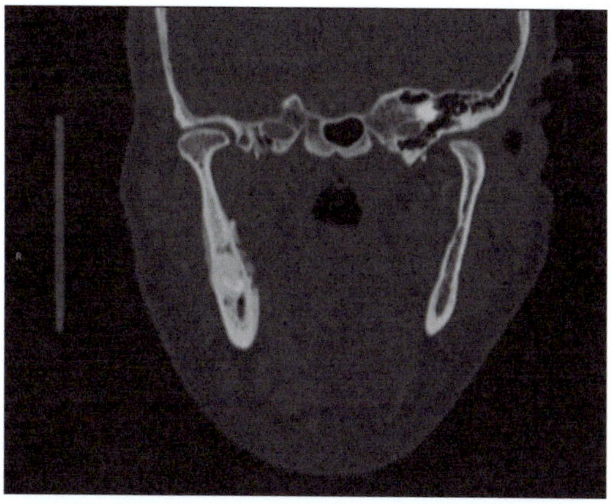

Fig. 11.4 CT scan obtained immediately following the panoramic radiograph

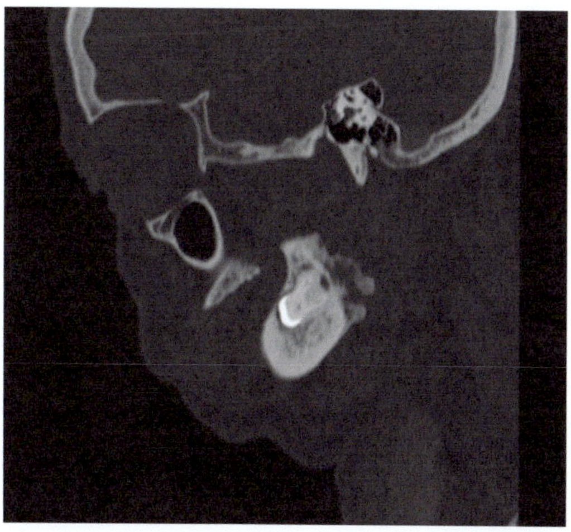

Fig. 11.5 CT scan obtained immediately following the panoramic radiograph

A biopsy of the area was completed which demonstrated devitalized bone with saprophytic bacterial colonies and acute inflammatory infiltrate, consistent with acute osteomyelitis. It is important to note how the extensive periosteal bone formation is easily identified on CT and difficult to appreciate on the panoramic radiograph.

11.6 Jaw Tumors and Cysts

Jaw tumors and cysts are a broad group of pathologic conditions which can manifest as radiodense, radiolucent, or mixed lesions in the maxillofacial skeleton. One of the hallmarks of jaw tumors and cysts is their relatively asymptomatic growth. Only when they become very large, become superinfected, result in pathologic fracture, or obstruct/offend the patient's activities of daily living do patients typically become symptomatic. However, due to the rarity of jaw tumors and cyst in the general population, the US Food and Drug Administration only recommends panoramic exams to be completed on new patients with the following criteria: (1) child with transitional dentition, (2) adolescent with permanent dentition, and (3) adult who is dentate or partially edentulous [27]. Additionally panoramic radiographs are recommended for new and recall adolescent patients with permanent dentition to assess developing third molars [27]. There is no current recommendation for use of panoramic radiography as a screening tool for jaw tumors. Due to the asymptomatic nature of jaw tumors and cysts, it is imperative to take a thorough careful history and perform a physical exam to identify patients appropriate for additional imaging (Figs. 11.6, 11.7 and 11.8).

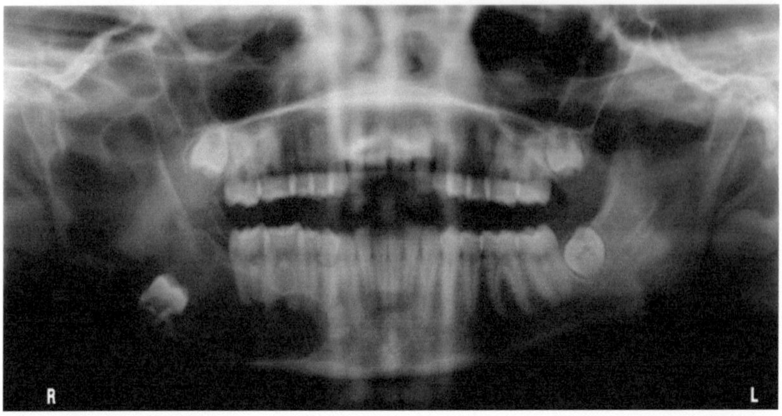

Fig. 11.6 Panoramic radiograph displays a well-circumscribed multilocular radiolucent lesion in the right mandible associated with an impacted right mandibular third molar. Following a biopsy, the diagnosis was consistent with odontogenic keratocyst

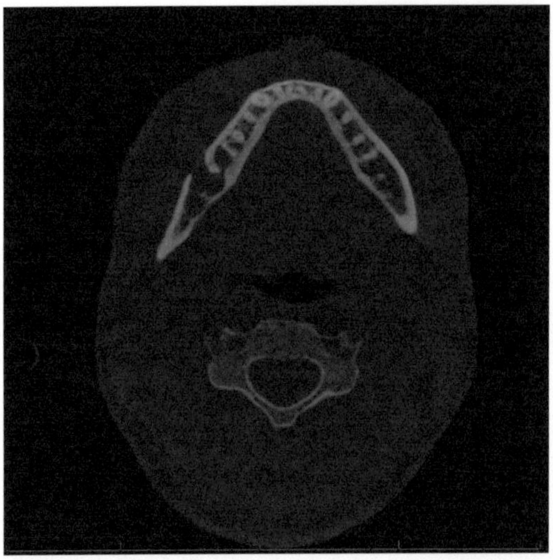

Fig. 11.7 CBCT shows a multilocular radiolucency in the right mandible with buccal cortical erosion. A subsequent biopsy was consistent with odontogenic keratocyst

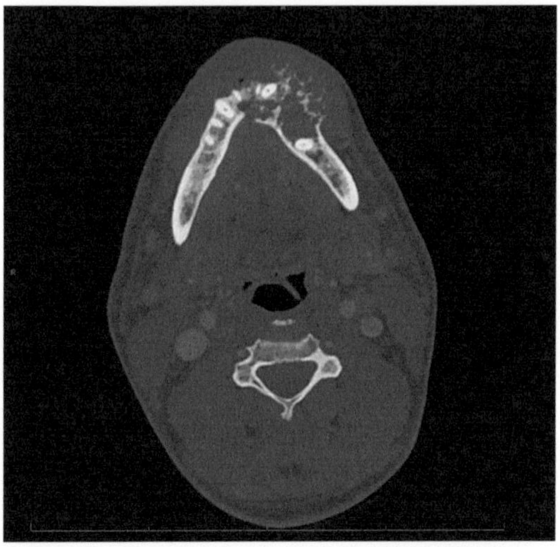

Fig. 11.8 Axial contrast-enhanced CT demonstrates an ill-defined destructive anterior mandibular lesion with cortical breakthrough. Lesion is mixed density and associated with facial asymmetry. Biopsy provided the diagnosis of ameloblastoma (follicular acanthomatous type)

11.7 Osteoradionecrosis

Osteoradionecrosis (ORN) of the jaw is a serious complication of ionizing radiation to the head and neck. ORN is classically defined as an area of exposed, necrotic bone that has been exposed to ionizing radiation and fails to heal within 3–6 months [28]. However, there have also been cases with radiographic evidence of necrosis with intact overlying mucosa present [28]. Various other local risk factors which have been linked to ORN include initial tumor depth of invasion, trauma, and trauma from dental treatment. Systemic factors that increase risk include smoking, alcohol consumption, and immunodeficiency [29]. Smoking and trauma to the area of the jaw previously exposed to ≥60 Gy of ionizing radiation are associated with increased ORN risk and carry the highest predictive factor. A 1-year incidence of 23% increase in risk of developing ORN in this population has been documented [30] (Figs. 11.9 and 11.10).

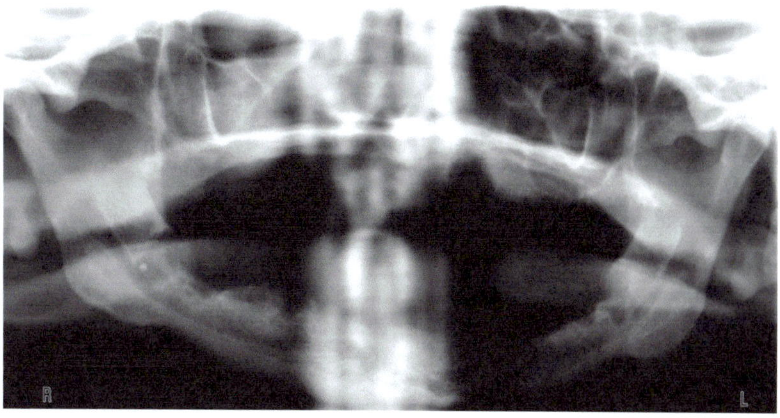

Fig. 11.9 Panoramic radiograph displaying lytic lesion changes associated with the maxilla and mandible in a patient who underwent radiation therapy (70 Gy of ionizing radiation over a 7-week course) for tonsillar squamous cell carcinoma

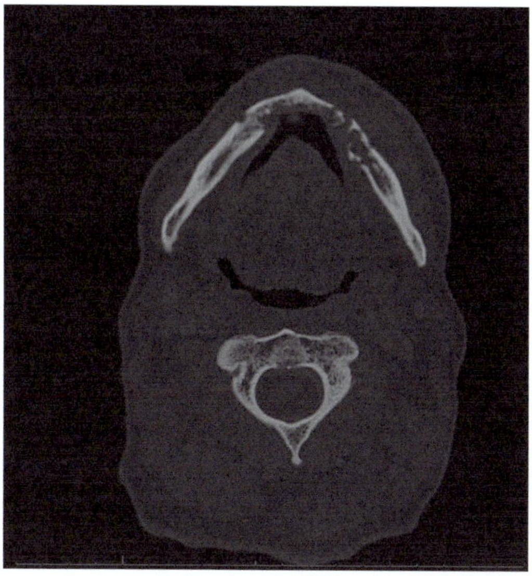

Fig. 11.10 Axial CT demonstrating a lytic lesion in the anterior left mandible with loss of the lingual cortical plate. There is simultaneous erosion of the buccal cortical plate in the left parasymphysis region of the jaw

11.8 Medication-Related Osteonecrosis of the Jaw

Medication-related osteonecrosis of the jaw (MRONJ) is a debilitating condition that can arise in patients who previously took or are currently taking antiresorptive or antiangiogenic agents, without a history of radiation therapy. Bisphosphonates are a family of widely used antiresorptive medications that act at a cellular level to target and inhibit osteoclast function. These medications have been established as the standard of care, first-line treatment regimen for hypercalcemia of malignancy, multiple myeloma, breast cancer, and metastatic bone lesions [31]. Bisphosphonates are also the current treatment of choice for managing osteoporosis [31]. Antiresorptive medication use have been shown to predispose patients to osteonecrosis of the jaw (ONJ), particularly in the presence of local risk factors [31]. Medications other than bisphosphonates have been implicated in the disease process of MRONJ. Denosumab is an antiresorptive monoclonal antibody that acts as an anti-RANKL antibody. Denosumab has the same mechanism of action as OPG, blocking RANK/RANKL interaction [32]. It has been reported that the risk of developing MRONJ in osteoporotic patients taking denosumab is 0.01–0.03%, while in cancer patients, this risk increases to 1–2% [33]. Antiangiogenic medications have also been correlated with developing MRONJ. These are sophisticated pharmacologic targets of vascular endothelial growth factor (VEGF) receptors [34] with a goal to prevent metastatic spread of cancer through the blood and lymphatics [35]. More common now is the use of antiangiogenic medications such as tyrosine kinase inhibitors that block the VEGF receptor and the downstream signaling pathways (i.e., sunitinib) and monoclonal antibiotics that bind VEGF (i.e., bevacizumab) [35] (Figs. 11.11, 11.12 and 11.13).

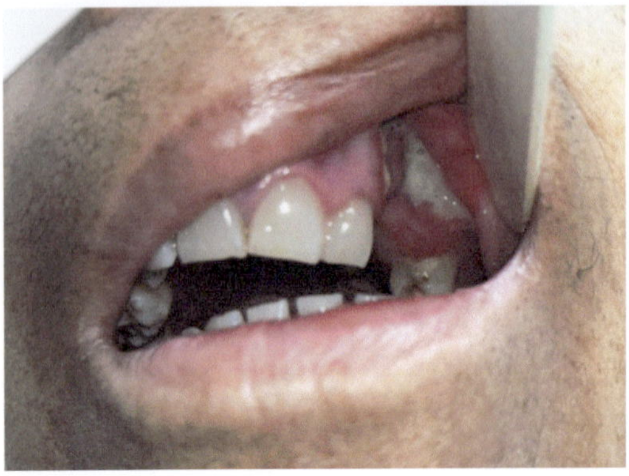

Fig. 11.11 Exposed bone in the left maxilla following the extraction of the maxillary left canine and first premolar tooth in a patient with a history of breast primary metastatic carcinoma with a history of using a bisphosphonate

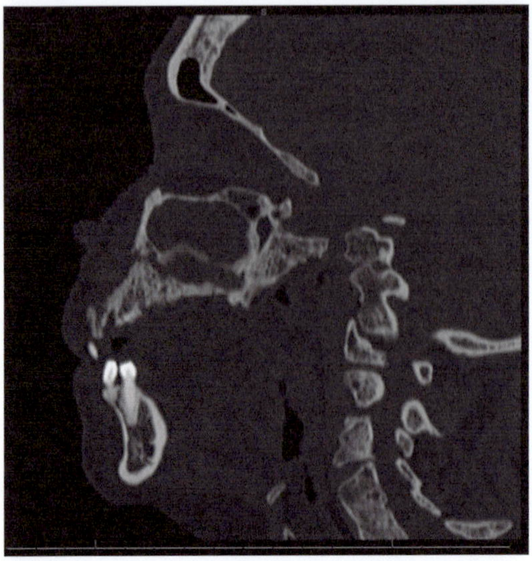

Fig. 11.13 CT demonstrates heterogeneous demineralization of the maxilla with a serpiginous osseous defect along the base of the maxillary sinus

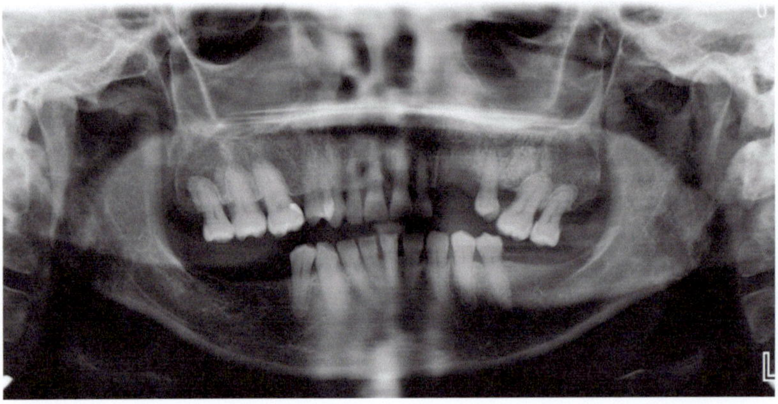

Fig. 11.12 Panoramic radiograph displaying sclerosis of the maxillary alveolar ridge with incomplete bony healing 1 year after extraction of left maxillary canine and first premolar. Note the opacification of maxillary sinus. A biopsy of the involved area was taken which reported osteonecrosis, acute osteomyelitis, and dense bacterial colonization consistent with the diagnosis of MRONJ

11.9 Conclusion

Imaging for the pathologic conditions of osteomyelitis, jaw tumors, ORN, and MRONJ, particularly for the diagnostic assessment, can be focused on the use of panoramic radiographs and CT. It is important to remember that when dealing with infection or tumor spread into the soft tissue, medical-based CT scans are superior to CBCT. These provide the ability to better assess the soft tissue and provide the opportunity to use intravenous contrast dye as indicated. When bone-only imaging is required, CBCT is an excellent choice secondary to its extremely fine resolution and reduced radiation dose. Imaging modalities such as MRI, nuclear medicine studies, and ultrasound are important adjuncts but should not be considered as a first-line tool for diagnosis of the discussed conditions in most situations. Thorough history taking and clinical examination of patients often provide clues to abnormalities which can trigger the decision to pursue imaging, as its use is not recommended as a screening tool.

References

1. Li X, Sun Y, Chen J, et al. A 3-dimensional scaffolding system recapitulates the hierarchical osteon structure. ACS Omega. 2024;9(40):41368–77.
2. Khosla S. Minireview: the OPG/RANKL/RANK system. Endocrinology. 2001;142(12):5050–5.
3. Karimi D, Osella G, Bacchetta J, et al. A multi-center observation study on medication-related osteonecrosis of the jaw (MRONJ) in patients with osteoporosis, and other non-malignant bone diseases, in northwestern Italy over 16 years. Biomedicine. 2024;12(10):2179.
4. Ayalon-Dangur I, Simanovich E, Zilber S, et al. Long-term effectiveness of zoledronic acid in patients with Paget's disease of bone – a retrospective cohort study. Endocrine. 2024;85(2):873–82.
5. Reid IR, Miller PD, Brown JP, Kendler DL, Fahrleitner-Pammer A, Valter I, et al. Effects of denosumab on bone histomorphometry: the FREEDOM and STAND studies. J Bone Miner Res. 2010;25(10):2256–65.
6. Eriksen EF. Cellular mechanisms of bone remodeling. Rev Endocr Metab Disord. 2010;11(4):219–27.
7. Bordukalo-Nikšić T, Kufner V, Vukičević S. The role of BMPs in the regulation of osteoclasts resorption and bone remodeling: from experimental models to clinical applications. Front Immunol. 2022;13:869422.
8. Yang H, Kim H, Park K, et al. Deep learning for automated detection of cyst and tumors of the jaw in panoramic radiographs. J Clin Med. 2020;9(6):1839.
9. Choi JW. Assessment of panoramic radiography as a National Oral Examination Tool: review of the literature. Imaging Sci Dent. 2011;41(1):1.
10. Benavides E, Koivisto R, Vu T. Optimizing radiation safety in dentistry. J Am Dent Assoc. 2024;155(4):280.
11. MacDonald D, Telyakova V. An overview of cone-beam computed tomography and dental panoramic radiography in dentistry in the community. Tomography. 2024;10(8):1222–37.
12. Vishwanath V, Sudhakar A, Nair P, et al. The role of imaging in head and neck cancer: an overview of different imaging modalities in primary diagnosis and staging of the disease. J Contemp Brachytherapy. 2020;12(5):512–8.
13. Driessen DAJJ, Eisenblaetter M, Serres SR, et al. High-accuracy nodal staging of head and neck cancer with USPIO-enhanced MRI. Investig Radiol. 2022;57(12):810–8.
14. Banjare AK, Dandapat S, Patra A, et al. Role of the FDG pet CT scan in pretreatment evaluation of oral carcinomas. Indian J Otolaryngol Head Neck Surg. 2024;76(6):5346–52.
15. Nocini R, Franchi L, Ferri A, et al. Image-based artificial intelligence models in the diagnosis and classification of vascular anomalies of the soft tissue in the head and neck. Comput Methods Programs Biomed. 2025;259:108525.
16. Sievert M, Müller A, Fischer M, et al. Sonographie des halses – Differenzialdiagnostische Aspekte. HNO. 2023;71(11):750–62.
17. Guerrisi A, Cantisani V, Giganti F, et al. Quantitative ultrasound radiomics analysis to evaluate lymph nodes in patients with cancer: a systematic review. Ultraschall Med. 2024;45(6):586–96.
18. Edwards MK, Daniels RH, Crowell MD. Inappropriate use of thyroid ultrasound: a systematic review and meta-analysis. Endocrine. 2021;74(2):263–9.
19. Leenhardt L, Erdogan MF, Hegedüs L, et al. 2013 European Thyroid Association Guidelines for cervical ultrasound scan and ultrasound-guided techniques in the postoperative management of patients with thyroid cancer. Eur Thyroid J. 2013;2(3):147–59.
20. Michaelsen SH, Rasmussen MH, Lindebjerg B, et al. The detection of pathological parathyroid glands is facilitated by identifying vascular features on ultrasound: the potential benefit of a low-frequency vascular probe. Endocrine. 2024;86(3):1131–9.
21. Chou SE, Yeh ML, Tsai CS, et al. Addressing the challenges of missed parathyroid glands in ultrasonography for secondary hyperparathyroidism: a retrospective observational study. Ann Surg Treat Res. 2024;107(3):136.
22. Li X, Wang T, Lin H, et al. Imaging-based diagnosis and classification of radioactive iodine-induced sialadenitis. Oral Dis. 2023;30(7):4303–11.
23. Lianou AD, Papadopoulos V, Ioannidis G, et al. The importance of elastography in the early diagnosis of highly differentiated parotid tumors: a case report. Maedica (Bucur). 2024;19(3):652.
24. Mousa HA. Bone infection. East Mediterr Health J. 2003;9(1–2):208–14.
25. Yfanti Z, Papadopoulou A, Karaliotas C, et al. Radiologic findings of osteonecrosis, osteoradionecrosis, osteomyelitis, and jaw metastatic disease with cone beam CT. Eur J Radiol. 2024;173:111387.
26. Tong ACK, Wu PC, Lee SY, et al. Osteomyelitis with proliferative periostitis: an unusual case. Oral Surg Oral Med Oral Pathol Oral Radiol Endod. 2006;102(5):e64–7.
27. Dental radiographic examinations recommendations for patient selection and limiting radiation exposure. https://www.fda.gov/media/84818/download.
28. Store G, Boysen M. Mandibular osteoradionecrosis: clinical behaviour and diagnostic aspects. Clin Otolaryngol Allied Sci. 2000;25:378–84.
29. Lee IJ, Koom WS, Lee CG, et al. Risk factors and dose-effect relationship for mandibular osteoradione-

crosis in oral and oropharyngeal cancer patients. Int J Radiat Oncol Biol Phys. 2009;75(4):1084–91.
30. Möring MM, Mast H, Wolvius EB, Verduijn GM, Petit SF, Sijtsema ND, et al. Osteoradionecrosis after postoperative radiotherapy for oral cavity cancer: a retrospective cohort study. Oral Oncol. 2022;133:106056.
31. Ruggiero SL. Bisphosphonate-related osteonecrosis of the jaw (BRONJ): initial discovery and subsequent development. J Oral Maxillofac Surg. 2009;67:13–8.
32. Shibahara T. Antiresorptive agent-related osteonecrosis of the jaw (ARONJ): a twist of fate in the bone. Tohoku J Exp Med. 2019;247:75–86.
33. Khan AA, Morrison A, Kendler DL, et al. Case-based review of osteonecrosis of the jaw (ONJ) and application of the international recommendations for management from the International Task Force on ONJ. J Clin Densitom. 2017;20:8–24.
34. Kuroshima S, Sasaki M, Sawase T. Medication-related osteonecrosis of the jaw: a literature review. J Oral Biosci. 2019;61:99–104.
35. Lombard T, Neirinckx V, Rogister B, Gilon Y, Wislet S. Medication-related osteonecrosis of the jaw: new insights into molecular mechanisms and cellular therapeutic approaches. Stem Cells Int. 2016;2016:8768162.

Imaging Neoplastic and Non-neoplastic Conditions in Neck and Cervical Region

12

Ghabi A. Kaspo and Gary D. Klasser

12.1 Introduction

Neck and facial pain can arise from various conditions, ranging from musculoskeletal disorders and nerve dysfunction to neoplastic processes. Understanding the different etiologies of pain in this region is critical for accurate diagnosis and appropriate treatment. This chapter explores both neoplastic and non-neoplastic causes of neck and facial pain, focusing on mechanisms, clinical presentations, and diagnostic approaches, including the utility of imaging.

Neck masses in adults should be considered potentially malignant until proven otherwise, as they are often the first sign of head and neck cancer [1, 2]. Accurate diagnosis requires a thorough history, physical examination, and targeted imaging [3, 4].

Clinical factors such as patient age, mass duration, and size can help predict neoplasia [5]. Sudden-onset, intermittent, sharp facial pain without improvement may indicate occult malignancy [6]. While most persistent neck masses in adults are neoplasms, clinicians should also consider non-neoplastic causes such as infection, particularly in children [4, 7].

12.2 Non-neoplastic Causes of Neck and Facial Pain

12.2.1 Musculoskeletal Causes

Neck and facial pain can have various non-neoplastic causes, including musculoskeletal, neurological, and systemic conditions [8, 9]. Other musculoskeletal causes include cervical muscle strain, disc herniation, and whiplash injuries [10]. Neurological conditions like trigeminal neuralgia and cluster headaches can also contribute to facial pain [11]. The cervical spine and stomatognathic system are closely associated with craniofacial pain, though more high-quality studies are needed to clarify this relationship [12]. Central sensitization may explain the connection between cervical and temporomandibular nociceptive neurons and primary headaches [13]. In children, it is crucial to distinguish between structural and non-structural causes of facial pain for appropriate treatment [4].

G. A. Kaspo (✉)
Henry Ford Health Systrem, Henry Ford Hospital, Department of Otolaryngology, Royal Oak, Michigan, USA

Wayne State University, Department of Psychiatry, Detroit, Michigan, USA
e-mail: drkaspo@facialpainclinic.com

G. D. Klasser
Louisiana State University Health Sciences Center, School of Dentistry, Department of Diagnostic Sciences, New Orleans, LA, USA
e-mail: gklass@lsuhso.edu

G. A. Kaspo, G. D. Klasser (eds.), *Orofacial and Head Pain*,
https://doi.org/10.1007/978-3-032-08275-6_12

12.2.2 Neurological Causes

Neurological disorders can contribute to neck and facial pain by affecting the nerves that supply these regions. Trigeminal neuralgia is a severe condition characterized by intense, electric shock-like facial pain due to irritation of the trigeminal nerve [14]. Occipital neuralgia results from compression or irritation of the occipital nerves, causing sharp, radiating pain from the neck to the scalp and face. Glossopharyngeal neuralgia is a rare disorder that presents with severe throat, ear, and jaw pain, typically triggered by swallowing or talking. Cervical radiculopathy, which occurs when nerve roots in the cervical spine are compressed, can lead to pain radiating from the neck to the head, face, and arms [15, 16].

12.2.3 Inflammatory and Systemic Causes

Inflammatory and systemic conditions can also contribute to neck and facial pain. Rheumatoid arthritis (RA), an autoimmune disorder, can cause chronic inflammation of the cervical vertebrae, leading to pain and stiffness [17, 18]. Fibromyalgia, a chronic pain syndrome, results in widespread musculoskeletal pain, including the neck and face [11, 19]. Myofascial pain syndrome, characterized by trigger points in the masticatory and neck muscles, often refers pain to the jaw, temples, and face [20]. Cervicogenic headaches, which originate from dysfunction in the cervical spine, frequently radiate to the head and face [12]. Meningitis, an infection that inflames the meninges, can cause severe neck pain, stiffness, and associated headaches [21].

12.3 Neoplastic Causes of Neck and Facial Pain

12.3.1 Head and Neck Cancers

Neoplastic conditions of the head and neck can present with persistent pain due to tumor invasion, nerve compression, or local inflammation [6]. Glossopharyngeal cancer arises in the oropharynx, particularly at the base of the tongue, tonsils, or posterior pharyngeal wall. Patients often experience throat pain radiating to the ear and jaw, along with difficulty swallowing and voice changes [22]. This cancer can also cause glossopharyngeal neuralgia, resulting in sharp, stabbing pain in the throat and tongue.

Hypopharyngeal cancer affects the lower pharynx near the larynx and is associated with persistent neck pain that radiates to the jaw or ear [23, 24]. Patients often report a sensation of a lump in the throat and progressive dysphagia. Nasopharyngeal cancer can cause facial pain, headaches, and ear symptoms due to involvement of the trigeminal nerve, along with nasal obstruction and epistaxis.

Thyroid cancer, particularly in advanced stages, may present with neck pain radiating to the jaw and ears, along with hoarseness and difficulty swallowing [25]. Salivary gland tumors, which affect the parotid, submandibular, or minor glands, can lead to facial pain, weakness, and numbness if they invade surrounding nerves. Parapharyngeal space tumors can compress the glossopharyngeal or vagus nerve, leading to pain, dysphagia, and referred ear pain [23, 26].

12.3.2 Metastatic and Systemic Cancers

Metastatic cancers commonly spread to the cervical lymph nodes, with primary sources including lung and breast. These cancers often cause persistent, deep aching pain due to tumor invasion of nerves or blood vessels [27]. Skull base tumors, such as chordomas, chondrosarcomas, and meningiomas, can lead to facial pain, headaches, and cranial nerve deficits. Involvement of cranial nerves V, IX, and X can result in facial numbness, dysphagia, and hoarseness [28].

12.4 Diagnostic Approach

12.4.1 Clinical Evaluation

A thorough clinical evaluation is essential for identifying the underlying cause of neck and facial pain [29]. A detailed history should include the duration, nature, and progression of symptoms, along with associated neurological deficits and systemic signs such as weight loss, fever, or night sweats. Physical examination should assess cranial nerve function, TMJ status, and lymph nodes and include the oropharyngeal region [30].

12.4.2 Imaging and Testing

Imaging plays a crucial role in diagnosis. Magnetic resonance imaging (MRI) and CT scans are used to detect structural abnormalities, tumor extent, and nerve involvement. PET-CT scans help identify metastatic disease [31, 32]. For suspected neoplastic conditions, biopsy and histopathological analysis are required for definitive diagnosis. Electromyography (EMG) and nerve conduction studies may be useful in evaluating neural involvement in non-neoplastic conditions.

12.5 Management Strategies

12.5.1 Non-neoplastic Pain Management

Management for non-neoplastic conditions varies depending on the underlying cause. Medications such as NSAIDs, muscle relaxants, anticonvulsants (for neuropathic pain), and corticosteroids (for inflammatory conditions) are commonly used [33]. Physical therapy is beneficial for musculoskeletal conditions like TMJ dysfunction and cervical strain. Interventional treatments, including Botox injections, nerve blocks, and radiofrequency ablation, may be considered for persistent neuropathic pain [34, 35].

12.5.2 Neoplastic Pain Management

For neoplastic conditions, surgical resection remains the primary treatment for localized tumors. Radiotherapy and chemotherapy are employed for inoperable or metastatic cancers [36]. Palliative care focuses on pain control through opioids, nerve blocks, and supportive therapies in advanced malignancies [37, 38].

12.6 Conclusion

Neck and facial pain can result from a wide range of conditions, including musculoskeletal disorders, neurological dysfunction, inflammatory diseases, and malignancies [4, 8]. A thorough clinical evaluation, appropriate imaging, and timely intervention are crucial for differentiating non-neoplastic from neoplastic causes. By understanding the diverse sources of pain in this region, clinicians can provide targeted, effective management strategies to improve patient outcomes [39].

References

1. Marshall JA, Mahanna GK. Cancer in the differential diagnosis of orofacial pain. Dent Clin N Am. 1997;41(2):355–65.
2. Pynnonen MA, Gillespie MB, Roman B, Rosenfeld RM, Tunkel DE, Bontempo L, et al. Clinical practice guideline: evaluation of the neck mass in adults. Otolaryngol Head Neck Surg. 2017;157(2_suppl):S1–S30.
3. Stern I, Greenberg MS. Clinical assessment of patients with orofacial pain and temporomandibular disorders. Dent Clin N Am. 2013;57(3):393–404.
4. Horswell BB, Sheikh J. Evaluation of pain syndromes, headache, and temporomandibular joint disorders in children. Oral Maxillofac Surg Clin North Am. 2018;30(1):11–24.
5. Bhattacharyya N. Predictive factors for neoplasia and malignancy in a neck mass. Arch Otolaryngol Head Neck Surg. 1999;125(3):303–7.
6. Van Abel KM, Starkman S, O'Reilly AG, Price DL. Craniofacial pain secondary to occult head and neck tumors. Otolaryngol Head Neck Surg. 2014;150(5):813–7.
7. Quail G. Facial pain – a diagnostic challenge. Aust Fam Physician. 2015;44(12):901–4.
8. Manusov EG, Johnson R. Orofacial pain: diagnosis and treatment. Am Fam Physician. 1992;45(2):773–82.
9. Lilly GE. Head- and neck pain of non-dental origin. Fogorv Sz. 1998;91(11):337–46.
10. Karnath BM, editor. Identifying the musculoskeletal causes of neck pain. The Journal of Musculoskeletal Medicine; Darien. 2012;29(3):82–6.
11. Friedman MH, Nelson AJ Jr. Head and neck pain review: traditional and new perspectives. J Orthop Sports Phys Ther. 1996;24(4):268–78.

12. Armijo Olivo S, Magee DJ, Parfitt M, Major P, Thie NM. The association between the cervical spine, the stomatognathic system, and craniofacial pain: a critical review. J Orofac Pain. 2006;20(4):271–87.
13. Graff-Radford SB. Facial pain, cervical pain, and headache. Continuum (Minneap Minn). 2012;18(4):869–82.
14. Robertson C. Cranial Neuralgias. Continuum (Minneap Minn). 2021;27(3):665–85.
15. Allam AK, Larkin MB, Sharma H, Viswanathan A. Trigeminal and glossopharyngeal neuralgia. Neurol Clin. 2024;42(2):585–98.
16. Khan M, Nishi SE, Hassan SN, Islam MA, Gan SH. Trigeminal neuralgia, glossopharyngeal neuralgia, and myofascial pain dysfunction syndrome: an update. Pain Res Manag. 2017;2017:7438326.
17. Oberstein EM, Carpintero M, Hopkins A. Neck pain from a rheumatologic perspective. Phys Med Rehabil Clin N Am. 2011;22(3):485–502. ix
18. Klasser GD, Balasubramaniam R, Epstein J. Topical review-connective tissue diseases: orofacial manifestations including pain. J Orofac Pain. 2007;21(3):171–84.
19. Totsch SK, Sorge RE. Immune system involvement in specific pain conditions. Mol Pain. 2017;13:1744806917724559.
20. Golhar S. Correlation between myofascial pain dysfunction syndrome and cervical pain: a review. In: Modern research in dentistry; 2020.
21. VanDemark M. Acute bacterial meningitis: current review and treatment update. Crit Care Nurs Clin North Am. 2013;25(3):351–61.
22. Reiter S, Gavish A, Winocur E, Emodi-Perlman A, Eli I. Nasopharyngeal carcinoma mimicking a temporomandibular disorder: a case report. J Orofac Pain. 2006;20(1):74–81.
23. Carroll C, Jagatiya M, Kamel D, Siddiqi J. A parapharyngeal space schwannoma arising from the vagus nerve: a case report. Int J Surg Case Rep. 2017;41:22–5.
24. Macfarlane TV, Wirth T, Ranasinghe S, Ah-See KW, Renny N, Hurman D. Head and neck cancer pain: systematic review of prevalence and associated factors. J Oral Maxillofac Res. 2012;3(1):e1.
25. Romero-Reyes M, Salvemini D. Cancer and orofacial pain. Med Oral Patol Oral Cir Bucal. 2016;21(6):e665–e71.
26. Dimitrijevic MV, Jesic SD, Mikic AA, Arsovic NA, Tomanovic NR. Parapharyngeal space tumors: 61 case reviews. Int J Oral Maxillofac Surg. 2010;39(10):983–9.
27. Amit M, Eran A, Billan S, Fridman E, Na'ara S, Charas T, et al. Perineural spread in noncutaneous head and neck cancer: new insights into an old problem. J Neurol Surg B Skull Base. 2016;77(2):86–95.
28. Grisold W, Grisold A. Cancer around the brain. Neurooncol Pract. 2014;1(1):13–21.
29. Alexander E. History, physical examination, and differential diagnosis of neck pain. Phys Med Rehabil Clin N Am. 2011;22:383.
30. Bender SD. Assessment of the orofacial pain patient. Dent Clin N Am. 2018;62:525.
31. Petrou M, Mukherji SK. Extracranial head and neck neoplasms: role of imaging. In: Cancer Treat Res, vol. 143; 2008. p. 93–117.
32. Junn JC, Soderlund KA, Glastonbury CM. Imaging of head and neck cancer with CT, MRI, and US. Semin Nucl Med. 2021;51(1):3–12.
33. Busse JW, Casassus R, Carrasco-Labra A, Durham J, Mock D, Zakrzewska JM, et al. Management of chronic pain associated with temporomandibular disorders: a clinical practice guideline. BMJ. 2023;383:e076227.
34. Madhuri DH, Suresh A, Tikoo P, Ankit K, Subham P, Kemmu A. Pain relief and efficacy of surgical vs nonsurgical management of TMJ disorders: a systematic review. J Pharm Bioallied Sci. 2024;16(Suppl 4):S3071–3.
35. Argueta-Figueroa L, Flores-Mejía LA, Ávila-Curiel BX, Flores-Ferreyra BI, Torres-Rosas R. Nonpharmacological interventions for pain in patients with temporomandibular joint disorders: a systematic review. Eur J Dent. 2022;16(3):500–13.
36. Yoon SY, Oh J. Neuropathic cancer pain: prevalence, pathophysiology, and management. Korean J Intern Med. 2018;33(6):1058–69.
37. Connolly I, Zaleon C, Montagnini M. Management of severe neuropathic cancer pain: an illustrative case and review. Am J Hosp Palliat Care. 2013;30(1):83–90.
38. Paice JA. Mechanisms and management of neuropathic pain in cancer. J Support Oncol. 2003;1(2):107–20.
39. Byrd HF, Kohutek ZA. Painful realities: navigating the complexities of head and neck cancer pain. Oral Dis. 2024; https://doi.org/10.1111/odi.15150.

Imaging for Neurogenous Issues 13

Iram F. Zaman, Ali Ghanem, Mohamed Ali Garada, and Utkarsh Agarwal

13.1 Introduction

Cranio-orofacial neuralgias are pain disorders caused by dysfunction in the nerves of the face and head, with trigeminal neuralgia being the most common. Despite having a serious impact on patients' quality of life, cranio-orofacial neuralgias are underrecognized and often misdiagnosed, frequently being mistaken for dental pathologies. Thus, patients with neuralgias of the face and head often experience delayed diagnoses and therapies—sometimes receiving inappropriate treatments and unnecessary dental procedures. In this chapter, we provide a comprehensive summary of both common and rare cranio-orofacial disorders, outlining the main clinical features and key diagnostic strategies with emphasis on neuroimaging studies. Improved clinician understanding of these serious neuro-pathologies is critically needed so that patients can receive accurate, timely, and effective treatment.

13.2 Trigeminal Neuralgia

Trigeminal neuralgia (TN) is a cranial nerve disorder characterized by recurrent, brief episodes of sudden, sharp pain in the distribution of one or more of the divisions of the trigeminal nerve. The estimated annual prevalence of TN is three to five per 100,000 individuals, and while TN can affect individuals across all age groups, the peak incidence typically occurs between the ages of 37 and 67 years [1]. However, the mean age of onset varies depending on the etiology of TN, and women are more frequently affected than men, with a female-to-male ratio of 2:1.5. Notably, the pain associated with TN typically occurs on one side of the face, usually the right side, and bilateral trigeminal involvement is rare—observed in less than 5% of patients [2–5].

Although the onset of pain from TN is usually abrupt, some patients may experience a prodrome consisting of dull, lingering pain lasting for minutes to hours or a persistent constant ache before the appearance of the characteristic sharp,

I. F. Zaman (✉)
Department of Neurology, Wayne State University School of Medicine, Detroit, MI, USA

Department of Neurology & Ophthalmology, Michigan State University College of Human Medicine, East Lansing, MI, USA

Department of Neurology, Henry Ford Health System, Detroit, MI, USA
e-mail: Izaman1@hfhs.org

A. Ghanem
Department of Neurology, Henry Ford Health System, Detroit, MI, USA
e-mail: aghanem2@hfhs.org

M. A. Garada
Henry Ford Hospital, Detroit, MI, USA
e-mail: agarada1@hfhs.org

U. Agarwal
Henry Ford Health – Henry Ford Hospital, Detroit, MI, USA
e-mail: uagarwa1@hfhs.org

G. A. Kaspo, G. D. Klasser (eds.), *Orofacial and Head Pain*,
https://doi.org/10.1007/978-3-032-08275-6_13

episodic pain. This prodromal pain, which may be described as toothache-like, can persist for months or even years before evolving into stabbing, paroxysmal pain [6]. Given the location and nature of the pain, many patients undergo extensive dental evaluations, and in some cases, tooth extractions, before the correct diagnosis of TN is made [2–4]. But overall, for most patients, the hallmark of TN is the sudden onset of sharp pain, often described as an electric shock-like or stabbing sensation. This pain is severe and occurs in brief episodes, each lasting only a few seconds to several minutes. In severe cases, patients may experience up to a dozen attacks per day.

Physiologically, the maxillary division (V2) of the trigeminal nerve is the most commonly affected in patients with TN, followed by the mandibular division (V3) or a combination of V2 and V3, with the ophthalmic division (V1) being the least commonly involved. When pain is confined to a single division, it typically remains localized to that area without radiating to other regions. However, in rare cases, the pain may radiate to other divisions [4, 7–9]. Within each division, the associated pain tends to have a specific region of onset, with common sites including the gingiva, lips, cheeks, and alae of the nose, and in some cases, two sites may be affected simultaneously.

One unique feature of TN is that pain onset can occur due to triggering factors. Up to 90% of patients report that pain can be induced when "trigger zones" are stimulated (e.g., nasal wing, lips, chin, cheeks, and alveolar gingiva), with common triggering activities including jaw movement, chewing, eating, swallowing, drinking, talking, gently touching the face, shaving, tooth brushing, and washing or drying the face. Between pain episodes, most patients experience a pain-free interval. However, some patients have reported persistent, less intense pain lasting from several minutes to several hours. This longer-duration pain is often described as dull, burning, or tingling, in contrast to the typical sharp, paroxysmal pain characteristic of TN. Episodes of sharp pain may last for months to years, with spontaneous remission occurring in some individuals. The duration of remission can vary, and sharp pain may recur after an interval of months or years.

In patients for whom the ophthalmic division (V1) is involved, mild lacrimation is common, but conjunctival injection is rare. Because short-lasting, unilateral, neuralgiform headache with conjunctival injection, tearing, and rhinorrhea (SUNCT) can manifest with similar signs and symptoms, these two disorders may be confused for one another. However, lacrimation in TN is generally mild, with no associated conjunctival injection, pupil size changes, nasal stuffiness, or ptosis as seen in SUNCT. Also, the duration of pain associated with V1 TN is usually shorter than what is seen in patients with SUNCT, with attacks typically lasting 5–28 s in TN compared to 80–140 s in SUNCT [4, 7].

Lastly, on sensory examination, patients with TN typically have normal sensation in the areas served by the trigeminal nerve. However, up to 25% of patients may have sensory abnormalities, with hypoesthesia being the most common, followed by hyperesthesia, allodynia, and hypoalgesia [4].

13.2.1 Diagnosis

A definitive diagnosis of TN is primarily based on clinical criteria determined by the International Classification of Headache Disorders, 3rd edition (ICHD-3) as outlined below [2]:

- Recurrent paroxysms of unilateral facial pain in the distribution(s) of one or more divisions of the trigeminal nerve (with no radiation beyond) and fulfilling *all* of the following pain characteristics:
  - Lasting from a fraction of a second to 2 min
  - Severe intensity
  - Electric shock-like, shooting, stabbing, or sharp in quality
  - Pain precipitated by innocuous stimuli within the affected trigeminal distribution
- Presentation is not better accounted for by another ICHD-3 diagnosis

13.2.2 Evaluation

Patients with suspected TN should undergo further evaluation to determine the underlying cause of pain (Fig. 13.1), and investigation typically involves neuroimaging, particularly magnetic resonance imaging (MRI). Notably, our ability to etiologically subclassify TN through neuroimaging has become more refined as imaging modalities have improved. Using a set of three different high-resolution imaging sequences has been shown to be effective for detecting vascular contact with the trigeminal nerve root as well as any associated distortion, displacement, indentation, or atrophy in the body of the nerve [10]. These sequences include three-dimensional (3D) T2-weighted imaging, 3D time-of-flight, and MR angiography (MRA) along with 3D T1-weighted gadolinium. On imaging, flattening and atrophy of the trigeminal nerve are considered sensitive indicators of clinically relevant neurovascular compression in patients with TN. However, clinicians should keep in mind that a clinical diagnosis of TN must precede MRI evaluation, as neurovascular compression at the brainstem may be an incidental finding of no clinical significance [11, 12].

For identifying the offending vessel possibly causing nerve compression, MRA is recommended. The most sensitive imaging technique is 3D multimodal image fusion, which combines 3D time-of-flight MRA with high-resolution T2-weighted imaging. This provides a high-resolution view of the cranial nerves in the cerebrospinal fluid and effectively differentiates vessels from nerves. This imaging modality not only identifies any possible compression, but also assesses the degree of morphological changes in the nerve resulting from the compression [13, 14]. However, for identifying secondary TN, which is caused by other identifiable structural anomalies or lesions, MRI sequences with gadolinium are sufficient to reveal evidence of issues such as central demyelination in the brainstem pontomedullary junction as well as any potential compression of the trigeminal nerve complex at the cerebellopontine angle [10].

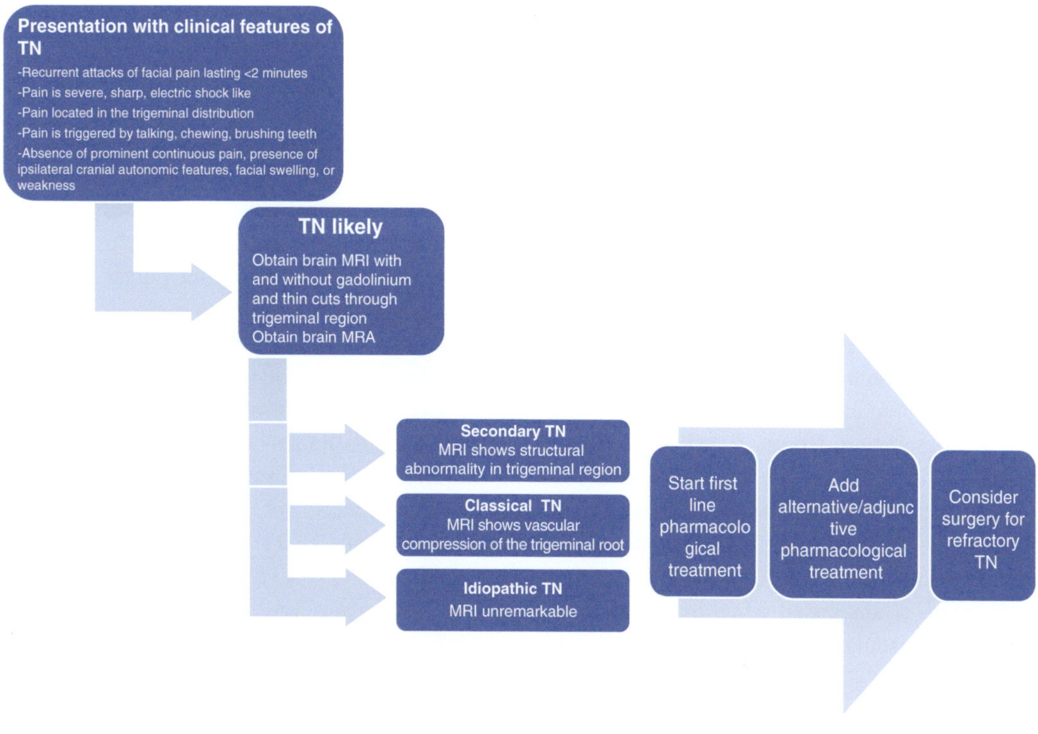

Fig. 13.1 Algorithm for evaluation and treatment of patients with trigeminal neuralgia

Table 13.1 Clinical and paraclinical descriptions of the various forms of trigeminal neuralgia

	Idiopathic TN	Classical TN	Secondary TN
Trigeminal pain	Unilateral pain	Unilateral pain	Unilateral or bilateral pain
Cause	Unknown	Vascular compression of trigeminal root	Cerebellopontine angle mass/tumor, brainstem tumor, multiple sclerosis, Sjögren disease, lupus, sarcoidosis
Trigeminal reflex test	Normal	Normal	Abnormal
Imaging features on MRI and MRA	Normal or vascular loop adjacent to or in contact with the trigeminal nerve not causing compression or other morphologic change	Distortion, dislocation, flattening, or atrophy of the trigeminal root due to vascular compression	Structural lesions along the trigeminal nerve pathway, cerebellopontine junction, brainstem

Abbreviations: *MRI* magnetic resonance imaging. *MRA* magnetic resonance angiograph, *TN* trigeminal neuralgia

Trigeminal reflex testing is a neurodiagnostic procedure sometimes used to evaluate trigeminal nerve function (motor and sensory). But this approach is seldom used since MRI has become the preferred method for determining the underlying cause of TN. However, trigeminal reflex testing may be useful for patients with TN who are unable to undergo MRI, or when MRI is nondiagnostic. Notably, trigeminal reflex test results are often normal in patients with idiopathic and classical TN, but can be abnormal in patients with secondary TN [15].

13.2.3 Classification

TN is classified into three categories based on the underlying cause: idiopathic, classical (or primary), and secondary (Table 13.1).

Idiopathic TN is the diagnosis when patients display the characteristic pain of TN with no clear underlying cause identified on neuroimaging or other testing. However, MRI may show a blood vessel touching but not compressing the symptomatic trigeminal nerve in patients with idiopathic TN, and the significance of this observation is not clear. Classical TN, on the other hand, is diagnosed when imaging reveals clear neurovascular compression of the trigeminal nerve resulting in morphological changes such as nerve displacement and atrophy. The nerve entry zone of the trigeminal nerve is most commonly involved in classical TN, and compression at this site is more likely to result in symptoms. But importantly, neurovascular contact with no obvious morphological changes is frequently seen on imaging in individuals with no TN symptoms, underscoring the importance of determining a clinical TN diagnosis before imaging and the significance of clear morphological changes observed on MRI. Also, patients with classical TN are more likely to experience a prodrome of dull pain before the onset of sharp paroxysms as well as continuous or longer-duration dull pain between episodes of sharp pain. According to the ICHD-3, classical TN may be subclassified as either purely paroxysmal TN or classical TN with concomitant continuous pain [2]. Lastly, patients with secondary TN have a discrete, identifiable cause other than neurovascular compression (Fig. 13.2), such as benign and malignant tumors, multiple sclerosis, arteriovenous malformations, vascular aneurysms, metastases, tuberculosis, and other etiologies (Table 13.1). Patients with secondary TN are more likely to present with sensory abnormalities and have a younger mean age of onset [4].

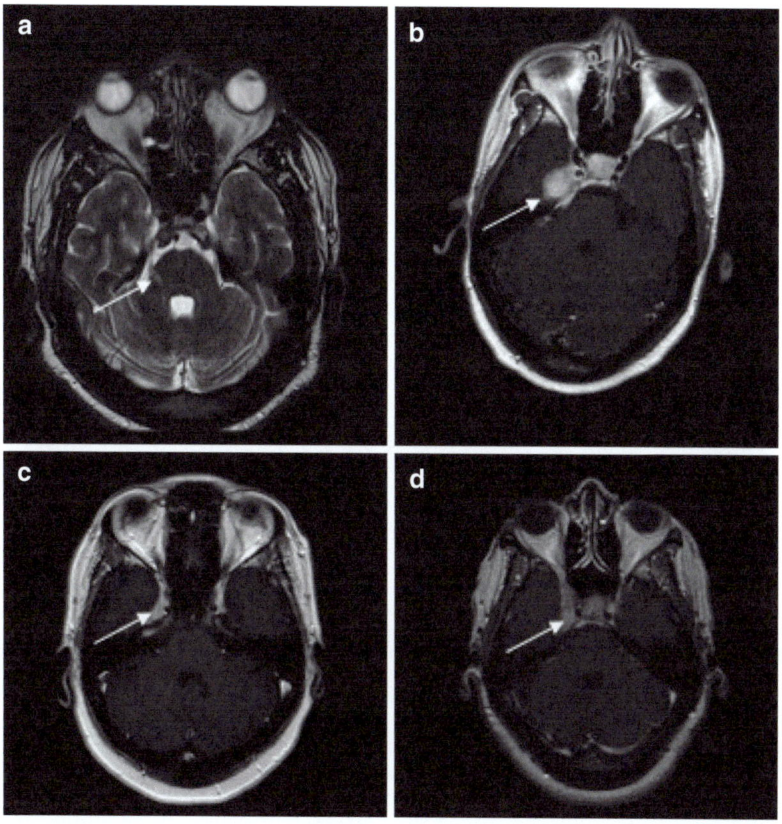

Fig. 13.2 Axial brain magnetic resonance imaging (MRI) of patients with secondary trigeminal neuralgia. (**a**) T2-weighted lesion (arrow) at the level of the trigeminal nucleus in the brainstem of a patient with multiple sclerosis. (**b**) T1-weighted imaging with gadolinium showing a neurosarcoidosis lesion (arrow) in the right cavernous sinus and Meckel's cave mimicking meningioma. (**c**) T1-weighted imaging with gadolinium showing a neurosarcoidosis lesion (arrow) in the right cavernous sinus and Meckel's cave mimicking trigeminal schwannoma. (**d**) T1-weighted imaging with gadolinium showing an enhanced neurosarcoidosis lesion in the right cavernous sinus and Meckel's cave region (arrow)

13.3 Glossopharyngeal Neuralgia

Glossopharyngeal neuralgia (GN) is an orofacial pain syndrome characterized by paroxysms of stabbing pain along the distribution of the glossopharyngeal nerve and often accompanied by pain in areas innervated by the vagus nerve [2, 16]. GN is a rare condition that has a significantly lower incidence than TN and occipital neuralgia (ON). The underlying mechanism leading to GN typically involves dysfunction of the glossopharyngeal nerve, which is usually due to identifiable causes, particularly neurovascular compression, but many instances are idiopathic [2].

GN typically affects individuals over the age of 20, with most patients being in their 50s and 60s. While GN has no clear gender predominance, some studies have noted a slight female predominance. Individuals with GN commonly present with sharp, shooting, or electric shock-like pain in the head and neck region that lasts only a few seconds. The onset of pain can be sudden and unpredictable, occurring sporadically throughout the day, including during sleep. The frequency of GN episodes can vary widely, ranging from several dozen to several hundred instances per day, and in most cases, the pain resolves abruptly, with complete remission between episodes. However, some patients may experience mild lingering discomfort between episodes [16–18]. Pain associated with GN most commonly occurs in the ear and throat and is typically localized to the ear, throat, mandible, tonsils, and the base of the tongue. However, pain from GN can radiate from the mouth or throat to the ear, and vice versa, sometimes involving multiple areas simultaneously, such as the ear and pharynx, with pain radiating to other parts of the face, eyes, or even the shoulders. A small proportion of patients have reported experiencing uncomfortable irritation weeks or months before the onset of the sharp pain that characterizes GN. Physiological processes such as swallowing, chewing, yawning, speaking, and touching can provoke episodes, and in some individuals, the pain may spontaneously resolve over a period of months to years [2, 17, 18].

Although pain from GN can occur on either side of the face, studies have suggested a slightly higher frequency of pain occurring on the left side. Some patients may even experience pain on both sides of the face, and the co-occurrence of GN and TN is increasingly being reported [17, 19]. Due to the overlapping clinical features of these two distinct neuropathies, GN is often misdiagnosed as TN, particularly when the pain involves the mandible or radiates to the face. When pain primarily affects the ear, distinguishing GN from nervus intermedius neuralgia can also be challenging. Furthermore, because of the close proximity of the vagus nerve's somatic sensory fibers to those of the glossopharyngeal nerve in the larynx, distinguishing GN from neuralgia of the superior laryngeal branch of the vagus nerve can also be difficult [17, 19]. Given the anatomical relationship between the glossopharyngeal and vagus nerves, some patients with GN may also experience symptoms associated with vagus nerve stimulation, such as cough, hoarseness, and syncope [19].

A wide range of conditions can lead to GN, including neurovascular compression, neoplasms, infections, inflammatory processes, structural abnormalities, and trauma [17]. GN is thus classified into three forms based on the underlying etiology: classic, secondary, and idiopathic. While the classic form is attributed to neurovascular compression of the glossopharyngeal nerve, GN due to other identifiable causes such as infections, multiple sclerosis, and tumors is classified as secondary. When no identifiable cause is found, the condition is termed idiopathic GN. The blood vessel most commonly involved in the neurovascular compression associated with classic GN is the posterior inferior cerebellar artery, followed by the anterior inferior cerebellar artery, vertebral artery, and superior cerebellar artery [17, 19, 20].

13.3.1 Diagnostic Imaging

MRI is the preferred modality for identifying glossopharyngeal nerve compression in patients who are experiencing overt symptoms, and typically, T2-weighted MRI and MRA are performed together. The T2-weighted sequence helps identify structural abnormalities and is crucial for ruling out secondary causes of GN. When neurovascular compression is the underlying cause of pain, MRA is then used to visualize the involved vessels. In addition to T2-weighted imaging, a specialized sequence known as constructive interference in steady state (CISS) is often required to clearly visualize the glossopharyngeal nerve and to provide a detailed evaluation of the individual cranial nerves in relation to the other cranial nerves and blood vessels. CISS is a form of steady-state free precession imaging that produces high-resolution images of the cranial nerves, brainstem, cerebellum, and surrounding vascular structures. Note that the terminology used to describe this sequence may vary depending on the MRI vendor, and other names for the CISS sequence include FIESTA (fast imaging employing steady-state acquisition), TrueFISP (true fast imaging with steady-state precession), and other similar variations. Regardless, for superior visualization of the veins and arteries, high-resolution 3D MRA time-of-flight is preferred over conventional MRA because the blood moving within the vessels generates high contrast with the surrounding stationary tissues, making this approach ideal for evaluating vascular anatomy. But when infectious or inflammatory causes of compression are suspected, contrast-enhanced MRI sequences should be used to provide a truly comprehensive assessment. Importantly, not all neurovascular compressions lead to overt symptoms, and asymptomatic neurovascular compression is commonly seen during routine imaging, presenting somewhat of a diagnostic challenge. If the compression is not leading to displacement or atrophy of the nerve, it is unlikely to cause any symptoms. While patients with neurovascular compressions but no symptoms may not have any overt pathology, thorough documentation of the finding is critical in the event that disease does develop in the future. However, compressions are more likely to cause symptoms when they are located within the "transition zone," where the central and peripheral myelin sheaths meet [20–22].

In summary, GN is a rare, painful orofacial neuropathy characterized by sharp, stabbing pain along the areas innervated by the glossopharyngeal nerve. Importantly, GN may be confused with TN—a more common neuropathy that causes similar symptoms—and precise diagnostic imaging of the nerves and vessels is essential to distinguish GN from other neuropathies and to determine the underlying cause. Although most patients with GN have a form of neurovascular compression, GN may also be caused by infectious and inflammatory processes or may have no identifiable underlying cause at all. Overall, because GN is so rare, we have a poor understanding of the predictors associated with disease, long-term outcomes from medical and surgical therapies, and the risks of recurrence. Notably, studies evaluating the psychosocial and quality-of-life impacts of GN on patients are needed to provide insights for improving patient care.

13.4 Nervus Intermedius (Geniculate) Neuralgia

Nervus intermedius neuralgia (NIN), also referred to as geniculate neuralgia, is a rare craniofacial pain syndrome attributed to irritation or dysfunction of the nervus intermedius—the sensory and parasympathetic component of the facial nerve (cranial nerve VII). This nerve transmits sensation from the external auditory canal, posterior auricle, tympanic membrane, and parts of the oropharynx. The cause of pain in most patients with NIN is vascular compression of the root entry zone of cranial nerves VII and VIII by structures such as the anterior inferior cerebellar artery, the posterior inferior cerebellar artery, and the branches of the vertebral arteries [23]. Misdiagnosis of NIN is common because associated symptoms are similar to other dental, otologic, and temporomandibular disorders.

13.4.1 Clinical Presentation

Patients with NIN typically report sudden, severe, stabbing, or electric shock-like pain deep in the ear, often radiating to the auditory canal, mastoid region, or oropharynx. Attacks last from several seconds to a few minutes and may be triggered by chewing, swallowing, talking, yawning, or touching the external auditory canal. A dull, persistent ache may occur between paroxysms, and the pain may be accompanied by dysfunction of lacrimation, taste, and salivation [2, 23]. In some cases, NIN coexists with other cranial neuralgias, most often GN. Importantly, the pain associated with NIN can have a very serious impact on patients' quality of life, and suicidal ideation due to the intensity of disabling ear pain has been reported.

The ICHD-3 [2] defines NIN as follows:

- Paroxysmal attacks of unilateral pain in the distribution of nervus intermedius (auditory canal, auricle, in the region of the mastoid process, and occasionally the soft palate) and fulfills **all** the following characteristics:
  - Lasting from a few seconds to minutes
  - Severe in intensity
  - Shooting, stabbing, or sharp in quality
  - Precipitated by stimulation of a trigger area in the posterior wall of the auditory canal and/or periauricular region
- Not better accounted for by another ICHD-3 diagnosis

13.4.2 Diagnosis

The diagnosis of NIN is clinical, requiring careful attention to the patient's history and exclusion of more common causes of otalgia. Critically, neurologic and otolaryngologic evaluation is essential. Also, dentists may be the first clinicians that patients with NIN seek care from, particularly when symptoms mimic dental or temporomandibular joint pathology.

High-resolution MRI with CISS or FIESTA (fast imaging employing steady-state acquisition) sequences involving thin-slice images ($\leq$1 mm) through the cerebellopontine angle can aid in identifying neurovascular compression at the facial nerve root entry zone. One study described the radiologic and intraoperative correlates in patients who were treated surgically, identifying the anterior inferior cerebellar artery as the most common cause of nerve compression [24]. Intraoperative findings in patients with NIN often confirm the anatomical relationship between offending vessels and the nervus intermedius/facial nerve complex, supporting the neurovascular compression model of pathophysiology [24]. But clinicians should note that a significant proportion of individuals with a vascular loop compressing the nerve may not have any pain symptoms at all, highlighting the critical importance of clinical evaluation.

Another consideration when evaluating patients with possible NIN is to differentiate this specific disorder from other forms of neuralgia that may have overlapping distribution of pain and areas of enervation. GN, which predominantly manifests as ear pain, is an important differential diagnosis to consider in patients with craniofacial pain, especially during exploration of the posterior cranial fossa (both on imaging or intraoperatively). Similarly, TN is often similar to NIN in terms of pain characteristics and therefore should also be investigated and ruled out.

13.5 Superior Laryngeal Neuralgia

Superior laryngeal neuralgia (SLN) is a craniofacial pain syndrome characterized by paroxysmal, severe pain in the lateral anterior neck, submandibular region, and occasionally the ear, corresponding to the sensory distribution of the internal branch of the superior laryngeal nerve. Despite increased awareness surrounding this disorder, SLN continues to be underdiagnosed because it is an uncommon condition with symptoms that are similar to more prevalent pain disorders. Advancements in neuroimaging techniques have significantly improved our ability to identify the underlying causes of SLN and guide therapeutic interventions, transforming the diagnostic approach and treatment strategies for patients with SLN [25–27].

13.5.1 Epidemiology

The exact prevalence of SLN is unknown, mainly because this condition is probably underdiagnosed and often misclassified. However, based on limited studies, the estimated prevalence is thought to be 0.2–0.4 cases per 100,000 individuals, with a female-to-male ratio of approximately 2:1 [26]. The peak incidence of SLN occurs in the fifth and sixth decades of life [26, 27]. Multiple risk factors preclude the development of SLN, including history of neck trauma, history of intubation, and thyroid disorders.

13.5.2 Neuroanatomy

The superior laryngeal nerve is a branch of the vagus nerve (cranial nerve X) that originates from the inferior vagal ganglion. After its origin, this nerve descends posterolaterally to the internal carotid artery and divides into two primary branches [28, 29]. The internal branch is primarily sensory and provides innervation to the laryngeal mucosa superior to the vocal folds, the inferior surface of the epiglottis, and portions of the aryepiglottic fold. The internal branch runs deep to the thyrohyoid muscle, piercing the thyrohyoid membrane approximately 2–3 mm from the insertion of this muscle on the thyroid cartilage. The external branch is primarily motor, supplying the cricothyroid muscle and inferior pharyngeal constrictor. This branch runs alongside the superior thyroid artery before terminating in the cricothyroid muscle.

13.5.3 Pathophysiology and Etiology

The pathophysiological mechanisms underlying the development of SLN include direct neural compression, neurovascular conflict, and inflammatory processes [25–27]. Direct neural compression refers to mechanical compression of the internal branch of the superior laryngeal nerve, particularly at anatomical bottlenecks where the nerve traverses fascial planes or rigid structures. Neurovascular conflict is defined as pulsatile compression of the internal branch by adjacent vascular structures—typically the superior thyroid artery or linguofacial trunk. Lastly, inflammatory processes include perineural inflammation secondary to infection, autoimmune conditions, or local tissue reaction.

Traumatic causes of SLN include neck trauma with direct nerve injury, iatrogenic injury during endotracheal intubation, post-surgical scarring following thyroidectomy, injury from carotid endarterectomy or cervical spine procedures, and fractures of the hyoid bone or thyroid cartilage. Inflammatory causes of SLN include upper respiratory tract infections, laryngopharyngeal reflux disease, and autoimmune conditions affecting the larynx. Compressive causes of SLN include thyroid nodules or goiter, cervical osteophytes, and carotid artery ectasia or aneurysm. Neoplastic causes of SLN include laryngeal carcinoma, thyroid neoplasms, metastatic disease affecting cervical lymph nodes, and paragangliomas. Although many etiologies for the development of SLN are known, clinicians should be aware that approximately 40–50% of patients with SLN have no identifiable etiology, making this entity somewhat challenging to identify [26–28].

13.5.4 Clinical Presentation

Patients with SLN typically present with paroxysmal, lancinating, electric shock-like pain in a unilateral distribution ranging from seconds to minutes. Painful episodes often affect the anterolateral neck and correspond to the level of the thyrohyoid membrane, sometimes radiating to the ipsilateral submandibular region and ear. The pain associated with SLN typically ranges from moderate to severe, with reported pain being typically 7–10 on a 10-point pain scale. Common triggers for painful episodes include swallowing, coughing, yawning, or neck rotation toward the affected side. Oftentimes, patients report vocal changes during painful episodes, painful swallowing, and foreign body sensations in the throat [26–28].

13.5.5 Diagnosis

Based on the ICHD-3, SLN is diagnosed when all of the following are present [2]:

1. At least three attacks of unilateral pain fulfilling the following criteria 2 and 3.
2. Pain located in the lateral aspect of the throat, submandibular region, or under the ear.
3. Pain has at least three of the following characteristics: (i) recurring in paroxysmal attacks lasting seconds to minutes; (ii) severe intensity; (iii) shooting, stabbing, or sharp quality; and (iv) precipitated by swallowing, talking, coughing, or yawning.
4. No clinically evident neurological deficit.
5. Pain is temporarily relieved by local anesthetic block of the superior laryngeal nerve. Not better accounted for by another ICHD-3 diagnosis.

13.5.6 Imaging

MRI is the preferred initial imaging modality for the evaluation of SLN. On MRI, the internal branch of the superior laryngeal nerve appears as a thin, linear T2-hyperintense structure coursing from the vagus nerve and passing deep to the thyrohyoid muscle, piercing the thyrohyoid membrane. MRI is best used to detect structural lesions (tumors and vascular malformations), inflammatory conditions, and nerve root compression. Abnormal findings include focal thickening of the nerve, increased T2 signal intensity suggesting edema or inflammation, and enhancement following contrast administration indicating disruption of the blood-nerve barrier.

Abnormal imaging findings due to neurovascular compromise include [29–31] abnormal course of the lingual artery with compression at the level of the hyoid bone, loop or ectasia of the superior thyroid artery contacting the superior laryngeal nerve, vascular calcifications or atherosclerotic plaques in proximity to the nerve course, and vascular malformations adjacent to the nerve pathway. Abnormal imaging findings with structural abnormality as the etiology are [29–31] superior thyroid notch variants, calcification of the superior cornu of the thyroid cartilage, asymmetry or thickening of the thyrohyoid membrane, hypertrophy of the thyrohyoid muscle, and fibrosis or scarring from previous procedures. Abnormal imaging findings associated with neoplastic lesions to be considered are [29–31] laryngeal tumors with extra-laryngeal extension, thyroid masses impinging on the nerve course, paragangliomas or schwannomas of the vagus nerve, and metastatic cervical lymphadenopathy.

13.5.7 Prognosis

The long-term prognosis for patients with SLN can be variable. Approximately 15–20% of patients will experience spontaneous remission of SLN, particularly when inflammatory processes are implicated. Around 40–60% of patients experience satisfactory control with pharmacological therapy. But only around 10–15% remain refractory to all therapeutic modalities [24, 32, 33].

13.6 Occipital Neuralgia

Occipital neuralgia (ON) is a distinct neuropathic pain syndrome described as a paroxysmal, sharp, stabbing pain in the distribution of the greater occipital nerve, lesser occipital nerve, or third occipital nerve. The pain typically originates in the suboccipital region and radiates to the vertex of the skull. While the pain associated with ON often manifests unilaterally, bilateral involvement is not uncommon. ON is an important clinical entity within the broader spectrum of craniofacial pain disorders and headache syndromes, which all require specific diagnostic approaches [34].

13.6.1 Epidemiology

The prevalence of ON is not well established, partly because this condition is difficult to diagnose and is frequently misclassified. ON accounts for approximately 8–10% of facial neuralgias, with a slight female predominance represented by a female-to-male ratio of roughly 3:1 [34]. Peak incidence occurs in the fourth and fifth decades of life. However, ON may affect individuals of any age [34].

13.6.2 Neuroanatomy

The greater occipital nerve originates from the dorsal ramus of the C2 spinal nerve, with contributions from C3. It courses through the semispinalis capitis muscle before emerging superolaterally, ascending along the posterior scalp and providing sensory innervation to it.

The lesser occipital nerve originates from the ventral rami of C2 and C3 spinal nerves and ascends along the posterior aspect of the sternocleidomastoid muscle to supply the lateral aspects of the occipital region and the superior portion of the ear.

The third occipital nerve arises from the dorsal ramus of C3, supplying a relatively small area of the lower occipital scalp and upper neck.

13.6.3 Pathophysiology and Etiology

The pathophysiological mechanisms underlying ON involve neural inflammation, mechanical compression, or direct injury to the occipital nerves [35]. Traumatic causes include whiplash injuries, direct trauma, and iatrogenic injury following surgical procedures involving the posterior cranial fossa or cervical spine. Compressive causes include entrapment at muscular, fascial, or vascular sites. This commonly involves compression at the semispinalis capitis, where the greater occipital nerve penetrates the muscle. However, it may also be due to entrapment between the inferior oblique and semispinalis capitis muscles, compression at the trapezius muscle insertion, or fascial band compression. Inflammatory or infectious causes of ON include C1-C2 facet joint arthropathy, vasculitis affecting the occipital vessels, or upper cervical spine infections. Neoplastic causes are a much less common pathophysiology contributing to the development of ON but should always be considered. Most commonly, they are schwannomas of the occipital nerves, C2 myelomas, metastatic disease, or meningiomas or neuromas affecting the upper cervical nerve roots. Although many causes for the development of ON are well known, approximately 22–30% of patients with ON have no identifiable etiology, which is an important consideration for clinicians evaluating patients with unexplained pain of the head and neck [34].

13.6.4 Clinical Presentation

Patients with ON typically present with sharp or paroxysmal pain in the occipital region, oftentimes with pain radiating from the suboccipital area to the vertex. Pain may extend to the frontal, temporal, or periorbital regions via trigeminocervical complex connections. Painful episodes have a variable duration and can range from as short as seconds to multiple days. The pain associated with ON typically ranges from moderate to severe, with pain ratings reported typically as 7–10 on a 10-point numerical rating scale. Associated symptoms may include scalp dysesthesia or hypersensitivity, photophobia, phonophobia during pain exacerbations, ipsilateral lacrimation or conjunctival injection, and limited range of motion in the cervical spine. Aggravating factors that can exacerbate ON include neck movements, particularly extension and rotation, pressure on occipital nerve trigger points, sustained poor head posture, stress, and fatigue.

13.6.5 Diagnosis

The diagnosis of ON is primarily clinical, being supported by medical history, physical examination, and response to diagnostic nerve blocks [2]. According to the ICHD-3, ON is diagnosed when all of the following criteria are met [2]:

1. Unilateral or bilateral pain that includes ***all*** of the following criteria 2 through 5.
2. Pain is located within the distribution of the greater, lesser, or third occipital nerves.
3. Pain has at least two of the following characteristics: (i) recurring in paroxysmal attacks lasting from seconds to minutes; (ii) severe intensity; or (iii) shooting, stabbing, or sharp in quality.
4. Pain is associated with both of the following: (i) dysesthesia or allodynia apparent during innocuous stimulation of the scalp or hair; and (ii) either or both of the following—tenderness over the affected nerve branches and trigger points at the emergence of the greater occipital nerve or in the area of distribution of C2.
5. Pain is temporarily relieved by a local anesthetic block of the affected nerve.
6. Not better accounted for by any other ICHD-3 diagnosis.

13.6.6 Clinical Examination

The following are the key signs and symptoms that are characteristic of ON: tenderness on palpation over the affected nerve, positive Tinel's sign (paresthesia or pain elicited by tapping over the nerve), hyperalgesia or allodynia in the affected dermatomes, limited range of motion in the cervical spine, trigger points in the suboccipital musculature, and reduced sensation in the distribution of the affected nerve(s) (less common).

13.6.7 Diagnostic Studies

The gold standard confirmatory test for ON involves the injection of a local anesthetic (e.g., 1–2% lidocaine) at the affected nerve site. Significant pain reduction (> 50%) following the block strongly supports the diagnosis of ON [34]. Electrodiagnostic studies may have limited utility in routine diagnosis but may help exclude other neuropathic conditions.

13.6.8 Imaging

Imaging studies play an essential role in the diagnostic workup of patients displaying the symptoms of ON, although they are not sufficient for a direct diagnosis. Rather, imaging can rule out secondary causes of occipital pain, identify structural abnormalities that might be compressing or irritating the occipital nerves, and guide interventional or surgical treatments [34]. Brain and cervical spine MRI is the preferred initial imaging modality and is used to detect structural lesions (tumors and vascular malformations), inflammatory conditions, cervical disc disease or herniation, nerve root compression, atlanto-axial pathology, and muscle hypertrophy affecting the occipital nerves. Special sequences such as STIR (short-TI inversion recovery) may help visualize nerve inflammation. Computed tomography is superior for evaluating bony abnormalities and helpful in visualizing cervical osteophytes, fractures, C1-C2 joint arthropathy, or foraminal stenosis.

Plain radiographs have limited utility but may show degenerative changes in the cervical spine, cervical instability on flexion/extension views, or atlantoaxial subluxation [35].

13.6.9 Prognosis

The long-term prognosis of patients with ON is variable. Approximately 40–50% of patients experience significant improvement with conservative care. Interventional procedures provide moderate to substantial relief in 60–80% of patients, although repeat procedures are often necessary [34]. Surgical outcomes are less predictable, with success rates ranging from 40% to 80% depending on patient selection criteria and surgical technique. Recurrence rates following all treatment modalities remain high, at about 30–50% at 2 years [36].

13.7 Auriculotemporal Neuralgia

Auriculotemporal neuralgia is an uncommon, yet clinically distinct, craniofacial pain syndrome characterized by paroxysmal stabbing pain in the preauricular and temporal regions. It results from dysfunction or irritation of the auriculotemporal nerve, a branch of the mandibular division of the trigeminal nerve (V3). This nerve carries sensory fibers to the anterior ear, temporal scalp, and parotid region, and it may also carry parasympathetic fibers from the otic ganglion to the parotid gland [37].

13.7.1 Clinical Presentation

Patients with auriculotemporal neuralgia typically report sudden, sharp, or burning pain localized anterior to the ear and radiating toward the temporal or mandibular region. Attacks are brief—lasting seconds to minutes—and may be triggered by chewing, talking, jaw movement, or touching the skin over the temple. Some patients may have a dull, lingering ache that persists between paroxysms. However, symptoms are rarely accompanied by autonomic features such as tearing or facial flushing [38].

Notably, auriculotemporal neuralgia is often misdiagnosed as temporomandibular joint dysfunction, dental pathology, or even TN, as neighboring nerves can produce similar pain patterns. However, the hallmark of auriculotemporal neuralgia remains well-localized pain over the auriculotemporal nerve distribution with reproducibility upon palpation near the tragus or mandibular ramus [39].

13.7.2 Pathophysiology

Most auriculotemporal neuralgia diagnoses are idiopathic, with no obvious cause. However, structural abnormalities causing nerve entrapment should be explored [42], since the auriculotemporal nerve has been reported to become entrapped while traversing the lateral pterygoid muscle [39, 40]. Other reported causes of auriculotemporal neuralgia include nerve compression by synovial cyst [41], middle meningeal artery malformation/aneurysm [42], mandible condylar fracture [43], and tumoral perineural invasion [44]. Cross-talk between trigeminal and autonomic fibers, particularly parasympathetic efferents traveling with the auriculotemporal nerve, may also contribute to the autonomic features of the pain associated with this condition, as well as the overlapping phenotype with cluster-like syndromes. This specific pain disorder likely reflects a convergence of structural, inflammatory, and neurovascular factors, consistent with the heterogeneity seen across other idiopathic facial neuralgias [37].

13.7.3 Diagnosis

The diagnosis of auriculotemporal neuralgia is clinical and based on the characteristic symptomatology and careful mapping of the pain distribution. Provocation of pain with palpation of the nerve near the tragus is a key finding. MRI and computed tomography are useful for excluding secondary structural causes such as tumors, trauma, or temporomandibular joint pathology. Also, a diagnostic local anesthetic block can support the diagnosis and offer temporary relief [37, 38].

References

1. De Toledo IP, Conti Réus J, Fernandes M, Porporatti AL, Peres MA, Takaschima A, et al. Prevalence of trigeminal neuralgia: a systematic review. J Am Dent Assoc. 2016;147(7):570–6.e2.
2. Headache classification Committee of the International Headache Society (IHS) the international classification of headache disorders, 3rd edition. Cephalalgia. 2018;38, 1:1–211.
3. Jainkittivong A, Aneksuk V, Langlais RP. Trigeminal neuralgia: a retrospective study of 188 Thai cases. Gerodontology. 2012;29(2):e611–7.
4. Maarbjerg S, Gozalov A, Olesen J, Bendtsen L. Trigeminal neuralgia–a prospective systematic study of clinical characteristics in 158 patients. Headache. 2014;54(10):1574–82.
5. Katusic S, Beard CM, Bergstralh E, Kurland LT. Incidence and clinical features of trigeminal neuralgia, Rochester, Minnesota, 1945–1984. Ann Neurol. 1990;27(1):89–95.
6. Fromm GH, Graff-Radford SB, Terrence CF, Sweet WH. Pre-trigeminal neuralgia. Neurology. 1990;40(10):1493–5.
7. Pareja JA, Barón M, Gili P, Yangüela J, Caminero AB, Dobato JL, et al. Objective assessment of autonomic signs during triggered first division trigeminal neuralgia. Cephalalgia. 2002;22(4):251–5.
8. Peet MM, Schneider RC. Trigeminal neuralgia; a review of six hundred and eighty-nine cases with a follow-up study of sixty five per cent of the group. J Neurosurg. 1952;9(4):367–77.
9. Maarbjerg S, Di Stefano G, Bendtsen L, Cruccu G. Trigeminal neuralgia – diagnosis and treatment. Cephalalgia. 2017;37(7):648–57.
10. Bendtsen L, Zakrzewska JM, Heinskou TB, Hodaie M, Leal PRL, Nurmikko T, et al. Advances in diagnosis, classification, pathophysiology, and management of trigeminal neuralgia. Lancet Neurol. 2020;19(9):784–96.
11. Cruccu G, Finnerup NB, Jensen TS, Scholz J, Sindou M, Svensson P, et al. Trigeminal neuralgia: new classification and diagnostic grading for practice and research. Neurology. 2016;87(2):220–8.
12. Zakrzewska JM, Linskey ME. Trigeminal neuralgia. BMJ. 2014;348:g474.
13. Liang C, Yang L, Reichardt W, Zhang B, Li R. Different MRI-based methods for the diagnosis of neurovascular compression in trigeminal neuralgia or hemifacial spasm: a network meta-analysis. J Clin Neurosci. 2023;108:19–24.
14. Leal PR, Hermier M, Souza MA, Cristino-Filho G, Froment JC, Sindou M. Visualization of vascular com-

pression of the trigeminal nerve with high-resolution 3T MRI: a prospective study comparing preoperative imaging analysis to surgical findings in 40 consecutive patients who underwent microvascular decompression for trigeminal neuralgia. Neurosurgery. 2011;69(1):15–25. discussion 6
15. Bendtsen L, Zakrzewska JM, Abbott J, Braschinsky M, Di Stefano G, Donnet A, et al. European academy of neurology guideline on trigeminal neuralgia. Eur J Neurol. 2019;26(6):831–49.
16. Xu R, Xie ME, Jackson CM. Trigeminal neuralgia: current approaches and emerging interventions. J Pain Res. 2021;14:3437–63.
17. Rushton JG, Stevens JC, Miller RH. Glossopharyngeal (vagoglossopharyngeal) neuralgia: a study of 217 cases. Arch Neurol. 1981;38(4):201–5.
18. Martínez-González JM, Martínez-Rodríguez N, Calvo-Guirado JL, Brinkmann JC, Dorado CB. Glossopharyngeal neuralgia: a presentation of 14 cases. J Oral Maxillofac Surg. 2011;69(6):e38–41.
19. Han A, Montgomery C, Zamora A, Winder E, Kaye A, Carroll C, et al. Glossopharyngeal neuralgia: epidemiology, risk factors, pathophysiology, differential diagnosis, and treatment options. Health Psychol Res. 2022;10(5):36042.
20. Gaul C, Hastreiter P, Duncker A, Naraghi R. Diagnosis and neurosurgical treatment of glossopharyngeal neuralgia: clinical findings and 3-D visualization of neurovascular compression in 19 consecutive patients. J Headache Pain. 2011;12(5):527–34.
21. Haller S, Etienne L, Kövari E, Varoquaux AD, Urbach H, Becker M. Imaging of neurovascular compression syndromes: trigeminal neuralgia, Hemifacial spasm, vestibular Paroxysmia, and glossopharyngeal neuralgia. AJNR Am J Neuroradiol. 2016;37(8):1384–92.
22. Garcia M, Naraghi R, Zumbrunn T, Rösch J, Hastreiter P, Dörfler A. High-resolution 3D-constructive interference in steady-state MR imaging and 3D time-of-flight MR angiography in neurovascular compression: a comparison between 3T and 1.5T. AJNR Am J Neuroradiol. 2012;33(7):1251–6.
23. Tang IP, Freeman SR, Kontorinis G, Tang MY, Rutherford SA, King AT, et al. Geniculate neuralgia: a systematic review. J Laryngol Otol. 2014;128(5):394–9.
24. Tubbs RS, Mosier KM, Cohen-Gadol AA. Geniculate neuralgia: clinical, radiologic, and intraoperative correlates. World Neurosurg. 2013;80(6):e353–7.
25. Baugh RF, Baugh A, Bunge F. Superior laryngeal nerve syndrome and the evaluation of anterior neck pain. Am J Otolaryngol. 2012;33(4):481–3.
26. Shephard MK, Macgregor EA, Zakrzewska JM. Orofacial pain: a guide for the headache physician. Headache. 2014;54(1):22–39.
27. Narouze SPJ. Orofacial pain. 4th ed. Philadelphia: Elsevier; 2018.
28. Bacchi G, Miani P, Piemonte M. Surgical anatomy of the superior laryngeal nerve. Rev Laryngol Otol Rhinol (Bord). 1990;111(2):157–9.
29. Chhabra A, Bajaj G, Wadhwa V, Quadri RS, White J, Myers LL, et al. MR Neurographic evaluation of facial and neck pain: Normal and abnormal Craniospinal nerves below the Skull Base. Radiographics. 2018;38(5):1498–513.
30. Jagadeesan JRG, Ruan DT. Imaging of the recurrent laryngeal nerve. Springer; 2016.
31. Yousry I, Camelio S, Schmid UD, Horsfield MA, Wiesmann M, Brückmann H, et al. Visualization of cranial nerves I-XII: value of 3D CISS and T2-weighted FSE sequences. Eur Radiol. 2000;10(7):1061–7.
32. van Tilburg CWJ. Percutaneous pulsed radiofrequency treatment in a patient with chronic bilateral painful glossopharyngeal neuropathy. Am J Case Rep. 2020;21:e920579.
33. Orestes MI, Chhetri DK. Superior laryngeal nerve injury: effects, clinical findings, prognosis, and management options. Curr Opin Otolaryngol Head Neck Surg. 2014;22(6):439–43.
34. Choi I, Jeon SR. Neuralgias of the head: occipital neuralgia. J Korean Med Sci. 2016;31(4):479–88.
35. Blake P, Burstein R. Emerging evidence of occipital nerve compression in unremitting head and neck pain. J Headache Pain. 2019;20(1):76.
36. Robinson IS, Salibian AA, Alfonso AR, Lin LJ, Janis JE, Chiu ES. Surgical Management of Occipital Neuralgia: a systematic review of the literature. Ann Plast Surg. 2021;86(3S Suppl 2):S322–S31.
37. O'Neill F, Nurmikko T, Sommer C. Other facial neuralgias. Cephalalgia. 2017;37(7):658–69.
38. Pinto MJ, Guerrero AL, Costa A. Botulinum toxin as a novel therapeutic approach for auriculotemporal neuralgia. Headache. 2021;61(2):392–5.
39. Shimokawa T, Akita K, Sato T, Ru F, Yi SQ, Tanaka S. Penetration of muscles by branches of the mandibular nerve: a possible cause of neuropathy. Clin Anat. 2004;17(1):2–5.
40. Loughner BA, Larkin LH, Mahan PE. Nerve entrapment in the lateral pterygoid muscle. Oral Surg Oral Med Oral Pathol. 1990;69(3):299–306.
41. Ansari H, Robertson CE, Lane JI, Viozzi CF, Garza I. Auriculotemporal neuralgia secondary to TMJ synovial cyst: a rare presentation of a rare entity. Headache. 2013;53(10):1662–5.
42. Anil A, Peker T, Turgut HB, Gülekon IN, Liman F. Variations in the anatomy of the inferior alveolar nerve. Br J Oral Maxillofac Surg. 2003;41(4):236–9.
43. Schmidseder R, Scheunemann H. Nerve injury in fractures of the condylar neck. J Maxillofac Surg. 1977;5(3):186–90.
44. Schmalfuss IM, Tart RP, Mukherji S, Mancuso AA. Perineural tumor spread along the auriculotemporal nerve. AJNR Am J Neuroradiol. 2002;23(2):303–11.

Imaging for Central Nervous System Issues

14

Mirela Cerghet and Zahid Iqbal

14.1 Introduction

Central facial pain or neuropathic facial pain is caused by a lesion or dysfunction in the central nervous system (CNS). A lesion in the CNS causing facial pain can occur at any level of somatosensory pathway, from the spinal trigeminal nucleus up to the cerebral cortex. Common sites to cause facial pain include the brainstem (lateral aspect of medulla, base of pons) or thalamic nuclei in the lateral and posterior thalamus [1]. Many neurological disorders can cause central pain syndrome, including stroke, multiple sclerosis, tumors, epilepsy, brain or spinal cord trauma, or Parkinson's disease [2–5].

M. Cerghet (✉)
Henry Ford Health, Department of Neurology, Wayne State University, Detroit, MI, USA

School of Medicine, Department of Neurology and Ophthalmology, Michigan State University, East Lansing, MI, USA
e-mail: mcerghe1@hfhs.org

Z. Iqbal
Henry Ford Health, Department of Neurology, Wayne State University, Detroit, MI, USA
e-mail: ziqbal1@hfhs.org

14.2 Central Facial Nerve Pain and Altered Sensation

Central facial neuropathic pain can vary in intensity, can be mild or excruciating, and can be intermittent or continuous. Patients may describe the pain as burning sensation, freezing-type dysesthesia, numbness or tingling, cramps, pressing/aching, or bursts of sharp pain [6]. Some patients have difficulties describing the pain, others may report more than one type of pain.

Some patients have continuous pain that can be exacerbated by certain triggers; others have intermittent pain, in paroxysmal runs also exacerbated by certain triggers. As triggers, light touch, draft/air movement, cold, certain movements (chewing, talking), or distress have been reported.

Patients with central neuropathic pain can report pain over a certain facial area or the entire half of their face, sometimes from the head to the craniocervical region. Patients may also have pain/numbness over the ipsilateral or contralateral body depending on the localization of a CNS lesion.

Central neuropathic pain can develop at the onset of acute CNS lesion or can develop weeks to months after loss of sensation or numbness due to a lesion in somatosensory pathways.

A diagnosis of central neuropathic facial pain should be suspected in patients who develop unilateral or bilateral facial pain after having a demyelinating or ischemic CNS event.

G. A. Kaspo, G. D. Klasser (eds.), *Orofacial and Head Pain*,
https://doi.org/10.1007/978-3-032-08275-6_14

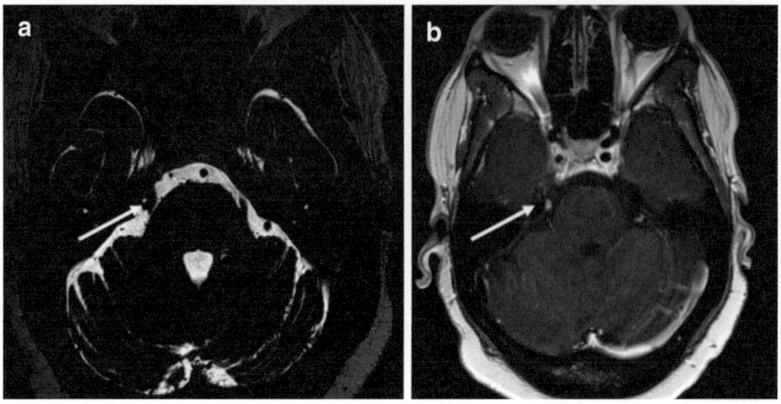

Fig. 14.1 The right superior cerebellar artery (arrow) courses superior to the cisternal portion of the right trigeminal nerve complex, and a vein abuts the lateral aspect of the right trigeminal nerve. (**a**) MRI T2-weighted image and (**b**) MRI T1-weighted imaging with gadolinium contrast

Central neuropathic pain post-stroke is described as unilateral facial pain associated with impaired sensation, caused by a stroke with onset within 6 months after the event [7]. According to the International Classification of Headache Disorders, 3rd edition (ICHD-3) [8], the diagnostic criteria for central post-stroke pain include facial and/or head pain; a confirmed ischemic or hemorrhagic stroke; evidence of causation demonstrated by pain developing within 6 months of the stroke and imaging showing a vascular lesion in an appropriate site; and pain that is not better accounted for by another headache syndrome.

Central neuropathic pain attributed to multiple sclerosis is characterized by bilateral or unilateral craniocervical pain, with or without sensory changes, associated with a demyelinating lesion in the somatosensory pathways. Per ICHD-3, diagnostic criteria include facial and/or head pain; a diagnosis of multiple sclerosis supported by MRI evidence of a demyelinating lesion in the brainstem or ascending projections of the trigeminal nuclei; pain that has developed in temporal relation to the demyelinating lesion or that has led to the diagnosis of multiple sclerosis; and pain that is not better explained by another headache syndrome.

Evaluation of central neuropathic facial pain starts with physical examination and neurological examination. Findings on direct examination suggesting other etiologies of facial pain may point to a different diagnosis.

Neuroimaging is the next step in evaluating central neuropathic pain. Magnetic resonance imaging (MRI) of the brain with and without gadolinium contrast is the preferred method for evaluation. A computed tomography scan (CT) of the head is an alternative if a patient is unable to undergo MRI. However, CT of the head is less sensitive than an MRI in evaluating potential causes of central facial neuropathic pain. Additionally, magnetic resonance angiography is the preferred test for evaluation of neurovascular compression of the trigeminal root associated with trigeminal facial pain (Fig. 14.1).

MRI findings in central neuropathic facial pain include acute or chronic ischemic or demyelinating lesions of the trigeminal nuclei or their projections to the cortex [9–11].

14.3 Multiple Sclerosis

Multiple sclerosis (MS) is a demyelinating, inflammatory and neurodegenerative disorder of the central nervous system [12]. MS demyelinating lesions occur in the brain, optic nerve, and spinal cord. Pain in MS can occur as an acute syndrome, due to an attack of the disease, or can be chronic, with chronic pain resulting from MS reported in 50–75% of patients [11]. Central neuropathic pain is one of the types of pain reported in MS and is due to demyelinating lesions affecting the somatosensory network.

Central dysesthetic pain, trigeminal neuralgia, and Lhermitte's sign have been grouped in central neuropathic pain syndromes in MS [13].

14.3.1 Central Dysesthesia in Multiple Sclerosis

Central dysesthetic pain is rarely the presenting symptom in MS, and lifetime prevalence in MS was reported between 12% and 28% [13, 14]. Pain is described as burning, aching, prickling, stabbing with toothache, and sensory loss noted on examination [14]. Central dysesthetic pain is mostly constant but can also be intermittent, present daily being either unilateral or bilateral. It involves mostly the extremities and does not follow a dermatomal distribution. Atypical facial pain frequently confused with trigeminal neuralgia was reported. The pain is mostly continuous, and there is sensory deficit on facial examination. Although pathophysiology of central dysesthesia is poorly understood, pain is presumed to arise from lesions in the somatosensory pathways of the spinal thalamocortical system [15]. MRI in MS patients with central dysesthetic pain showed demyelinating plaques in the periventricular area, thalamus, and spinal cord [13–15] (Fig. 14.2).

14.3.2 Trigeminal Neuralgia in Multiple Sclerosis

Trigeminal neuralgia (TN) or tic douloureux is a facial pain frequently mistaken for dental pain by patients [16]. TN is 20 times or more common in patients with MS compared to the general population [11, 17]. In 15% of patients, TN can precede the diagnosis of MS [18]. TN pain is described as sudden, brief, severe stabbing, or shock-like facial pain [19]. It is one of the most severe and difficult pains to treat in MS. Facial pain comes in paroxysmal attacks that last seconds and the attacks can happen multiple times a day. The attacks can be triggered by talking, chewing, touching the face or hair, or even by wind blowing across the face.

In MS, TN has similar features with classic/idiopathic TN. It is unilateral, affects more the right side of the face, and presents most commonly within the distribution of the second and third trigeminal branch as compared to the first branch. In MS, 18% of patients can have bilateral TN [13, 19], and while it occurs at an earlier age, onset is more common between 40 and 50 [19]. The prevalence of TN in MS increases with disease duration, age, and disability [18].

TN in MS is associated with a demyelinating lesion in the brainstem at the root entry zone of the trigeminal nerve in the pons [13, 19]. MRI of the brain with and without gadolinium is the preferred test to evaluate for demyelinating lesions. T2-weighted images and FLAIR images can identify demyelinating lesions in the ventrolateral pons, which locate the pathways between the trigeminal root entry zone and trigeminal nuclei (Fig. 14.3). Other brainstem lesions may be found and can be responsible for trigeminal sensory disturbance in patients with MS (Fig. 14.2). MRI is also important in assessing the anatomy and the relationship of blood vessels with the trigeminal nerve, thereby excluding the presence of vascular compression of the trigeminal nerve at root entry.

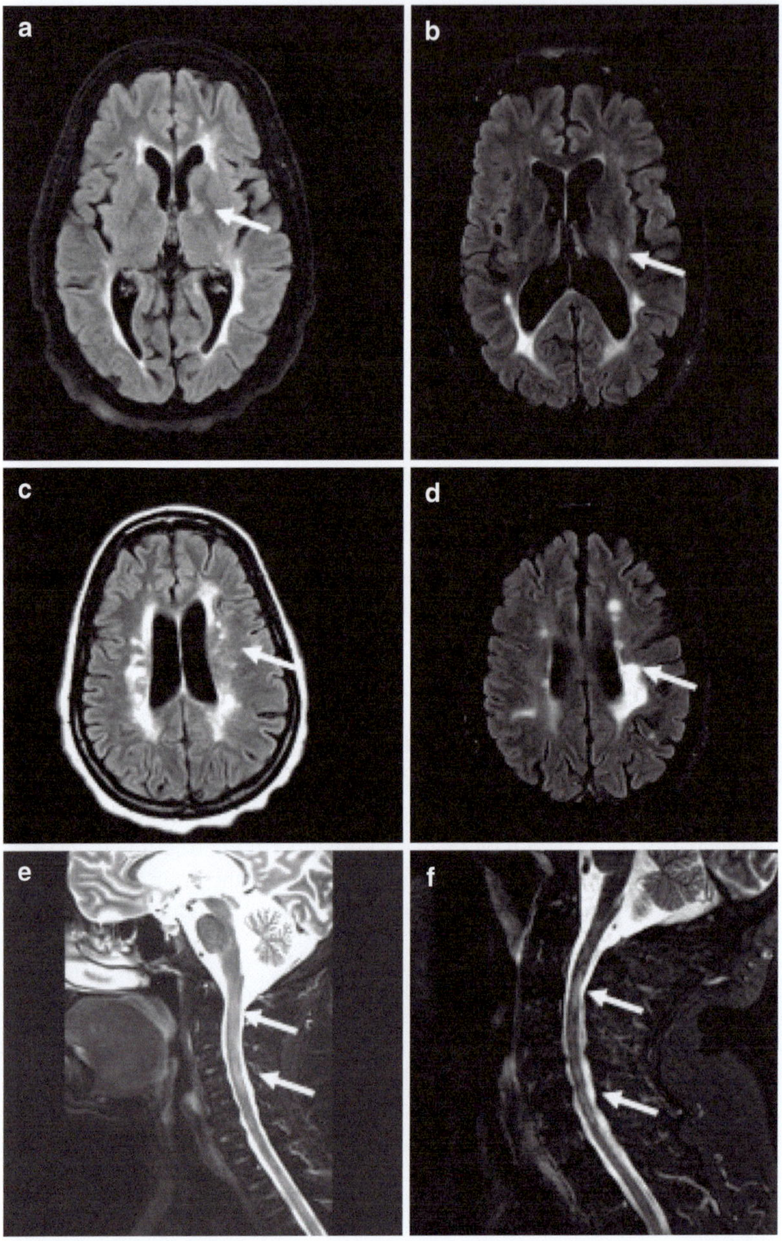

Fig. 14.2 MR images of patients with multiple sclerosis. Axial FLAIR images show foci of hyperintense signal (arrow) in the thalamus (**a**, **b**) and periventricular area (**c**, **d**). Sagittal T2 images of the cervical spine shows T2 hyperintense signal consistent with demyelinating plaques (**e**, **f**)

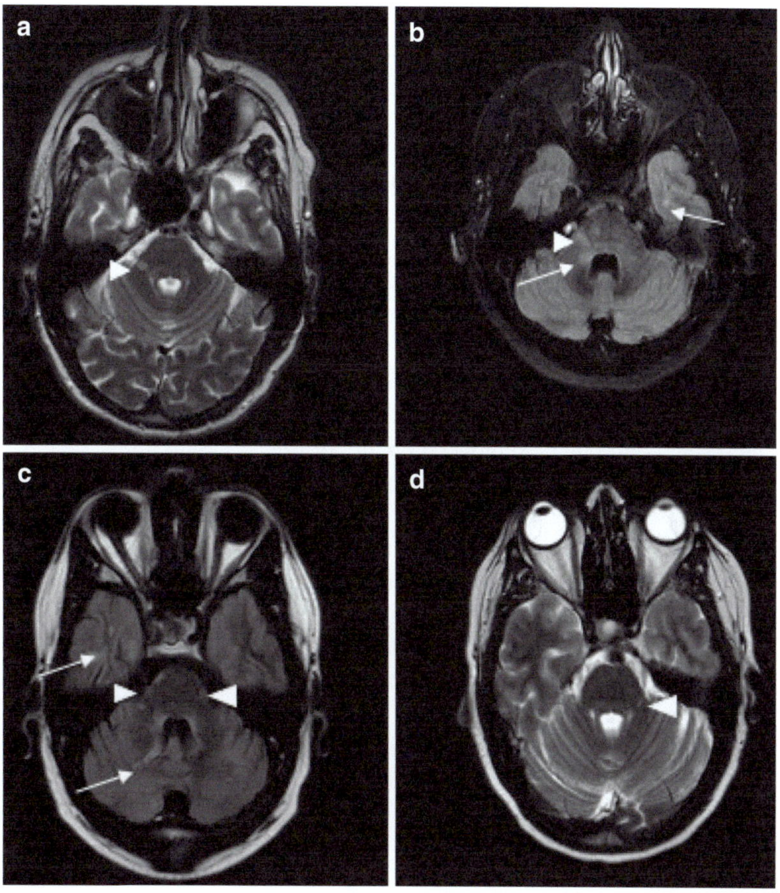

Fig. 14.3 Axial brain MRI at the level of the trigeminal nucleus in the brainstem of patients with multiple sclerosis. (**a**) T2-weighted lesion (arrowhead) showing evidence of demyelination in a patient with right trigeminal neuralgia. (**b**) Fluid attenuated inversion recovery (FLAIR) sequence demonstrating a right trigeminal nucleus lesion (arrowhead) and other demyelinating lesions (white arrow). (**c**) FLAIR sequence images of demyelinating lesions in a patient with bilateral trigeminal neuralgia (arrowhead) and other demyelinating lesions (white arrows). (**d**) T2-weighted lesion (arrowhead) showing evidence of demyelination in a patient with left trigeminal neuralgia

14.4 Cerebrospinal Fluid

Spontaneous intracranial hypotension, which is caused by cerebrospinal fluid (CSF) leaks, presents with various symptoms, including orthostatic headaches and audiovestibular disturbances.

This condition can mimic other headache disorders, resulting in diagnostic challenges.

Imaging techniques such as MRI, CT myelography, and radionuclide cisternography are essential for diagnosis and locating leaks [21, 22]. Moreover, connective tissue abnormalities may contribute to dural weakness and leak development [20].

14.5 Movement Disorders

Movement disorders are a group of clinically, pathologically, and sometimes genetically heterogeneous neurological conditions characterized by the hallmark features of impaired planning, control, and/or execution of movement [23]. However, patients with various movement disorders often also have non-motor symptoms, such as pain in the orofacial region, a condition that can substantially affect quality of life [24–26]. Importantly, current evidence suggests that orofacial manifestations of movement disorders are frequently underdiagnosed or largely mislabeled under the umbrella category of more common temporomandibular disorders (TMDs), which can lead to delayed treatment or unnecessary interventions [27].

14.5.1 Orofacial Pain in Parkinson Disease

Parkinson disease (PD) is a neurological disorder characterized by motor symptoms such as tremor, rigidity, bradykinesia, and postural instability. However, non-motor features, including orofacial and head pain, are increasingly recognized as significant contributors to reduced quality of life in patients with PD [24]. Orofacial pain affects approximately 40%–60% of patients with PD, yet this aspect of the disease remains underreported and undertreated [28]. In fact, pain may precede motor symptoms by several years [30]. The multifactorial nature of pain in patients with PD stems from direct disease pathophysiology and the secondary consequences of motor dysfunction. Orofacial pain in patients with PD manifests through several pathways [28, 30]:

1. Central Parkinsonian pain: This pain is described as deep, aching, or burning sensations in the face and oral cavity that does not follow the typical neuroanatomical distributions. Pain arises secondary to central dopaminergic deficiency and may often fluctuate with medication cycles.
2. Musculoskeletal pain: This pain commonly manifests as being secondary to a TMD. It often occurs with mastication and is associated with limited jaw opening and jaw deviation upon mouth opening. Some motor features of PD, such as rigidity, bradykinesia, and tremor, increase the risk of TMD.
3. Radicular/neuropathic pain: This manifestation is a sharp, shooting pain following trigeminal nerve distribution. This pain may seem to mimic trigeminal neuralgia, but it is distinctive in its association with the motor symptoms of PD.

Several clinical features may help distinguish PD-related orofacial pain from other causes [28, 29]:

1. Temporal correlation with medication cycles: Pain often worsens during periods in which the patient is not actively taking pharmacotherapy for PD and improves with reintroduction of medication.
2. Asymmetry: Pain frequently mirrors the asymmetrical pattern of motor symptoms.
3. Pain quality fluctuation: Pain may transition between dull, aching, and sharp stabbing sensations.
4. Sensory abnormalities: Altered perception, hyperalgesia, or allodynia in the orofacial region may arise.
5. Associated motor symptoms: Tremor, rigidity, or bradykinesia in orofacial musculature may appear during pain episodes.

Treating patients who have orofacial pain within the context of PD warrants an ample interdisciplinary approach. Optimizing dopaminergic medications is key, as pain often fluctuates with medication cycles. Pharmacological management of orofacial pain should include careful consideration of analgesics with particular attention to potential drug interactions, targeted use of muscle relaxants for dystonia-related pain, and appropriate neuropathic pain agents such as gabapentin or pregabalin for central pain mechanisms. Orofacial interventions may also play a crucial therapeutic role and may include custom oral appliances addressing bruxism and abnormal muscle activity, modified occlusal therapy accounting for changing motor function, and implementation of simplified oral hygiene protocols with more frequent preventive visits. Fixed rather than removable prosthetics should be considered when appropriate, and dental treatment timing should be coordinated with medication cycles to maximize patient comfort and therapeutic adherence.

14.5.2 Orofacial Pain in Dystonia

Orofacial dystonia, particularly oromandibular dystonia (OMD), is a unique and often under-recognized group of movement disorders that can manifest as orofacial pain and dysfunction [30]. Clinicians should be able to differentiate between various conditions that might manifest similarly, such as TMD, myofascial pain, and even atypical facial pain. Patients with OMD may present with a variety of symptoms and concerns, and jaw pain is one of the main presenting features. In fact, most patients with OMD report jaw pain as their primary symptom. This pain is often the result of prolonged dystonic muscle contractions affecting the masticatory muscles, leading to pain and functional impairment [30]. Clinicians should be aware that OMD can coexist with TMD and a diagnosis of myofascial pain or temporomandibular joint (TMJ) arthralgia [31]. This overlap may cause challenges in distinguishing between the conditions.

Other common clinical features of OMD include dental attrition, hyposalivation, and masseter hypertrophy, all of which are significant indicators of muscular hyperactivity or dystonic movements. Additionally, some patients may display abnormal oral habits, such as cheek biting or abnormal tongue movement, which can exacerbate pain and contribute to further diagnostic complexity [31]. Psychosocial factors are also an important consideration in the diagnosis of OMD. In one study, 83% of patients with OMD had a comorbid psychological condition, including anxiety and depression [31]. While the precise relationship between psychosocial stress and the development of OMD remains unclear, clinicians must consider these factors when assessing and treating patients [30]. Sensory tricks (geste antagoniste) are simple physical actions or touches that can temporarily alleviate dystonic movements, and these are highly suggestive of OMD [32]. The presence of sensory tricks adds specificity to the diagnosis of OMD, distinguishing this disorder from other conditions such as tardive dyskinesia, for which such tricks are generally not effective and not observed [31, 32].

14.5.3 Orofacial Pain in Bruxism

Bruxism is a stereotyped movement disorder characterized by grinding or clenching of the teeth, often but not always occurring during sleep [33]. When manifesting during sleep, bruxism involves strong contractions of the jaw muscles, which can be rhythmic or continuous isometric contractions lasting from several seconds to as long as 10 min each night. The pathophysiology of bruxism is unknown, but various factors have been associated with this condition. The most cogent hypotheses describe bruxism as a neuromotor dysregulation disorder [33]. The clinical features of orofacial pain in patients with bruxism include a range of symptoms affecting the masticatory system. Patients often report jaw pain, muscle tenderness, and headaches, particularly upon waking, when bruxism occurs during sleep [33, 34]. Other symptoms include tooth wear, hypersensitivity of the teeth, and pain or discomfort in the TMJ.

References

1. Cohen SP, Mao J. Neuropathic pain: mechanisms and their clinical implications. BMJ. 2014;348:f7656.
2. Foley PL, Vesterinen HA, Laird BJ, et al. Prevalence and natural history of pain in adults with multiple sclerosis: systemic review and meta-analysis. Pain. 2013;154(5):632–42.
3. Anosike KC, Rajaram Manoharan SVR. Central post-stroke pain syndrome. In: Stat Pearls [internet]. Treasure Island (FL): Stat Pearls Publishing; 2025. https://www.ncbi.nlm.nih.gov/books/NBK604196/.
4. Timarova G, Steno A. Late-onset jaw and teeth pain mimicking trigeminal neuralgia associated with chronic vagal nerve stimulation: case series and review of literature. BMC Neurol. 2017;17:113.
5. Dzhafarov V, Rzaev J, Moysak G, et al. Facial pain as an initial manifestation of intramedullary spinal cord tumor: a case report and literature review. Surg Neurol Int. 2020;11:173.
6. Nicholson BD. Evaluation and treatment of central pain syndrome. Neurology. 2004;63950:S30–6.
7. Dev P, Kumar Singh A, Kumar D, et al. Persistent facial pain in post-stroke patients, a hospital-based cohort study, experience from North India. Heliyon. 2024;10(7):e28557.
8. Headache Classification Committee of the International Headache Society (IHS). The interna-

tional classification of headache disorders 3rd edition. Cephalalgia. 2018;38:1–211.
9. Goel R, Kumar S, Pamwar A, et al. Pontine infarct presenting with atypical dental pain: a case report. Open Dent J. 2015;9:337–9.
10. Shi Y, Feng Z, Ju Y, et al. Pain mimicking trigeminal neuralgia in patients with acute ischemic stroke of the brainstem. Neuropsychiatr Dis Treat. 2022;18:1237–48.
11. Racke KM, Frohman EM, Frohman T. Pain in multiple sclerosis: understanding pathophysiology, diagnosis and management through clinical vignettes. Front Neurol. 2022;12:799698. https://doi.org/10.3389/fneur.2021.799698.
12. Cree BAC, Oksenberg JR, Hauser SL. Multiple sclerosis: two decades of progress. Lancet Neurol. 2022;21(3):211–4.
13. Nurmikko TJ, Gupta S, MacIver K. Multiple sclerosis-related central pain disorders. Curr Pain Headache Rep. 2010;14:189–95.
14. Osterberg A, Boivie J, Thuomas KA. Central pain in multiple sclerosis-prevalence and clinical characteristics. Euro J Pian. 2005;9:531–42.
15. Truini A, Barbanti P, Pozzilli C, et al. A mechanism-based classification of pain in multiple sclerosis. J Neurol. 2013;260:351–67.
16. Cruccu G. Trigeminal neuralgia. Continuum (Minneap Minn). 2017;23(2):396–420.
17. Houshi S, Tavallai MJ, Barzegar M, et al. Prevalence of trigeminal neuralgia in multiple sclerosis: a systematic review and meta-analysis. Mult Scler Relat Disord. 2022;57:103472. https://doi.org/10.1016/j.msard.2021.103472.
18. Fallata A, Salter A, Tyry T, et al. Trigeminal neuralgia commonly precedes the diagnosis of multiple sclerosis. Int J MS Care. 2017;19:240–6.
19. Di Stefano G, Maarbjerg S, Truini A. Trigeminal neuralgia secondary to multiple sclerosis: from the clinical picture to the treatment options. J Headache Pain. 2019;20(1):20. https://doi.org/10.1186/s10194-019-0969-0.
20. Mokri B. Headaches caused by decreased intracranial pressure: diagnosis and management. Curr Opin Neurol. 2003;16(3):319–26.
21. Urbach H. Intracranial hypotension: clinical presentation, imaging findings, and imaging-guided therapy. Curr Opin Neurol. 2014;27(4):414–24.
22. Schievink WI. Spontaneous spinal cerebrospinal fluid leaks. Cephalalgia. 2008;28(12):1345–56.
23. Chaudhuri KR, Ondo WG, Logishetty K, Reddy P, Sherman R. Handbook of movement disorders. Springer; 2009.
24. Poewe W. Non-motor symptoms in Parkinson's disease. Eur J Neurol. 2008;15:14–20.
25. Kuyper DJ, Parra V, Aerts S, et al. Nonmotor manifestations of dystonia: a systematic review. Mov Disord. 2011;26(7):1206–17.
26. Louis ED. Non-motor symptoms in essential tremor: a review of the current data and state of the field. Parkinsonism Relat Disord. 2016;22:S115–8.
27. Balasubramaniam R, Ram S. Orofacial movement disorders. Oral Maxillofac Surg Clin North Am. 2008;20(2):273–85.
28. Verhoeff MC, Koutris M, Tambach S, et al. Orofacial pain and dysfunction in patients with Parkinson's disease: a scoping review. Eur J Pain. 2022;26(10):2036–59.
29. Tseng M-T, Lin C-H. Pain in early-stage Parkinson's disease: implications from clinical features to pathophysiology mechanisms. J Formos Med Assoc. 2017;116(8):571–81.
30. Saraf U, Chandarana M, Divya K, Krishnan S. Oromandibular dystonia–a systematic review. Ann Indian Acad Neurol. 2022;25(1):26–34.
31. Handa S, Shaefer JR, Keith DA. Oromandibular dystonia and temporomandibular disorders. J Am Dent Assoc. 2022;153(9):899–906.
32. Ramos VFML, Karp BI, Hallett M. Tricks in dystonia: ordering the complexity. J Neurol Neurosurg Psychiatry. 2014;85(9):987–93.
33. Shetty S, Pitti V, Satish Babu C, et al. Bruxism: a literature review. J Indian Prosthodont Soc. 2010;10:141–8.
34. Bulanda S, Ilczuk-Rypuła D, Nitecka-Buchta A, et al. Sleep bruxism in children: etiology, diagnosis, and treatment—a literature review. Int J Environ Res Public Health. 2021;18(18):9544.

15 Imaging for Neurovascular Disorders Presenting as Orofacial Pain

Dace Zvirbulis

15.1 Introduction

Headache is a common presenting symptom in any healthcare setting with an estimated global prevalence of 52% [1, 2]. Healthcare providers seeing patients with headache complaints have to distinguish between a primary or secondary headache. Most headaches are primary headache disorders. Only a small percentage of patients presenting with complaints of headaches have serious secondary causes for the headache [1, 3].

Obtaining a detailed history, including pain severity, quality, duration, location, and accompanying symptoms, and performing a head, neck, and neurologic examination can help to distinguish between primary headache disorder and headache as a symptom of another disease. Primary headache disorders are diagnosed based on a clinical presentation using diagnostic criteria of the International Headache Society (ICHD-3). In general, there is no need for neuroimaging in patients presenting with primary headache disorder [4]. Neuroimaging should be considered in patients presenting with atypical headache features to rule out secondary causes.

Most commonly used imaging modalities in evaluation of patients presenting with complaint of headache are computed tomography (CT), also known as computerized axial tomography (CAT) scan, and magnetic resonance imaging (MRI).

CT scan is recommended for evaluating patients with acute thunderclap headache, suspected paranasal sinus pathology, and head trauma and in patients where MRI is contraindicated [5].

CT has high sensitivity to detect acute intracranial hemorrhage, including subarachnoid hemorrhage. It is also the preferred imaging modality to evaluate any bone pathology.

The main advantage of CT scans is availability and fast scanning times. A disadvantage of using CT scans in the evaluation of headache includes the patient's exposure to radiation, which increases the risk of future malignancies, especially if patients receive repeated CT scans [6, 7]. Non-contrast CT scan of the head can miss vascular diseases (aneurysms, arteriovenous malformations (AVM), cerebral venous sinus thrombosis, cervical artery dissection, and vasculitis), posterior fossa or cervical medullary lesions, neoplasms, signs of infection, and signs of low or high spinal fluid pressure.

In the majority of cases, MRI is the preferred imaging technique for evaluating patients with headache since MRI scan can provide better soft tissue resolution without exposure to radiation.

Disadvantages of MRI use include the need for more detailed patient screening to exclude contraindications such as magnetic metal in the body or implanted devices that are not compatible

D. Zvirbulis (✉)
Wayne State University, Department of Psychiatry, Detroit, Michigan, USA
e-mail: dzvirbu1@hfhs.org

G. A. Kaspo, G. D. Klasser (eds.), *Orofacial and Head Pain*,
https://doi.org/10.1007/978-3-032-08275-6_15

with MRI. MRI scans are also more expensive and require longer testing times, limiting their use in claustrophobic patients.

15.2 Primary Headache Disorders

There are three main types of primary headaches: migraine, tension-type headache, and trigeminal autonomic cephalalgias (Table 15.1). Numerous studies have demonstrated very few significant structural abnormalities on neuroimaging that would require further action.

15.2.1 Migraine

Migraine is the most common headache disorder seen in any healthcare setting. It is also one of the most disabling conditions affecting 12% of the population. Patients with migraine usually complain of moderate to severe unilateral or bilateral throbbing, pounding, or pulsating headache, associated with photophobia, phonophobia, and nausea and/or vomiting. Migraine headache is usually aggravated by any regular activity and lasts for 4 h or longer if untreated. Patients with migraine with aura also can experience reversible episodes of vision changes, numbness, tingling, or speech problems, typically lasting from 5 to 60 min. Significant MR imaging abnormalities are found in only 0.6–0.8% of patients with migraine headache [4, 8].

According to the American College of Radiology Appropriateness Criteria (ACR AC), neuroimaging is not necessary for patients with migraine headache, no red flags, and normal neurologic examination [2, 4].

15.2.2 Tension-Type Headache

Tension-type headache is the most common headache disorder with a lifetime prevalence of 30–78% [4]. Patients with tension-type headache usually complain of mild to moderate bilateral pressing or tightening pain, typically not associated with nausea or vomiting and not worsened by routine physical activity. Due to milder intensity and lack of accompanying disabling symptoms, most people with tension-type headache do not seek medical care and manage these at home.

Major structural abnormalities on neuroimaging are found only in 0.4% of patients presenting with tension-type headache [4, 8].

According to the ACR AC, neuroimaging is not necessary for patients with tension-type headache, no red flags, and normal neurologic examination [2, 4].

15.2.3 Trigeminal Autonomic Cephalalgias

Trigeminal autonomic cephalalgias (TACs) are a group of headache disorders characterized by

Table 15.1 Primary headache disorder characteristics

Primary headache disorder	Unilateral	Bilateral	Severity	Photophobia and phonophobia	Nausea and/or vomiting	Autonomic symptoms	Duration
Migraine	Yes	Yes	Moderate to severe	Yes—both together	Yes	Mild	4–72 h
Tension-type headache	No	Yes	Mild to moderate	1 or another	No	No	30 min to 7 days
Cluster headache	Yes	No	Extremely severe	No	No	Yes	15–180 min
Paroxysmal hemicrania	Yes	No	Severe	No	No	Yes	2–30 min
SUNCT and SUNA	Yes	No	Severe	No	No	Yes	1–600 s
Hemicrania continua	Yes	No	Moderate	Occasionally	No	Yes	Persistent

unilateral attacks of relatively short duration (except for hemicrania continua), associated with ipsilateral autonomic symptoms such as ptosis, miosis, lacrimation, rhinorrhea, and nasal congestion. TACs include cluster headache, paroxysmal hemicrania, short-lasting unilateral neuralgiform headache attacks with conjunctival injection and tearing (SUNCT), short-lasting unilateral neuralgiform headache with autonomic symptoms (SUNA), and hemicrania continua. These are relatively uncommon headache disorders.

Cluster headache is the most severe primary headache characterized by excruciating unilateral pain localized in the first division of the trigeminal nerve and associated with ipsilateral autonomic symptoms and restlessness, lasting 15–180 min.

Paroxysmal hemicrania symptoms are slightly less pronounced than in hemicrania continua, lasting for 2–30 min at a time.

SUNCT and SUNA episodes are very frequent and brief, lasting only 1–60 s, mimicking trigeminal neuralgia.

Hemicrania continua is a primary headache disorder characterized by continuous unilateral head pain, associated with ipsilateral autonomic symptoms, and responsive to indomethacin.

Diagnosis of TACs is clinical, mostly based on the history and physical examination. Neuroimaging is indicated in all patients presenting with TACs to rule out secondary etiology [2, 4, 9].

The differential diagnosis of TACs includes structural lesions affecting the trigeminal autonomic reflex, such as pituitary or hypothalamic lesions, cavernous sinus lesions, carotid or vertebral artery dissection, sphenoid sinus infection, and posterior fossa lesions.

According to the ACR AC, brain MRI without and with gadolinium, including detailed imaging of pituitary area and cavernous sinus, is the appropriate initial imaging for all patients presenting with symptoms of TACs [2, 4]. MR angiography (MRA) of the head without contrast or CT angiography (CTA) of the head with contrast is indicated as a follow-up evaluation in patients with suspected cerebrovascular lesions [10] or the presence of Horner's syndrome [2, 4].

In patients presenting with SUNCT- or SUNA-type episodes, MRI with thin-section multiplanar heavily T2-weighted steady-state free precession sequences (FIESTA, CISS) that provide excellent contrast resolution between CSF and the adjacent soft tissues is recommended to look for evidence of neurovascular compression [11].

CT venography or MR venography can be used as a follow-up study in cases of suspected cerebral venous thrombosis in patients presenting with hemicrania continua type of headache.

15.3 Secondary Headaches

Secondary headaches are headaches that are caused by underlying medical conditions. According to World Health Organization, 18% of the patients presenting to neurology clinics with complaint of headache have a secondary headache disorder. Medication overuse headache is the most common secondary cause, accounting for 7.4% [1]. Although secondary headaches are less common than primary headache disorders, it is still important to differentiate between these headache disorders in order to provide timely and appropriate treatment to the patient. According to the ICHD-3, to diagnose a secondary headache, the medical provider must identify a clear link between the headache and the underlying medical condition, often requiring clinical evaluation, laboratory tests, and/or imaging studies.

In 2003, the mnemonic SNOOP was introduced to use clinical clues as "red flags" to detect secondary headaches. This was later updated to SNNOOP10 to include more features to check for secondary causes of headache (Table 15.2). The presence of red flags indicates the need for further testing to rule out secondary causes [1]. 5.5% of patients presenting to an outpatient headache clinic and having "red flags" were found to have intracranial abnormalities on neuroimaging compared to 0.9–1.2% of patients without "red flags" [12].

Based on SNNOOP10, clinical features indicating a possible underlying disorder causing headache include sudden-onset headache that reaches maximum intensity in less than 5 min,

Table 15.2 SNNOOP10 list of "red flags"

Sign or symptom	Possible etiology
Systemic symptoms including fever	Infection, vasculitis, inflammatory disease
Neoplasm in history	Primary brain tumor, CNS lymphoma, metastasis
Neurologic deficit, including decreased consciousness	Vascular pathology, infection, neoplasm
Onset of headache is sudden	Subarachnoid hemorrhage and other cerebrovascular disorders
Older age (over 50)	Giant cell arteritis, cerebrovascular disorders, neoplasms, infection, trauma
Pattern change or recent onset of headache	Neoplasms, cerebrovascular disorder, vasculitis, intracranial hypertension or hypotension
Positional headache	Intracranial hypertension or hypotension
Precipitated by sneezing, coughing, or exercise	Chiari malformation, posterior fossa lesion, vascular malformation, intracranial hypertension or hypotension
Papilledema	Intracranial hypertension–either primary or secondary, neoplasms, cerebral venous thrombosis
Progressive headache and atypical presentations	Neoplasms, cerebral venous thrombosis, intracranial hypertension or hypotension
Pregnancy or postpartum	Cerebrovascular disorders, postdural headache, hypertension-related disorders, pituitary apoplexy
Painful eye with autonomic features	Pituitary region, hypothalamic or cavernous sinus lesion
Posttraumatic	Subdural hematoma
Pathology of the immune system such as HIV or immunosuppression	Opportunistic infections, neoplasm
Painkiller overuse/medication overuse headache	

new-onset headache after age of 50, change in previous headache character or pattern, headache that changes with positional change such as lying down or standing up, headache precipitated by Valsalva maneuver or physical activity, headache associated with systemic symptoms such as fever, headache associated with neurologic symptoms or signs including papilledema and seizures, and headache in patients with a history of malignancy or immunosuppression.

According to the ACR AC, MRI of the head without and with IV contrast, and CT of the head without contrast are appropriate initial imaging techniques in patients with headache and one or more "red flags" such as increasing headache frequency or severity, associated fever or neurologic deficit, history of cancer or immunocompromise, new-onset headache in individuals older than 50, and posttraumatic headache [4].

Although currently no specific data are available to favor one imaging modality over another, MRI of the head is the preferred initial imaging modality, especially in the outpatient setting, due to higher soft tissue resolution. Addition of intravenous contrast/gadolinium can be helpful to demonstrate breakdown in the blood-brain barrier due to neoplastic or inflammatory disease [4].

CT angiography of the head and neck, CT venography of the head, MR angiography of the head and neck without contrast, and MR venography of the head can be performed following initial evaluation with non-contrast CT of the head or MRI of the head if there are clinical or imaging findings suspicious for cerebrovascular disease [4].

15.3.1 Headache Associated with Systemic Symptoms Including Fever

Patients presenting with headache associated with systemic symptoms have to be evaluated for possible central nervous system (CNS) infection, systemic or CNS vasculitis, or inflammatory disease. CNS infections include meningitis, encephalitis, and brain abscess.

Patients with meningitis will usually present with systemic symptoms of fever, malaise, neck stiffness, and headache. Headache is present in 51.7–87% of patients with meningitis, and fever is present in 61.1–97% of cases [1]. Headache can be associated with photophobia and phonophobia, mimicking migraine-type headache. In addition to headache and systemic symptoms, patients with encephalitis and brain abscess can also present with focal neurologic deficits or seizures. It is important to obtain a detailed history, including previous headache history to assess for any changes in headache pattern or character. Although non-contrast CT will not reveal any abnormalities in patients with meningitis, the Infectious Disease Society of America recommends performing non-contrast CT scan prior to doing lumbar puncture (LP) to exclude cerebral edema or mass effect that would increase the risk for herniation during LP [13].

MRI of the brain usually is not required in patients with meningitis unless there are suspected complications of encephalitis or intracranial abscess. Brain MRI with and without contrast may show dural enhancement in patients with meningitis.

15.3.2 Headache in Patients with a History of Neoplasm

According to the ICHD-3 "headache attributed to intracranial neoplasia is caused by space-occupying intracranial neoplasms and has developed in temporal relation to development of the neoplasm, or related to its discovery; headache has significantly worsened in parallel with worsening of the neoplasm or improved in temporal relation to successful treatment of neoplasm; and has characteristics of being progressive, worse in the morning or when lying down, aggravated by Valsalva maneuvers, accompanied by nausea and/or vomiting."

The risk of finding a brain tumor in patients presenting with headaches, but without history of any neoplasm, is less than 0.1%, of which the majority present after the age of 50 [1]. According to studies, 32.2–71% patients with known brain tumors complain of headaches [14]. Both primary brain tumors and metastatic brain tumors are equally likely to cause headaches, often in association with other neurologic signs and symptoms. Intracranial metastasis is found in 32–54% of patients with known history of malignancy presenting with new-onset headache [1]. Lung cancer, breast cancer, and melanoma have the highest risk of intracranial metastasis [15].

The likelihood of headache is greater in children, young patients, and patients with rapid growth of the tumor, or posterior fossa or midline localization [14].

A low threshold for investigation is suggested in any patient with history of malignancy. Every oncology patient with new-onset headache should have MRI of the brain without and with contrast.

15.3.3 Headache Associated with Neurologic Deficit

In patients presenting with an acute-onset headache associated with sudden development of focal neurologic deficit, intracranial vascular pathology such as ischemic or hemorrhagic stroke or cerebral venous thrombosis (CVT) should be considered in the differential diagnosis.Headache occurs in 25% of episodes of acute stroke with a higher frequency in hemorrhagic than in ischemic stroke [5].

Non-contrast head CT can be performed as the initial imaging to rule out intracranial hemorrhage. Non-contrast head CT is not very sensitive to display hyper-acute ischemic stroke.Non-contrast MRI of the head with diffusion-weighted imaging (DWI) sequence is preferred for the evaluation of patients with acute ischemic stroke. CT perfusion scan can also be performed in the hyper-acute setting of ischemic stroke [16].

In patients presenting with headache associated with subacute or gradual development of focal neurologic deficit intracranial mass, cerebral venous sinus thrombosis, cerebral vascular malformations, vasculitis, or cerebral spinal fluid (CSF) pressure abnormalities should be ruled out.

Vasculitis is an inflammatory disease of blood vessel walls. Central nervous system (CNS) vasculitis can be primary or secondary to systemic vasculitis. Secondary vasculitis includes giant cell arteritis (GCA), systemic lupus erythematosus, rheumatoid arthritis, Sjogren syndrome, scleroderma, polyarteritis nodosa, microscopic polyangiitis, IgA arteritis, Kawasaki disease, Behcet's disease, drug- or radiation-induced vasculitis, or infectious vasculitis secondary to tuberculosis, varicella zoster, HIV, syphilis, or fungal infections [17].

Patients with vasculitis usually present with complaints of subacute-onset headache accompanied by focal neurologic signs and symptoms and cognitive changes.

GCA is the most common primary medium to large vessel systemic vasculitis in the western world. It typically affects patients over the age of 50 and presents with headache, episodes of vision changes, and systemic symptoms of malaise, night sweats, unintentional weight loss, and jaw claudication. Diagnosis requires clinical assessment, laboratory testing (sed rate, C-reactive protein), neuroimaging, and superficial temporal artery biopsy.

In patients with suspected CNS vasculitis, MRI of the head with and without contrast is the preferred initial imaging study [4]. CT of the head and MRI of the head may show multifocal ischemic and hemorrhagic infarcts of varying ages with micro hemorrhages. Post-contrast MRI may show leptomeningeal enhancement. After initial neuroimaging, CTA of the head and neck or MRA of the head and neck may be useful if vascular pathology is suspected. In patients with vasculitis, vascular imaging with either CTA of the head or MRA of the head without contrast can show multifocal narrowing, irregularities, and occlusions of blood vessels. MRI of the brain with high-resolution blood vessel wall imaging and contrast (SPACE, CUBE, VISTA sequences) can show eccentric blood vessel wall thickening and enhancement [4]. In patients with GCA, MRI of the brain with contrast with vessel wall imaging has high negative predictive value and can decrease the need for superficial temporal artery biopsy if the MRI is negative [18]. For small vessel vasculitis, both CTA and MRA of the head have limited resolution. Even digital subtraction angiography has a sensitivity of only 20–64% to detect CNS vasculitis [17]. Brain and blood vessel biopsy might be necessary for diagnosis.

In patients with GCA, duplex ultrasound of superficial temporal artery has moderate sensitivity (53.3%) and high specificity (9 1.1%) and can be performed to assess for increased diameter and hypoechoic wall thickening (halo sign) [19].

If CVT or stenosis is suspected, MR venography of the head is recommended. If there is contraindication to MRI, CT venography (CTV) of the head is an alternative.

15.3.4 Sudden-Onset "Thunderclap" Headache

Thunderclap headache is characterized by sudden severe head pain that reaches its maximum in less than 1 min or "worst headache of life." Most of the patients with thunderclap headache will present to the emergency department.

Thunderclap headache can be caused by subarachnoid hemorrhage (SAH) due to cerebral aneurysm rupture, reversible cerebral vasoconstriction syndrome (RCVS), CVT, cervical artery dissection, spontaneous intracranial hypotension, or pituitary apoplexy. Patients with RCVS can have repeated episodes of thunderclap-type headache.

SAH can be seen on non-contrast head CT as hypertensive blood in the basal cisterns and around the circle of Willis in 29–71% of adults presenting with sudden-onset thunderclap headache [17]. The sensitivity of non-contrast CT for acute subarachnoid hemorrhage is 92–95% during the first 12–24 h after the aneurysm rupture, and 82–84% afterward [5]. Non-contrast CT of the head performed within 6 h of headache onset has high negative predictive value in detecting aneurysmal SAH (99.9–100%) [4]. In patients presenting with sudden-onset thunderclap headache with negative non-contrast head CT, lumbar puncture should be performed to look for xanthochromia since smaller subarachnoid hemorrhages can be concealed by artifact and/or bone.

RCVS causes multifocal segmental cerebral artery vasoconstriction that starts in the distal small blood vessels and gradually progresses centripetally [20]. It can be triggered by serotoninergic, sympathomimetic, or immunosuppressant medications, illicit drugs such as cocaine, LSD, amphetamines, marijuana, caffeine, licorice, preeclampsia, eclampsia, high altitude, and neck or carotid artery surgeries. Patients with RCVS present with sudden-onset "thunderclap" headache, occasionally recurrent, associated with focal neurologic deficits and seizures. RCVS can mimic aneurysmal SAH. Stroke can develop a few days after initial presentation of RCVS.

Initial non-contrast head CT and brain MRI can be normal [20]. Over the next 2 weeks, up to 70% of patients with RCVS will develop convexity SAH without evidence of aneurysm on vascular imaging. Follow-up CT of the head without contrast and MRI of the brain without contrast can show multifocal watershed territory ischemic infarcts, lobar intracranial hemorrhages, and vasogenic edema [21]. Earliest ischemic or vasogenic edema lesions are usually located in the cortical-subcortical junction. Initial blood vessel imaging with CTA or MRA of the head done within the first week of symptom onset can be normal. Cerebral vasoconstriction reaches maximum on angiogram 2–3 weeks after clinical onset [20]. CTA or MRA of the head shows segmental narrowing and dilatation of arteries (string of beads). Repeat blood vessel imaging after a few days might show resolution of changes in some blood vessels with new constriction affecting more proximal blood vessels.

CVT can either cause sudden onset "thunderclap" or subacute/chronic headache.Headache is the most common symptom of CVT and can precede other symptoms by days or weeks [22]. In 40% of cases, headache is the only symptom [1].

The most important risk factor for CVT is female gender due to hormonal changes from oral contraceptive or hormonal replacement therapy use, or pregnancy causing a pro-coagulative state [22]. In elderly patients, malignancy and inherited thrombophilic conditions are the most common causes of CVT. Although nonspecific, headache in patients with CVT can either mimic migraine or hemicrania continua, or have features typical to intracranial hypertension.

Patients usually have constant unilateral or bilateral headache, fluctuating in intensity—worse at night or in recumbent position, also worsened by Valsalva maneuvers, associated with episodes of blurred or double vision and pulsatile tinnitus. Non-contrast CT head scans are normal in up to one-third of patients [22]. Occasionally, CT of the head can show dense delta sign on non-contrast imaging reflecting hyperdensity of venous thrombus. CT of the head with IV contrast can show an "empty delta" sign, reflecting enhancing dural collateral venous channels [17, 22]. In one-third of CVT cases, patients may develop venous infarct or hemorrhage [23]. MRI of the brain without contrast may show venous thrombus as a loss of flow void in the venous sinus on the T2-weighted images. MRI of the brain also may show venous infarcts and hemorrhage.

According to the ACR AC, CT of the head without IV contrast is an appropriate initial imaging, and CTA of the head with IV contrast may be performed in conjunction with non-contrast CT of the head, especially when the patient presents more than 6 h after the symptom onset, since the sensitivity of CT of the head for SAH diminishes over time [4].

CTA of the head can assess vessel diameters of 0.7 mm and larger and has 90–100% sensitivity for detecting aneurysms larger than 4 mm. MRA of the head has 95% sensitivity for detecting aneurysms larger than 4 mm, but it has more false positives when compared to CTA of the head [17]. Digital subtraction angiography (DSA) has the best spatial and temporal resolution and best sensitivity for detecting small aneurysms, and it might be useful in patients with SAH and negative CTA of the head since DSA can assess vessel diameters as small as 0.4 mm and also might be helpful in the workup of suspected RCVS, which primarily affects the smaller blood vessels [1, 17]. Disadvantages of DSA include need for specific technical expertise and possibility of developing stroke as a complication of the procedure.

MRI of the head can be obtained as a follow-up imaging study when there are clinical or imaging findings concerning aneurysm, arterial dissection, AVM, or RCVS [4].

CT venography or MR venography (MRV) of the head without and with contrast are recommended in all patients with suspected CVT to look for filling defects [4]. Non-contrast MRV is preferred in pregnancy and in patients with renal failure [17].

There is inadequate evidence to recommend the use of MRI of the head in the initial imaging evaluation of "thunderclap" headache. MRI of the head without and with IV contrast may be helpful in follow-up evaluation to assess for pituitary apoplexy, colloid cyst, or signs of spontaneous intracranial hypotension [4].

Cervical artery dissection (CAD) is characterized by an intramural hematoma of the internal carotid or the vertebral artery. It is a major cause of stroke in the young. Patients can present with complaints of headache, neck pain, and focal neurologic symptoms including Horner syndrome and cranial nerve palsies [24]. It is important to recognize cervical artery dissection early to initiate appropriate treatment. Cervical artery dissection is confirmed by neuroimaging showing the presence of at least one of the following: visualization of a mural hematoma, aneurysmal dilatation, long tapering stenosis, intimal flap, double lumen, and occlusion great than 2 cm above the carotid bifurcation revealing an aneurysmal dilatation or a long tapering stenosis after recanalization in the internal carotid or vertebral artery [24].

CTA of the head and neck can be done as a rapid initial imaging study. Occasionally, vertebral artery dissections can be missed on CTA. High-resolution MRI of the head and neck can better assess blood vessel walls and changes caused by the dissection.

15.3.5 New-Onset Headache After Age 50

There is a higher frequency of secondary headache in the older population. Infection is the most common cause, followed by headache attributed to neoplasms, or cerebrovascular disorders, including GCA.

MRI of the brain without and with contrast is an appropriate initial imaging choice in this population.

More detailed choice of neuroimaging for these conditions was discussed previously in this chapter.

15.3.6 Pattern Change or Recent Onset of Headache

Neuroimaging is indicated in patients with prior history of headache if they develop new headache features and/or focal neurologic signs. Recent increase in headache frequency, newly developed headache within the previous 3 months, or change in headache character can be the only signs of underlying secondary etiology presenting in up to 20% of patients [1].

According to the ACR AC, MRI of the head without and with contrast, MRI of the head without contrast, and CT of the head without contrast are all appropriate as initial imaging modalities in patients with change in headache pattern to rule out neoplasms, vascular or known vascular intracranial disorders [4].

15.3.7 Headache Precipitated by Sneezing, Coughing, or Exercise

Headaches associated with physical exertion or coughing can be primary or secondary. Additional testing is warranted to rule out structural lesions. Studies have shown that about half of the patients presenting with cough headache have structural lesions—either Chiari I malformation or space-occupying lesions in posterior fossa [25, 26]. In comparison, up to 80% of exercise- and sexual activity-induced headaches are primary. Secondary causes for exercise- and sexual activity-induced headaches include vascular malformations, SAH, RCVS, cervical artery dissection, hypertensive crisis, and hydrocephalus [25].

Headaches due to high or low CSF pressure also can be aggravated by cough or other Valsalva maneuvers.

In patients with Chiari I malformation, MRI of the brain will show cerebellar tonsillar herniation of 5 mm or greater below the foramen magnum, best seen on sagittal imaging [27]. It is important to remember that the prevalence of symptomatic Chiari malformation is different from the prevalence of image-defined Chiari malformation, and anatomic MRI of the brain findings do not correlate with the type and severity of headache [28]. Only one-third of MRI-detected cases are symptomatic [1]. Chiari malformation associated headache is caused by impairment of CSF flow at the level of foramen magnum. Motion-sensitive MRI techniques with CINE phase contrast are recommended to assess for CSF flow obstruction around the brainstem and at the level of the foramen magnum [28].

MRI of the brain without and with contrast is recommended to exclude hydrocephalus, mass, or signs of intracranial hypotension. CTA of the head or MRA of the head without contrast is recommended to assess for possible vascular malformations. CTA of the neck or MRA of the neck might be useful to assess for cervical artery dissection.

15.3.8 Headache Associated with Papilledema

A high prevalence of patients with papilledema has serious underlying intracranial pathology, causing intracranial hypertension resulting in papilledema. Intracranial hypertension can be either idiopathic, also known as pseudotumor cerebri, or secondary to structural brain lesions including mass, hydrocephalus, and CVT.

Idiopathic intracranial hypertension (IIH) is characterized as an elevation of CSF pressure of unknown cause above 250 mm water when measured in lateral decubitus position, with no identifiable secondary cause. IIH mostly affects young overweight women. Headache often is a presenting symptom of IIH and affects up to 90% of patients [4]. Headache tends to be positional, worse in recumbent position, at night, and worsened by Valsalva maneuvers. A lumbar puncture to document elevated opening pressure requires a diagnostic tool for the diagnosis of IIH [4]. Patients with intracranial hypertension can also experience episodes of vision changes, double vision, pulsatile tinnitus, nausea, or vomiting. Neuroimaging is required to exclude secondary causes.

According to the ACR AC, in patients presenting with headache with papilledema, MRI of the head without and with contrast, MRI of the head without IV contrast, and CT of the head without IV contrast are appropriate as initial imaging to rule out neoplasm and assess for signs of intracranial hypertension, followed by MRV or CTV of the head to assess for cerebral venous thrombosis or stenosis. MRV of the head with IV contrast is preferred over MRV of the head without contrast since the use of IV contrast helps delineate the venous sinus lumen and avoids some of the flow-related artifact encountered in non-contrast MRV techniques [4].

Non-contrast CT of the brain head can be helpful to evaluate for possible mass, cerebral edema, or hydrocephalus, especially prior to performing lumbar puncture to avoid brain herniation [4]. MRI of the head without IV and MRI of the head without and with IV contrast can help exclude secondary causes of elevated intracranial pressure and detect imaging signs that are associated with primary IIH, such as partially empty Sella, flattening of the posterior globe, optic nerve head protrusion, optic nerve sheath distention, optic nerve tortuosity, prominence of Meckel's cave, and slit-like ventricles [29, 30].

15.3.9 Progressive Headache and Headache with Atypical Presentation

Progressive headaches and headaches with atypical presentations are associated with an increased likelihood of major abnormalities in neuroimaging. Possible causes include neoplasms, cerebral venous sinus thrombosis, vasculitis, and headache secondary to intracranial hypertension or intracranial hypotension. According to the ACR AC, MRI of the head without and with contrast, MRI of the head without contrast, and CT of the head without contrast are all appropriate as initial imaging modalities in patients presenting with progressive headache or headache with atypical presentation.

15.3.10 Headache in Pregnancy or Puerperium

Pregnant individuals with new-onset, progressive headache or change in the previous headache pattern are more likely to have secondary intracranial pathology when compared with the general population [31]. Among pregnant women presenting with acute headache, 35% were found to have secondary headache, with most presentations during the third trimester [32].

Due to hypercoagulability and hormonal changes, pregnant patients are at high risk for developing subarachnoid hemorrhage, stroke, cerebral venous sinus thrombosis, idiopathic intracranial hypertension, pituitary apoplexy, hypertensive encephalopathy with reversible cerebral vasoconstriction syndrome, and/or posterior reversible encephalopathy syndrome in the setting of preeclampsia/eclampsia.

According to the ACR AC, MRI of the head without or CT of the head without contrast is usually an appropriate initial imaging for new-onset headache or pattern change during pregnancy or the postpartum period [4].

Non-contrast CT of the head can be performed in urgent situations where subarachnoid or intracranial hemorrhage is suspected. According to the ACR and the American College of Obstetricians and Gynecologists, the estimated radiation exposure is low for CT when the fetus is outside the field-of-view, and non-contrast CT scanning can be safely performed during any trimester of pregnancy [5, 32]. After initial CT of the head, concurrent or follow-up MRA of the head without contrast or CTA of the head with contrast is useful in suspected cases of intracranial aneurysm, arterial dissection, or RCVS [4]. Overall, MRI without contrast is preferred over CTA with contrast. CTV of the head with contrast or MRV of the head without contrast can be useful in the initial imaging evaluation of a new headache during pregnancy or postpartum. To rule out cerebral venous thrombosis, iodinated contrast agents are considered safer than gadolinium-based contrast agents with regard to potential effects on the fetus [4].

Due to higher tissue resolution, MRI of the brain without gadolinium is the preferred initial imaging modality to evaluate pregnant patients presenting with subacute headache onset or change in previous headache pattern or character [32].

15.3.11 Posttraumatic Headache

Headache is the most common symptom reported after head trauma. Up to 90% of patients with mild traumatic brain injury report headache [5]. According to the ICHD-3 criteria, posttraumatic headache starts within 7 days after the injury. It is classified as acute posttraumatic headache during the first 3 months after head trauma and as a persistent headache after 3 months. Non-contrast CT of the head can be performed in the emergency department to assess for intracranial hemorrhage or bone fracture [4].

The ACR AC recommends performing MRI of the brain without contrast or MRI of the brain without and with contrast for patients with traumatic brain injury with any new or progressive neurologic deficits or worsening cognition [4].

15.3.12 Headache in Immunocompromised Patients

Immunocompromised patients are at higher risk for intracranial infections such as toxoplasmosis, progressive multifocal leukoencephalopathy, and neoplastic disorders, including CNS lymphoma. MRI of the brain with and without contrast should be performed in these patients if they have developed new or progressively worsening headache [4].

15.4 Conclusion

Although most patients presenting with headaches have a primary headache disorder, imaging is an important component of the diagnostic assessment to exclude secondary causes that may require intervention and could result in significant morbidity or mortality.

It is very important to obtain a detailed headache history, including assessment for possible "red flags," and perform neurologic evaluation to look for focal neurologic deficits. Patients with primary headache disorder such as migraine or tension-type headache with normal neurologic examination do not need any further neuroimaging. Patients with TACs might benefit from neuroimaging since there are many secondary causes that could mimic TACs. Any patient presenting with complaints of new-onset headache or headache associated with any of the "red flags" should be screened and evaluated for possible secondary causes. Choice of specific neuroimaging modality should be based on the clinical scenario. ACR AC guidelines for neuroimaging in the headache setting provide evidence-based imaging recommendations for specific headache patterns in various clinical context (Table 15.3) (Figs. 15.1, 15.2, 15.3).

Table 15.3 ACR AC recommendations for neuroimaging modalities for patients presenting with headache

Headache variant	Initial imaging	Additional imaging
Sudden-onset severe headache	CT head without contrast	CT angiography of the head MRA angiography without contrast Digital subtraction angiography MRI of the head without and with contrast MRI of the head without contrast
Migraine with normal neurologic examination	None	None
Tension type headache with normal neurologic examination	None	None
Trigeminal autonomic cephalalgia/periorbital headache associated with autonomic symptoms	MRI of the head without and with contrast	CT angiography of the head and neck MR angiography of the head and neck without contrast CT venography of the head MR venography of the head with contrast
Headache with features of intracranial hypertension—Papilledema, worse with Valsalva	MRI of the head without and with contrast MRI of the head without contrast CT of the head without contrast	MRV of the head with IV contrast MRV of the head without contrast CTV of the head with contrast
Headache with features of intracranial hypotension	MRI of the head without and with contrast	MR myelography Dynamic CT myelography
Headache with new onset or pattern during pregnancy or peripartum period	MRI of the head without contrast CT of the head without contrast	MRV of the head without contrast CTV of the head with contrast
Headache associated with 1 or more of the following "red flags": Increasing frequency or severity, fever or neurologic deficit, history of cancer or immunocompromise, older age over 50, and posttraumatic	MRI of the head without and with contrast MRI of the head without contrast CT of the head without contrast	CT venography MR venography with contrast MR venography without contrast
Headache without any of the red flags	None	None

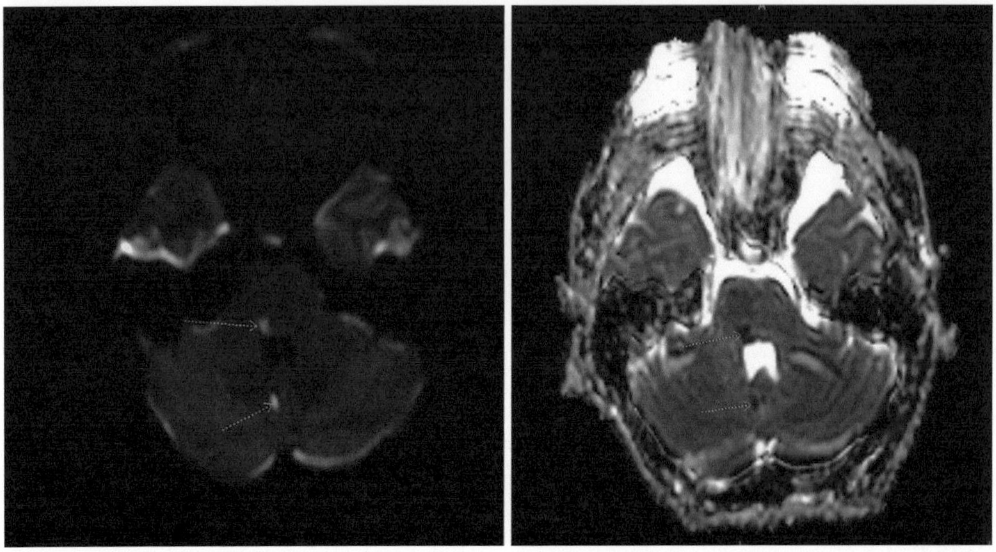

Fig. 15.1 MRI brain with diffusion-weighted imaging (DWI) demonstrates a tiny right paramedian pontine lacunar infarct. Additional focal infarcts are seen in the right paramedian vermis and inferior right cerebellar hemisphere. Corresponding areas of low signal intensity on the ADC map are consistent with acute, non-hemorrhagic infarcts estimated to be greater than 8 hours in duration. Clinical symptoms included new-onset headache, neck pain, and left-sided tingling and numbness, along with transient visual aura described as zigzagging, rainbow-colored streaks in the left eye, characteristic of an ocular migraine.

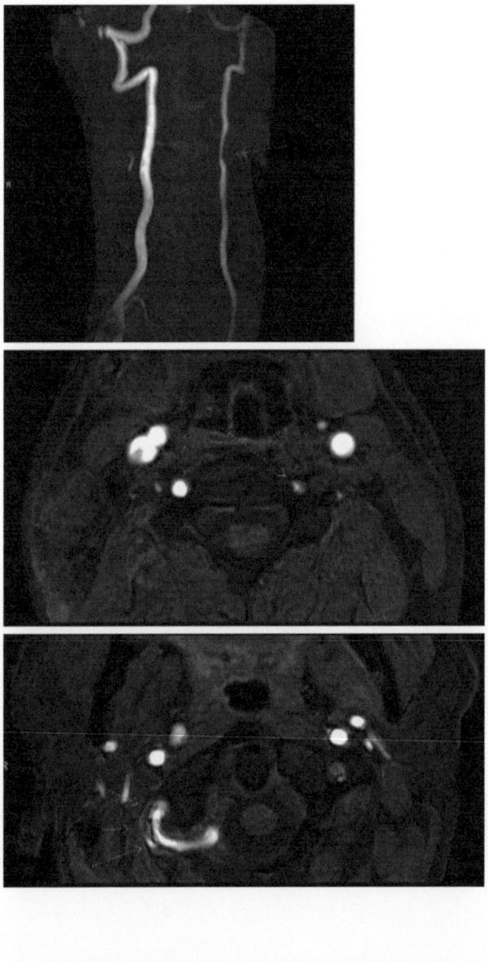

Fig. 15.2 MR angiography demonstrates a small, irregular left vertebral artery with a focal dissection extending from approximately C2 to C4, associated with intramural hematoma. A right vertebral artery dissection is also identified, involving the artery within the foramina transversarium at C1 and extending distally.

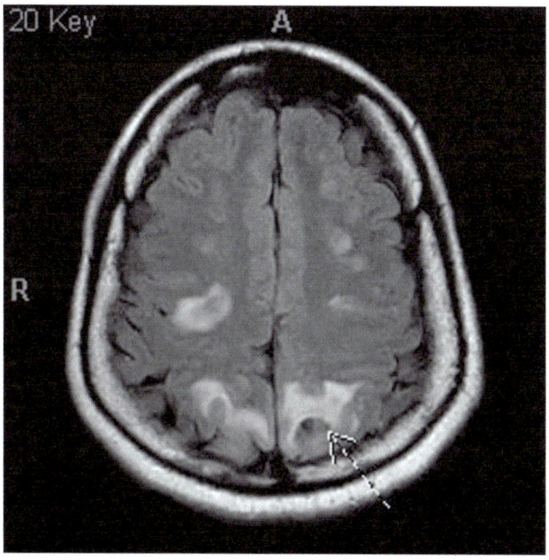

Fig. 15.3 MRI brain demonstrates relatively symmetric high signal intensity in the parietal-occipital regions and cerebellar hemispheres, with right greater than left involvement of the cortex and subcortical white matter in the frontal lobes. Findings are suggestive of eclampsia-related hypertensive encephalopathy (PRES). Clinical presentation included a postpartum day 8 patient with severe occipital headache, photophobia, visual disturbance, nausea, and witnessed generalized tonic-clonic seizures, with systolic blood pressure ranging from 140s to 170s.

References

1. Do TP, Remmers A, Schytz HW, Schankin C, Nelson SE, Obermann M, et al. Red and orange flags for secondary headaches in clinical practice: SNNOOP10 list. Neurology. 2019;92(3):134–44.
2. Stovner LJ, Hagen K, Linde M, Steiner TJ. The global prevalence of headache: an update, with analysis of the influences of methodological factors on prevalence estimates. J Headache Pain. 2022;23(1):34.
3. Mitsikostas DD, Ashina M, Craven A, Diener HC, Goadsby PJ, Ferrari MD, et al. European headache federation consensus on technical investigation for primary headache disorders. J Headache Pain. 2015;17:5.
4. Utukuri PS, Shih RY, Ajam AA, Callahan KE, Chen D, Dunkle JW, et al. ACR appropriateness criteria® headache: 2022 update. J Am Coll Radiol. 2023;20(5s):S70–s93.
5. Asadollahi S, Yousem DM, Nadgir R. Neuroimaging of headache: indications and controversies. Neurol Clin. 2022;40(3):471–89.
6. Einstein AJ. Medical radiation exposure to the U.S. population: the turning tide. Radiology. 2020;295(2):428–9.
7. Schultz CH, Fairley R, Murphy LS, Doss M. The risk of cancer from CT scans and other sources of low-dose radiation: a critical appraisal of methodologic quality. Prehosp Disaster Med. 2020;35(1):3–16.
8. Wang HZ, Simonson TM, Greco WR, Yuh WT. Brain MR imaging in the evaluation of chronic headache in patients without other neurologic symptoms. Acad Radiol. 2001;8(5):405–8.
9. Yildiz Goksel H, Bilgin S, Digre K, Cortez MM, Ozudogru SN. The critical role of neuroimaging in hemicrania continua: a systematic review and case series. Headache. 2024;64(6):674–84.
10. San-Juan D, Velez-Jimenez K, Hoffmann J, Martínez-Mayorga AP, Melo-Carrillo A, Rodríguez-Leyva I, et al. Cluster headache: an update on clinical features, epidemiology, pathophysiology, diagnosis, and treatment. Front Pain Res (Lausanne). 2024;5:1373528.
11. Cohen AS, Matharu MS, Goadsby PJ. Short-lasting unilateral neuralgiform headache attacks with conjunctival injection and tearing (SUNCT) or cranial autonomic features (SUNA)–a prospective clinical study of SUNCT and SUNA. Brain. 2006;129(Pt 10):2746–60.
12. Clarke CE, Edwards J, Nicholl DJ, Sivaguru A. Imaging results in a consecutive series of 530 new patients in the Birmingham Headache Service. J Neurol. 2010;257(8):1274–8.
13. Tunkel AR, Hasbun R, Bhimraj A, Byers K, Kaplan SL, Scheld WM, et al. 2017 Infectious Diseases Society of America's Clinical Practice Guidelines for Healthcare-Associated Ventriculitis and Meningitis. Clin Infect Dis. 2017;64(6):e34–65.
14. Hadidchi S, Surento W, Lerner A, Liu CJ, Gibbs WN, Kim PE, et al. Headache and brain tumor. Neuroimaging Clin N Am. 2019;29(2):291–300.
15. Lassman AB, DeAngelis LM. Brain metastases. Neurol Clin. 2003;21(1):1–23, vii.
16. Munich SA, Shakir HJ, Snyder KV. Role of CT perfusion in acute stroke management. Cor Vasa. 2016;58:e215–24.
17. Wang LL, Mahammedi A, Vagal AS. Imaging of headache attributed to vascular disorders. Neurol Clin. 2022;40(3):507–30.
18. Bley TA, Uhl M, Carew J, Markl M, Schmidt D, Peter HH, et al. Diagnostic value of high-resolution MR imaging in giant cell arteritis. AJNR Am J Neuroradiol. 2007;28(9):1722–7.
19. Gielis JF, Geelhoed R, Yogeswaran SK, Lauwers P, Van Schil P, Hendriks JMH. Evaluation of temporal artery duplex ultrasound for diagnosis of temporal arteritis. J Surg Res. 2021;261:320–5.
20. Singhal AB. Reversible cerebral vasoconstriction syndrome: a review of pathogenesis, clinical presentation, and treatment. Int J Stroke. 2023;18(10):1151–60.
21. Miller TR, Shivashankar R, Mossa-Basha M, Gandhi D. Reversible cerebral vasoconstriction syndrome, part 2: diagnostic work-up, imaging evaluation, and differential diagnosis. AJNR Am J Neuroradiol. 2015;36(9):1580–8.

22. Aliprandi A, Borelli P, Polonia V, Salmaggi A. Headache in cerebral venous thrombosis. Neurol Sci. 2020;41(Suppl 2):401–6.
23. Canedo-Antelo M, Baleato-González S, Mosqueira AJ, Casas-Martínez J, Oleaga L, Vilanova JC, et al. Radiologic clues to cerebral venous thrombosis. Radiographics. 2019;39(6):1611–28.
24. Engelter ST, Traenka C, Von Hessling A, Lyrer PA. Diagnosis and treatment of cervical artery dissection. Neurol Clin. 2015;33(2):421–41.
25. González-Quintanilla V, Madera J, Pascual J. Update on headaches associated with physical exertion. Cephalalgia. 2023;43(3):3331024221146989.
26. Riveira C, Pascual J. Is Chiari type I malformation a reason for chronic daily headache. Curr Pain Headache Rep. 2007;11(1):53–5.
27. Pascual J. Primary cough headache. Curr Pain Headache Rep. 2005;9(4):272–6.
28. Bezuidenhout AF, Chang YM, Heilman CB, Bhadelia RA. Headache in Chiari malformation. Neuroimaging Clin N Am. 2019;29(2):243–53.
29. Maralani PJ, Hassanlou M, Torres C, Chakraborty S, Kingstone M, Patel V, et al. Accuracy of brain imaging in the diagnosis of idiopathic intracranial hypertension. Clin Radiol. 2012;67(7):656–63.
30. Beier D, Korsbæk JJ, Bsteh G, Macher S, Marik W, Pemp B, et al. Magnetic resonance imaging signs of idiopathic intracranial hypertension. JAMA Netw Open. 2024;7(7):e2420138.
31. Robbins MS, Farmakidis C, Dayal AK, Lipton RB. Acute headache diagnosis in pregnant women: a hospital-based study. Neurology. 2015;85(12):1024–30.
32. Zamora C, Castillo M. Role of MRI and CT in the evaluation of headache in pregnancy and the postpartum period. Neurol Clin. 2022;40(3):661–77.

Future Directions in Orofacial and Head Pain Imaging

16

Kaan Orhan and Gurkan Unsal

16.1 Introduction

Orofacial and head pain arises from various etiologies, including temporomandibular disorders (TMDs), dental and periodontal pathology, sinus-related issues, neuropathic conditions, and systemic diseases affecting the craniofacial region [1, 2]. Previous chapters in this volume have detailed the current imaging modalities used to evaluate these conditions, from panoramic radiography and CBCT to MRI and nuclear imaging. While these tools provide valuable diagnostic information, they also have limitations, such as difficulty distinguishing referred sources of pain or detecting subtle anatomical changes [3, 4].

As the field progresses, emerging technologies offer promising areas for enhancing diagnostic precision and clinical decision-making. Innovations in artificial intelligence (AI), coupled with advanced imaging modalities and data analytics, stand to improve the ability to identify subtle pathologies, differentiate overlapping symptoms, and predict disease trajectories. AI-driven pattern recognition and predictive modeling can move care toward a more proactive model, where interventions are guided by data-based predictions rather than traditional reactive approaches [5–7].

In addition, new imaging techniques capable of capturing both structural and functional aspects of orofacial anatomy, as well as wearable devices that continuously monitor patient symptoms, may soon integrate seamlessly into clinical workflows [4]. This chapter explores these future directions, highlighting how refined imaging methods, improved computational tools, and innovative data integration strategies can reshape diagnostic approaches, guide personalized treatment planning, and ultimately enhance long-term patient outcomes.

16.2 Role of Artificial Intelligence in Precision Diagnosis

16.2.1 Predictive Algorithms and Diagnostic Support

Conventional approaches to orofacial pain diagnosis often rely on subjective patient reports and clinician experience. This can lead to diagnostic uncertainty, especially when distinguishing between closely related conditions such as odontogenic pain and TMD. AI addresses these

K. Orhan (✉)
Department of Oral and Maxillofacial Radiology, Faculty of Dentistry, Ankara University, Ankara, Türkiye

Medical Design Application and Research Center (MEDITAM), Ankara University, Ankara, Türkiye

G. Unsal
Department of Oral and Maxillofacial Radiology, Schulich School of Medicine & Dentistry, Western University, London, ON, Canada

G. A. Kaspo, G. D. Klasser (eds.), *Orofacial and Head Pain*,
https://doi.org/10.1007/978-3-032-08275-6_16

challenges by integrating data from diverse sources, imaging studies, validated TMD screener questionnaires, patient histories, clinical examinations, and even genetic or molecular information [4, 5, 8].

Preliminary models have demonstrated that AI-driven systems can achieve up to 86% accuracy in differentiating odontogenic from TMD-origin pain. Moreover, conversational AI tools, such as prototype chatbots, can correlate patient-reported symptoms with imaging findings to offer timely, evidence-based suggestions. For example, a virtual assistant named PAINe integrated a validated TMD Pain Screener and achieved 86% accuracy in this differentiation which shows the practicality of AI-enabled preliminary assessment [5]. As these models incorporate more comprehensive datasets (including CBCT and MRI results), they have the potential to refine differential diagnoses further, predict disease trajectories, and highlight risk factors for chronicity. Additionally, a systematic review has reported diagnostic accuracies ranging from 84% to 99.9% for various TMD conditions using AI, which indicates a strong potential despite the need for methodological improvements [9]. Machine learning models have also shown promise in classifying TMD subtypes, aiding non-specialists in diagnosis [10].

Beyond current capabilities, the next generation of AI-driven diagnostic support could apply advanced ensemble learning algorithms and incorporate real-time data streams, enabling a more proactive approach to patient management. These predictive algorithms can prompt earlier interventions, guide targeted preventive measures, and inform the selection of the most appropriate imaging modalities or therapies by detecting subtle morphological changes on CBCT or minor signal alterations on MRI. Ultimately, these tools can strengthen clinical confidence, reduce uncertainty, and improve patient outcomes. In headache medicine, similar AI and ML applications have been explored to classify disorders, predict treatment effects, and predict headaches, though larger datasets and improved validation are needed [4, 8, 11].

16.2.2 Integrating Functional Imaging with AI

While conventional imaging modalities capture structural details, functional imaging techniques like functional MRI (fMRI) [12] and diffusion tensor imaging (DTI) [13, 14] offer insights into the activity and integrity of pain-processing networks. For conditions such as TMD and primary headaches, these methods reveal altered neural connectivity patterns and microstructural changes associated with pain perception [5, 9].

AI can analyze these complex datasets to identify neural signatures that correlate with specific pain phenotypes, to help predict which patients may respond best to interventions. For instance, a patient whose fMRI patterns match those of individuals who have benefited from behavioral therapy or certain neuromodulatory treatments may be directed toward these modalities earlier, reducing the trial-and-error period. Similarly, understanding the microstructural abnormalities in trigeminal pathways via DTI could inform more precise interventions, such as targeted nerve blocks or pharmacological therapies. Support vector machine analyses of fMRI data have already shown potential in classifying pain-evoked brain activity in TMD, suggesting distinct central processing patterns [15]. In trigeminal neuralgia, AI-driven imaging analysis has identified critical neural substrates and improved diagnostic precision, as well as aided in predicting surgical outcomes [6, 12, 16, 17].

As these techniques transition from research into clinical practice, AI-enhanced functional imaging stands to become an important tool for precision medicine. Clinicians can minimize unnecessary procedures, reduce healthcare costs, and deliver more efficient, patient-centered care by predicting treatment responses and outcomes more accurately.

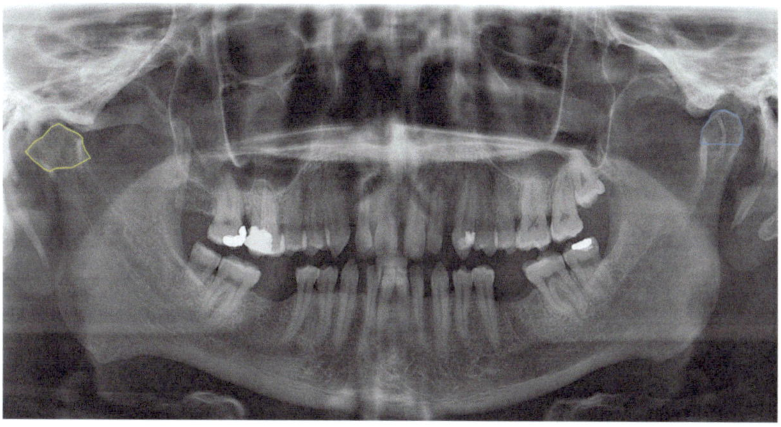

Fig. 16.1 Automated AI assessment of temporomandibular joint condyles on an orthopantomogram. The right condyle (yellow outline) displays flattening and trabecular rarefaction characteristic of osteoarthritis, whereas the left condyle (blue outline) retains normal morphology. Because panoramic radiography visualizes only hard tissue, segmentation is confined to osseous structures for AI-assisted TMJ pathology detection. These automated systems reduce inter-operator variability, standardize reporting, and ensure consistency in diagnostic workflows. In addition to identifying pathologies, advanced models can quantify lesion severity and predict the likelihood of progression, enabling clinicians to formulate more informed treatment plans and long-term management strategies. Recent advances include using a modified YOLOv5x architecture to segment maxillary sinuses and classify related pathologies with F1 scores up to 0.992 [19], and using CNN models to detect irreversible pulpitis in primary molars with high accuracy [20]

16.2.3 Automated Segmentation, Classification, and Interpretation

One of the significant bottlenecks in orofacial pain imaging is the manual interpretation of large, complex datasets. High-resolution volumetric imaging, such as CBCT, often demands considerable time and expertise to identify subtle pathologies. AI-based segmentation models, including deep convolutional neural networks (CNNs) and transformer-based architectures, can streamline this process by rapidly localizing and characterizing abnormalities, such as sinus mucosal thickening, subtle TMJ degenerative changes, or early dental lesions [18] (Fig. 16.1).

As AI becomes more deeply integrated into imaging software, clinicians may receive automated preliminary reports that highlight potential abnormalities, suggest differential diagnoses, and recommend further evaluations [5, 7]. Over time, these capabilities will extend beyond static interpretation to incorporate dynamic data and patient-specific factors, offering a comprehensive decision-support system. This evolution in workflow optimization promises to improve diagnostic speed, enhance accuracy, and ultimately support better patient outcomes.

16.3 Emerging Imaging Modalities and Their Future Integration

16.3.1 Advancements in CBCT

CBCT has become a popular imaging modality for evaluating the dentomaxillofacial region's hard tissue abnormalities. Ongoing improvements in detector technology and image reconstruction methods promise better spatial resolution and lower radiation exposure. When combined with AI algorithms, CBCT images can be processed to enhance soft-tissue contrast, improve bone quality assessments, and identify subtle joint or sinus pathologies that might not be detected by standard protocols (Fig. 16.2) [18, 19].

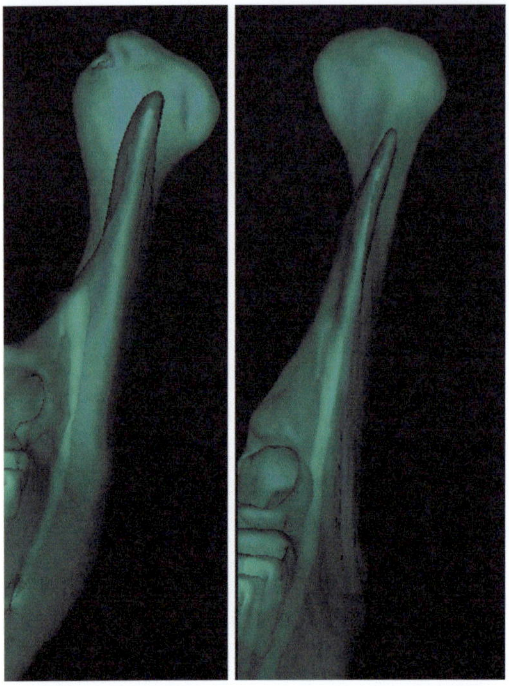

Fig. 16.2 Three-dimensional STL models of mandibular condyles derived from CBCT. An AI algorithm distinguishes an eroded condyle exhibiting cortical pitting and surface irregularity (left) from a healthy, smoothly contoured condyle (right), illustrating automated visualisation and classification of osseous degeneration

Enhanced CBCT analyses can inform early interventions in TMD patients, guide more precise surgical planning, and improve long-term prediction. Combining CBCT findings with patient-reported outcomes and biomechanical data, predictive models may determine which individuals are at risk for rapid degenerative changes or those who might benefit from non-invasive treatments like oral appliances and/or physical therapy [18].

16.3.2 Functional Imaging Modalities: fMRI and DTI

Although fMRI and DTI are currently more prevalent in research settings, these modalities may become more accessible in clinical practice as protocols shorten and costs decrease. AI-driven analyses can simplify the interpretation of complex functional datasets, making it practical for practitioners and orofacial pain specialists to incorporate functional imaging into their diagnostic toolkits. Such images can reveal the microstructural integrity of trigeminal nerve pathways and identify patterns of brain activity that correlate with pain intensity or frequency. For instance, a study by Hung et al. utilized pretreatment regional brain morphology, specifically cortical thickness and surface area measurements, to train machine learning models that accurately predicted pain relief in patients with trigeminal neuralgia undergoing Gamma Knife radiosurgery. Key predictors included features in the contralateral superior frontal gyrus and isthmus cingulate gyrus, underscoring the potential of these imaging biomarkers to guide personalized prognostication and improve the selection of surgical candidates [17].

This information could directly influence treatment recommendations. For example, if functional imaging suggests that a patient's trigeminal neuralgia is linked to a structural abnormality detectable by DTI, targeted surgical interventions or radiosurgery options may be more confidently pursued. With functional imaging integrated into routine care, clinicians can tailor treatment strategies based on objective neuroimaging biomarkers rather than relying solely on clinical symptoms [13, 14].

16.3.3 Non-ionizing and Emerging Imaging Alternatives

New imaging modalities that avoid ionizing radiation are gaining traction in orofacial pain diagnostics. Low-field MRI scanners, for instance, operate at reduced magnetic strengths compared to conventional MRI systems. This reduction can lower costs, increase portability, and potentially allow advanced imaging capabilities to reach community clinics that previously lacked the infrastructure for high-field MRI. While image resolution may initially be lower, ongoing improvements, such as AI-driven image denoising and resolution enhancement, are narrowing the performance gap [21, 22]. In conditions like

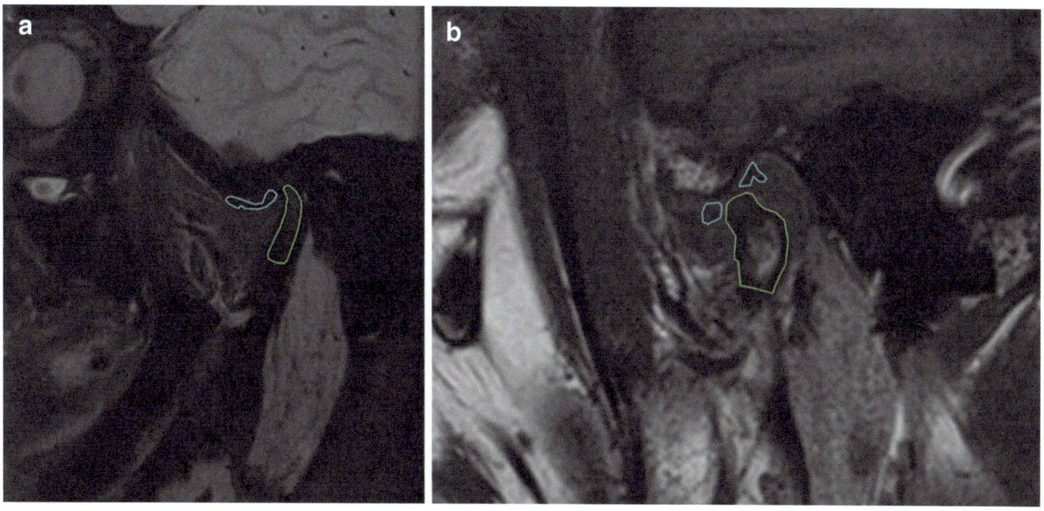

Fig. 16.3 Sagittal MRI sections of the TMJ with automatic segmentation for AI-based classification. (**a**) Anterior disc displacement without bony change: the segmented disc (blue) lies anterior to an intact condylar head (green). (**b**) Advanced osteoarthritis with disc perforation: irregular condylar cortex and discontinuous disc signal reveal severe joint degeneration. Segmentation provides precise anatomic localisation for subsequent automated analysis

TMD, where detailed bone imaging is often less critical than accurate assessment of soft tissues and joint structures, low-field MRI can offer sufficient diagnostic information with fewer logistical and economic barriers (Fig. 16.3).

Another promising modality is optoacoustic (photoacoustic) imaging, which uses light-induced ultrasound signals to provide both structural and functional information about vascular networks, inflammatory states, and other tissue characteristics. Because it does not employ ionizing radiation, optoacoustic imaging can be repeated safely over time, potentially aiding in the monitoring of disease progression or evaluating treatment responses [23, 24].

The combination of these emerging modalities with advanced AI algorithms can compensate for lower-resolution images and help highlight subtle abnormalities. Over time, the integration of non-ionizing imaging with AI-based enhancements may yield safer, more accessible, and more cost-effective diagnostic tools. These tools could be employed in ongoing patient follow-up, offering clinicians a means to track and adapt treatment strategies without subjecting patients to repeated ionizing radiation exposure. As research and technology continue to advance, these approaches have the potential to expand diagnostic options, improve patient outcomes, and streamline orofacial pain management. For example, deep learning-based super-resolution methods have enhanced MRI image quality in trigeminal neuralgia cases without altering surgical targeting parameters, thereby facilitating accurate, less resource-intensive diagnostic imaging [25].

16.4 Ethical, Practical, and Training Considerations

16.4.1 Data Privacy, Security, and Validation

The widespread adoption of AI in orofacial pain imaging relies on the collection and analysis of large datasets, raising critical concerns about patient privacy and data security. Techniques such as federated learning, where algorithms are trained on localized datasets without the transfer of identifiable patient information, offer a potential solution [26, 27]. These approaches help preserve patient confidentiality while mitigating biases that may arise from using small, homogeneous training samples. Ensuring that algorithms are validated across diverse, multicenter cohorts supports fairness and improves their generalizability, reducing the likelihood that specific populations receive less accurate or skewed diagnoses [28, 29].

In addition to privacy and fairness, regulatory and ethical frameworks must evolve to address questions of liability, transparency, and accountability. If an AI-driven tool suggests an incorrect diagnosis, determining who bears responsibility, the clinician who acted on the recommendation, the software developer, or the institution that supplied biased data, is complex. Clarifying these issues will require clear guidelines, rigorous validation standards, and ongoing oversight by professional organizations and regulatory agencies. As these standards and best practices emerge, clinicians and stakeholders must remain informed and adapt accordingly, ensuring responsible, secure, and equitable use of AI in orofacial pain diagnosis and management [28, 29].

16.4.2 Financial Considerations and Accessibility

The acquisition and maintenance of advanced imaging equipment and AI software may initially be cost-prohibitive. However, as computational technologies improve and commercial vendors introduce more affordable solutions, costs are likely to decline. Cloud-based analytics services may allow practices to access advanced AI models without significant upfront investment in hardware. Training clinicians and support staff to effectively use AI-based tools and interpret advanced imaging findings will be essential. Professional organizations and continuing education programs should adapt to this changing environment, ensuring that dental professionals possess the skills needed to integrate these technologies into their clinical routines [30, 31].

16.4.3 Interdisciplinary Collaboration and Team-Based Care

As advanced imaging modalities and AI-driven analytics reshape orofacial pain diagnosis; the clinical environment will likely become more interdisciplinary. Although dentists and orofacial pain specialists remain central to patient evaluation, the input of radiologists, data scientists, neurologists, and even genetic counselors will be increasingly valuable. Radiologists can help optimize image acquisition parameters for AI-driven analyses, while data scientists refine algorithms for better patient stratification and outcome prediction. Neurologists offer insights into complex pain mechanisms, and genetic counselors contribute perspectives on how molecular factors influence pain susceptibility and treatment responses [18, 32].

Effective collaboration also requires standardized protocols for data interpretation and sharing. Professional organizations and academic institutions can play a leading role by offering training programs that teach clinicians how to function effectively within multidisciplinary teams. In this emerging model, patients benefit from a coordinated, team-based approach, where multiple specialists combine their expertise to make well-informed, targeted treatment decisions [33, 34].

16.5 Future Trends in Predictive and Personalized Orofacial Pain Management

16.5.1 Real-Time Monitoring and Early Intervention

Wearable sensors, smartphone-based applications, and other continuous monitoring devices are beginning to play a role in tracking jaw movements, muscle activity, and physiological changes associated with orofacial pain conditions, such as TMD or migraine. Early prototypes already demonstrate the feasibility of capturing real-time data on jaw muscle tension or subtle changes in facial temperature. When these continuous data streams are integrated with AI-driven analytics, clinicians can identify early warning signs of an impending pain flare-up [4].

This proactive approach shifts the model of care from reactive to preventive. Instead of waiting for patients to report worsening symptoms, clinicians and patients could be alerted before pain escalates. For instance, if an AI algorithm detects an unusual increase in jaw muscle activity or a pattern correlating with prior migraine episodes, it could prompt timely interventions such as adjusting an oral appliance, prescribing a short course of medication, or recommending relaxation exercises. These early interventions have the potential to reduce pain severity, shorten flare-up duration, and improve overall quality of life. Moreover, AI-driven analysis of facial expressions in animal models has demonstrated the ability to capture neuropathic pain responses, offering insights that may inform future real-time monitoring approaches in human patients [35].

16.5.2 Multimodal Data Integration for Comprehensive Assessments

As data collection methods become more robust and diverse, clinicians can leverage an integrated approach to diagnosis and treatment planning. Currently, standard imaging techniques like CBCT and MRI provide detailed anatomical and sometimes functional information. Looking forward, additional modalities, such as ultrasound, low-field MRI, optoacoustic imaging, and advanced electrophysiological measurements, will improve the diagnostic landscape. These imaging outputs, combined with patient history, psychosocial assessments, and even genetic data, can construct a multi-dimensional patient profile, often referred to as a "pain phenotype" [6, 7, 10].

AI models, trained to fuse information from multiple sources, may surpass human capabilities in detecting subtle patterns and correlations. By synthesizing structural imaging (e.g., bony changes seen on CBCT), soft-tissue and disc positioning details (via MRI), vascular and inflammatory markers (via ultrasound or optoacoustic imaging), and neuromuscular activity (electromyography), clinicians can gain a deeper understanding of the underlying etiology of orofacial pain. This integration promotes a precision medicine framework, enabling individualized management strategies rather than relying on a "one-size-fits-all" approach [11, 18, 30].

16.5.3 Radiomics and "Omics" Integration for Personalized Therapies

Radiomics is an emerging field that involves the extraction of large numbers of quantitative features from medical images. Unlike traditional imaging assessments that rely on qualitative interpretation (e.g., "the condylar head appears flattened" or "there is mild mucosal thickening in the sinus"), radiomics transforms images into high-dimensional data sets. These data sets capture subtle differences in intensity, shape, texture, and spatial relationships of tissues or lesions. The goal is to identify imaging biomarkers and quantifiable features that correlate with disease severity, progression, or response to treatment [36–38].

For instance, radiomic analysis of the TMJ on CBCT or MRI may identify patterns that predict which patients with early arthritic changes will progress rapidly versus those who will remain stable. Similarly, radiomics applied to sinus imaging could differentiate between inflammatory changes that resolve with conservative management and those more likely to require surgical intervention. Over time, as radiomic methodologies become more refined and validated, they will help clinicians tailor treatments based on objective, reproducible metrics rather than subjective impressions [36–38].

In addition to radiomics, the integration of "omics" data, such as genomics, metabolomics, and microbiomics, further refines patient classification and prediction models. Clinicians can identify which patient subgroups are more susceptible to certain pain mechanisms or more responsive to specific interventions by correlating imaging-derived biomarkers with molecular and genetic signatures. For example, a patient with distinct imaging-based radiomic features might also exhibit a particular genetic profile that predisposes them to neuropathic pain. With this knowledge, clinicians could initiate preventive therapies early, adjust medication choices, or prioritize certain rehabilitation strategies [39, 40].

16.5.4 Patient Engagement and Technology Acceptance

As advanced imaging and AI-driven diagnostics become more prevalent, it is essential to involve patients in understanding these new methodologies. Patients may have concerns about how their data are used, the transparency of algorithmic decisions, or the implications of new imaging techniques for their care plans. Addressing these concerns can improve trust and adherence. Clear, patient-friendly explanations of how AI identifies subtle patterns in imaging data, or how wearable sensors predict flare-ups, can help alleviate anxiety about "black box" algorithms. Clinicians can use simple visual aids or mobile apps that summarize complex imaging findings in an accessible format, illustrating how data-driven insights guide decisions on therapy selection or timing [41].

Informed consent processes should incorporate explanations of data privacy measures, such as federated learning, to reassure patients that their information is protected [10, 26, 27]. It may also be beneficial to involve patients in the conversation about balancing innovation with safety and cost considerations, so they understand the value of these tools. Open communication fosters an environment where patients feel empowered and respected as partners in their care journey [41, 42]. Ultimately, patient acceptance and understanding of these technologies are integral to their success. As these tools guide more personalized and proactive interventions, patients who trust and embrace the technology are more likely to follow recommended treatments, attend regular follow-ups, and achieve better outcomes. Ensuring patient engagement remains a core objective as the field advances [41].

16.6 Conclusion

The future of orofacial and head pain imaging lies in the integration of advanced imaging modalities, AI-driven predictive models, and comprehensive data analysis. By leveraging functional imaging to map pain-processing networks, applying AI to streamline image interpretation, and developing predictive algorithms that anticipate disease progression and treatment outcomes, clinicians will be better equipped to offer individualized patient care.

The successful implementation of these technologies depends on ethical data management, appropriate regulatory frameworks, financial feasibility, and adequate professional training. Despite these challenges, the trajectory is clear: as imaging and AI tools become more sophisticated and accessible, clinicians will gain new opportunities to improve diagnostic accuracy, personalize interventions, and ultimately enhance patient quality of life.

References

1. Barad M, Romero-Reyes M. Orofacial pain. Continuum (Minneap Minn). 2024;30(5):1397–426.
2. Sharav Y, Haviv Y, Benoliel R. Orofacial migraine or neurovascular orofacial pain from pathogenesis to treatment. Int J Mol Sci. 2023;24(3):2456.
3. Katsuki M, Shimazu T, Kikui S, Danno D, Miyahara J, Takeshima R, et al. Developing an artificial intelligence-based headache diagnostic model and its utility for non-specialists' diagnostic accuracy. Cephalalgia. 2023;43(5):3331024231156925.
4. Stubberud A, Langseth H, Nachev P, Matharu MS, Tronvik E. Artificial intelligence and headache. Cephalalgia. 2024;44(8):3331024241268290.
5. de Araujo BMM, de Jesus Freitas PF, Deliga Schroder AG, Kuchler EC, Baratto-Filho F, Ditzel Westphalen VP, et al. PAINe: an artificial intelligence-based virtual assistant to aid in the differentiation of pain of odontogenic versus temporomandibular origin. J Endodont. 2024; https://doi.org/10.1016/j.joen.2024.09.008.
6. Battistelli M, Izzo A, D'Ercole M, D'Alessandris QG, Montano N. The role of artificial intelligence in the management of trigeminal neuralgia. Front Surg. 2023;10:1310414.
7. Daripa B, Lucchese S. Artificial intelligence-aided headache classification based on a set of questionnaires: a short review. Cureus. 2022;14(9):e29514.

8. Ihara K, Dumkrieger G, Zhang P, Takizawa T, Schwedt TJ, Chiang CC. Application of artificial intelligence in the headache field. Curr Pain Headache Rep. 2024;28(10):1049–57.
9. Jha N, Lee KS, Kim YJ. Diagnosis of temporomandibular disorders using artificial intelligence technologies: a systematic review and meta-analysis. PLoS One. 2022;17(8):e0272715.
10. Zatt FP, Cordeiro JVC, Bohner L, Souza BDM, Caldas VEA, Caldas RA. Using machine learning to classify temporomandibular disorders: a proof of concept. J Appl Oral Sci. 2024;32:e20240282.
11. Torrente A, Maccora S, Prinzi F, Alonge P, Pilati L, Lupica A, et al. The clinical relevance of artificial intelligence in migraine. Brain Sci. 2024;14(1):85.
12. Liang Y, Zhao Q, Hu Z, Bo K, Meyyappan S, Neubert JK, et al. Imaging the neural substrate of trigeminal neuralgia pain using deep learning. Front Hum Neurosci. 2023;17:1144159.
13. Owen SL, Heath J, Kringelbach ML, Stein JF, Aziz TZ. Preoperative DTI and probabilistic tractography in an amputee with deep brain stimulation for lower limb stump pain. Br J Neurosurg. 2007;21(5):485–90.
14. Huang X, Chen J, Liu S, Gong Q, Liu T, Lu C, et al. Impaired frontal-parietal control network in chronic prostatitis/chronic pelvic pain syndrome revealed by graph theoretical analysis: a DTI study. Eur J Neurosci. 2021;53(4):1060–71.
15. Harper DE, Shah Y, Ichesco E, Gerstner GE, Peltier SJ. Multivariate classification of pain-evoked brain activity in temporomandibular disorder. Pain Rep. 2016;1(3):e572.
16. Latypov TH, So MC, Hung PS, Tsai P, Walker MR, Tohyama S, et al. Brain imaging signatures of neuropathic facial pain derived by artificial intelligence. Sci Rep. 2023;13(1):10699.
17. Hung PS, Noorani A, Zhang JY, Tohyama S, Laperriere N, Davis KD, et al. Regional brain morphology predicts pain relief in trigeminal neuralgia. Neuroimage Clin. 2021;31:102706.
18. Orhan K, Sanders A, Unsal G, Ezhov M, Misirli M, Gusarev M, et al. Assessing the reliability of CBCT-based AI-generated STL files in diagnosing osseous changes of the mandibular condyle: a comparative study with ground truth diagnosis. Dentomaxillofac Radiol. 2023;52(7):20230141.
19. Altun O, Ozen DC, Duman SB, Dedeoglu N, Bayrakdar IS, Eser G, et al. Automatic maxillary sinus segmentation and pathology classification on cone-beam computed tomographic images using deep learning. BMC Oral Health. 2024;24(1):1208.
20. Ma T, Zhu J, Wang D, Xu Z, Bai H, Ding P, et al. Deep learning-based detection of irreversible pulpitis in primary molars. Int J Paediatr Dent. 2025;35(1):57–67.
21. Balaji S, Wiley N, Poorman ME, Kolind SH. Low-field MRI for use in neurological diseases. Curr Opin Neurol. 2024;37(4):381–91.
22. Ayde R, Vornehm M, Zhao Y, Knoll F, Wu EX, Sarracanie M. MRI at low field: a review of software solutions for improving SNR. NMR Biomed. 2025;38(1):e5268.
23. Mandras N, Pasqualini D, Roana J, Tullio V, Banche G, Gianello E, et al. Influence of photon-induced photoacoustic streaming (PIPS) on root canal disinfection and post-operative pain: a randomized clinical trial. J Clin Med. 2020;9(12):3915.
24. Zhou Y, Yi X, Xing W, Hu S, Maslov KI, Wang LV. Microcirculatory changes identified by photoacoustic microscopy in patients with complex regional pain syndrome type I after stellate ganglion blocks. J Biomed Opt. 2014;19(8):086017.
25. Hwang JH, Park CK, Kang SB, Choi MK, Lee WH. Deep learning super-resolution technique based on magnetic resonance imaging for application of image-guided diagnosis and surgery of trigeminal neuralgia. Life (Basel). 2024;14(3):355.
26. Rischke R, Schneider L, Muller K, Samek W, Schwendicke F, Krois J. Federated learning in dentistry: chances and challenges. J Dent Res. 2022;101(11):1269–73.
27. Schneider L, Rischke R, Krois J, Krasowski A, Buttner M, Mohammad-Rahimi H, et al. Federated vs local vs central deep learning of tooth segmentation on panoramic radiographs. J Dent. 2023;135:104556.
28. Copeland-Halperin LR, Oppikofer C. Artificial intelligence, data protection, privacy, and doxxing. Aesthet Surg J. 2024; https://doi.org/10.1093/asj/sjae219.
29. Martin KD, Zimmermann J. Artificial intelligence and its implications for data privacy. Curr Opin Psychol. 2024;58:101829.
30. Acharya S, Godhi BS, Saxena V, Assiry AA, Alessa NA, Dawasaz AA, et al. Role of artificial intelligence in behavior management of pediatric dental patients-a mini review. J Clin Pediatr Dent. 2024;48(3):24–30.
31. Vakay R, Alex G. Artificial intelligence: a mighty adjunct for caries detection. Compend Contin Educ Dent. 2024;45(2):110–2.
32. D'Souza RN, Colombo JS, Embree MC, Myers JM, DeRouen TA. Our essential and endangered dentist-scientist workforce. JDR Clin Trans Res. 2017;2(1):10–22.
33. Lobbezoo F, Parisius KGH, Verhoeff MC. Orofacial pain and dysfunction in patients with special needs, with a focus on interdisciplinarity. Pain. 2024;165(11S):S15–22.
34. Taqi M, Zaidi SJA, Siddiqui SU, Zia B, Khadija SM. Dental practitioners' knowledge, management practices, and attitudes toward collaboration in the treatment of temporomandibular joint disorders: a mixed-methods study. BMC Prim Care. 2024;25(1):137.
35. Andrade-Gonzalez RD, Perrusquia-Hernandez E, Montes-Angeles CD, Castillo-Diaz LA, Hernandez Campos ME, Perez-Martinez IO. Encoding signs of orofacial neuropathic pain from facial expressions in mice. Arch Oral Biol. 2022;135:105369.
36. Duyan Yuksel H, Orhan K, Evlice B, Kaya O. Evaluation of temporomandibular joint disc displacement with magnetic resonance imaging based

radiomics analysis. Dentomaxillofac Radiol. 2024; https://doi.org/10.1093/dmfr/twae066.
37. Ozturk EMA, Unsal G, Erisir F, Orhan K. Prediction of bone invasion of oral squamous cell carcinoma using a magnetic resonance imaging-based machine learning model. Eur Arch Otorrinolaringol. 2024;281(12):6585–97.
38. Tarakci OD, Kis HC, Amasya H, Ozturk I, Karahan E, Orhan K. Radiomics-based diagnosis in dentomaxillofacial radiology: a systematic review. J Imaging Inform Med. 2024; https://doi.org/10.1007/s10278-024-01307-3.
39. Ballard JL, Wang Z, Li W, Shen L, Long Q. Deep learning-based approaches for multi-omics data integration and analysis. BioData Min. 2024;17(1):38.
40. Kocak M, Akcali Z. Development trends and knowledge framework of artificial intelligence (AI) applications in oncology by years: a bibliometric analysis from 1992 to 2022. Discov Oncol. 2024;15(1):566.
41. Bahadir HS, Keskin NB, Cakmak ESK, Gunec G, Cesur Aydin K, Peker F. Patients' attitudes toward artificial intelligence in dentistry and their trust in dentists. Oral Radiol. 2024; https://doi.org/10.1007/s11282-024-00775-1.
42. Badawy W, Zinhom H, Shaban M. Navigating ethical considerations in the use of artificial intelligence for patient care: a systematic review. Int Nurs Rev. 2024; https://doi.org/10.1111/inr.13059.

Index

G. A. Kaspo, G. D. Klasser (eds.), *Orofacial and Head Pain*,
https://doi.org/10.1007/978-3-032-08275-6

D

E

F

MIX
Papier aus verantwortungsvollen Quellen
Paper from responsible sources
FSC® C105338

If you have any concerns about our products,
you can contact us on
ProductSafety@springernature.com

In case Publisher is established outside the EU,
the EU authorized representative is:
Springer Nature Customer Service Center GmbH
Europaplatz 3, 69115 Heidelberg, Germany

Printed by Libri Plureos GmbH
in Hamburg, Germany